Evaluation and Management of Adiposity

Evaluation and Management of Adiposity

Edited by Max Shaw

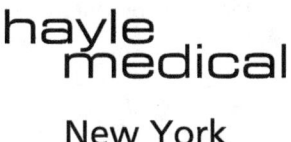

New York

Hayle Medical,
750 Third Avenue, 9th Floor,
New York, NY 10017, USA

Visit us on the World Wide Web at:
www.haylemedical.com

ISBN: 978-1-63241-873-9

Cataloging-in-Publication Data

Evaluation and management of adiposity / edited by Max Shaw.
   p. cm.
Includes bibliographical references and index.
ISBN 978-1-63241-873-9
1. Obesity. 2. Obesity--Evaluation. 3. Obesity--Treatment.
4. Metabolism--Disorders. I. Shaw, Max.
RC628 .E83 2020
616.398--dc23

Table of Contents

Preface

Adiposity or obesity is the clinical condition characterized by the accumulation of fat in the body, to the extent that it poses a negative effect on health. It increases the likelihood of developing cardiovascular diseases, obstructive sleep apnea, type 2 diabetes, certain cancers, osteoarthritis, etc. It is caused due to a combination of genetic susceptibility, excessive food intake and lack of physical activity. It can however be prevented through the right combination of personal choices and social changes. Changing the diet to reduce the consumption of energy-dense foods, increasing the intake of dietary fibers and regular exercising are the chief strategies for the management of obesity. This book consists of contributions made by international experts on adiposity. It discusses the fundamental as well as modern approaches in the evaluation and management of adiposity. For all readers who are interested in this medical condition, the case studies included in this book will serve as an excellent guide to develop a comprehensive understanding.

This book is a comprehensive compilation of works of different researchers from varied parts of the world. It includes valuable experiences of the researchers with the sole objective of providing the readers (learners) with a proper knowledge of the concerned field. This book will be beneficial in evoking inspiration and enhancing the knowledge of the interested readers.

In the end, I would like to extend my heartiest thanks to the authors who worked with great determination on their chapters. I also appreciate the publisher's support in the course of the book. I would also like to deeply acknowledge my family who stood by me as a source of inspiration during the project.

Editor

Obesity Peptide: Prokineticin

Canan Nebigil

Abstract

Obesity confers an increased risk for cardiovascular renal diseases, diabetes mellitus, nonalcoholic steatohepatitis, musculoskeletal disorders, and cancers. Prokineticin-2 is a peptide hormone, which exists as both a circulating hormone system and a local paracrine-signaling mechanism within various tissues including the brain, kidney, and adipose. It acts on the G-protein-coupled receptors (GPCRs) PKR1 and PKR2. The role of prokineticin-2 in the central nervous system is the control of food intake. Its anorexigenic effect is at least partly through the hypothalamic melanocortin system. Prokineticin-2 also prevents adipose tissue expansion by limiting preadipocyte proliferation and differentiation capacity. Prokineticin-2 signaling is important for insulin capillary passages. It also regulates heart and kidney development and function. Here, we discuss a new obesity peptide prokineticin signaling in central regulation of food intake, adipocyte tissue development, and cardiovascular function. Prokineticin may play a key role in the association between obesity and cardiovascular diseases. We also outline the potential of prokineticin receptor-1 as target for the treatment of obesity and cardiovascular diseases.

Keywords: prokineticin, GPCRs, obesity, diabetes, anorexigenic, angiogenic

1. Introduction

Obesity is a major health problem and an increased risk factor that worsens cardiovascular events leading to higher morbidity and mortality. [1] Several cardiovascular diseases can also occur due to structural and functional changes of the myocardium through excess fat deposition and other mechanisms related to obesity [2]. However, the mechanisms of relation between obesity and cardiovascular events are unclear. Nevertheless, pharmacological therapy for obesity has great potential to improve cardiovascular problems. Several anorexcigenic peptides have been studied as potential drugs in the treatment of obesity [3]. Recent evidence showed that some brain regions may not only be involved in food intake regulation but also play an important role in the regulation of cardiovascular blood homeostasis [4]. The rising prevalence of both obesity and heart failure make this association an important target for prevention. Therefore, it is important to determine the common mechanisms regulating both obesity and cardiovascular events. Identification of signaling pathways linking obesity and cardiovascular disease is important for the development of novel therapeutics. Here, we summarize the current information on the role of anorexigenic peptide prokineticin in obesity and cardiovascular renal diseases, emphasizing prokineticin receptor-1 signaling in these events.

2. Prokineticins and their receptors

Prokineticins are anorexigenic and angiogenic hormones. Because of the structural, signaling and functional similarities, prokineticins are considered as cytokines/chemokines [5]. They are released principally by macrophages and reproductive organs [6]. Recently, prokineticin is considered as an adipokine because a high level of prokineticins has been found in obese human WAT [7]. These small peptides (80–120 amino acids) are called prokineticins, because these molecules were first identified as potent contractile factors in the gastrointestinal tract [8]. Two isoforms of prokineticins have been identified: prokineticin-1 and prokineticin-2. Prokineticin-1 has been originally called as endocrine gland-derived vascular endothelial growth factor (EG-VEGF), [9] because of its functional similarity to VEGF. Prokineticin-2 is also called as Bv8. Both of these peptides are 45% identical with highly conserved N-terminal AVITGA motif essential for their biological activity [6, 10]. Prokineticin activity is mediated by two G-protein-coupled receptors, PKR1 and PKR2 [11].

2.1. Prokineticin-2 is an anorexigenic peptide

Circulating hormones and nutrients are integrated to mediate the regulation of short-term and long-term dietary intakes in the hypothalamus. A feeding and energy homeostasis control center in the hypothalamus is called as arcuate nucleus (ARC) [12, 13]. The ARC integrates most of the peripheral hormonal signals including leptin, insulin and ghrelin. The ARC has two major subpopulations of primary neurons that express neurohormones with opposing effects on food intake. ARC neurons that release the proopiomelanocortin (POMC)-derived peptide alpha-melanocyte-stimulating hormone (α-MSH) and cocaine- and amphetamine-regulated transcript (CART) peptide potently reduce food intake [13, 14]. However, neuro-peptide Y (NPY)-producing neurons in the ARC stimulate food intake.

Prokineticin-2 is involved in the control of food intake and of fat mass through actions in the ARC in the hypothalamus [15]. PKR1 receptor is expressed on both NPY/AgRP and POMC/CART neurons. Intracranial injection of prokineticin-2 in rats strongly decreases food intake. Controversy, anti-prokineticin-2 antibody increases food intake. Anorexigenic effect of pro-kineticin-2 is mediated at least partly via the hypothalamic ARC melanocortin system. Proki-neticin-2 increases the release of alpha-MSH from *ex vivo* hypothalamic explants. Recently,

PKR1 has been shown as the first non-melanocortin GPCR to be regulated by the melanocortin receptor accessory protein 2 (MRAP2). Indeed, MRAP2 significantly and specifically inhibits PKR1 signaling [16].

Peripheral administration of prokineticin-2 reduces food intake and body weight in both lean mice and diet-induced obesity models [17]. This effect of prokineticin-2 is not evident when appetite is increased or feeding behavior is promoted. Hypothalamic prokineticin-2 levels were found extremely high in the early neonatal period. However, a decreased level of prokineticin-2 was evident under fasting conditions [18]. Prokineticin-2-knockout mice became obese at the late age. Humans with the inactivating mutations of prokineticin-2 gene are also obese [17, 19]. The anorectic effects of prokineticin-2 are abolished by PKR1 antagonists and not observed in mice lacking PKR1 [17]. Thus, the anorectic effects of prokineticin-2 in the hypothalamus are mediated by PKR1.

2.2. Prokineticin in the development of obesity

The mechanisms underlying the development of obesity include the hypertrophy and/or hyperplasia of adipocytes, adipose tissue (AT) inflammation, impaired extracellular matrix remodeling and fibrosis together with an altered secretion of adipokines [20]. AT expansion involves two distinct mechanisms: an enlargement in adipose cells and an increase of adipocytes number [21]. Differentiated adipocytes are post-mitotic and therefore hyperplasia is the result of increased *de novo* adipocyte formation (adipogenesis). Impaired adipogenesis is associated with insulin resistance [22]. The balance between proliferation and differentiation of preadipocytes and adipocyte apoptosis or necrosis determines adipocyte number.

Prokineticin-2 levels were found to be high in obese human WAT [7]. Prokineticin-2 suppresses AT expansion by two distinct mechanisms: the central regulation of food intake and limiting preadipocyte proliferation and differentiation. The central regulation of body weight is counteracted by loss of PKR1 in adipose tissue in mice. Indeed, an abnormally excessive abdominal fat mass accumulation was observed in these mice where the PKR1 specifically deleted in the adipocytes (PKR1$^{ad-/-}$) [7]. The formation of new adipocytes in both PKR1 null and PKR1$^{ad-/-}$ mice was resulted from an acceleration of preadipocyte proliferation and differentiation. AT proliferative phenotype has switch to AT hypertrophic phenotype when these mice were treated with a high-fat diet, implicating high calorie intake is involved in the conversion of hyperplasia to hypertrophy. In isolated preadipocytes, PKR1 activation suppresses proliferation and adipogenic differentiation [38].

Both PKR1^{null} and PKR1$^{ad-/-}$ mice display abdominal obesity [7] However, only PKR1^{null} mice have peripheral obesity with a diabetes-like syndrome. Thus, non-adipocyte PKR1-mediated events contribute to the development of a diabetes-like syndrome. Indeed, endothelial-specific PKR1-knockout mice (PKR1$^{ec-/-}$) [23] had insulin resistance in adipocytes. In PKR1$^{ec-/-}$ adipocytes, insulin cannot promote normal fat storage, resulting in excess circulating free fatty acids that, in turn, further contribute into insulin resistance in muscle, leading to diabetes-like syndrome. However, it seems that PKR1 has no direct effect on fat deposition in adipocytes. PKR1$^{ad-/-}$ mice did not have severe accumulation of fat tissue in their adipocytes. Since adipocytes are not created from other adipocytes, but they arise from precursor cells (preadipocytes), PKR1 suppress the ability of these precursor cells to become adipocytes (**Figure 1**) [7]. The expansion and metabolism of the adipose tissue are the major problem in obesity.

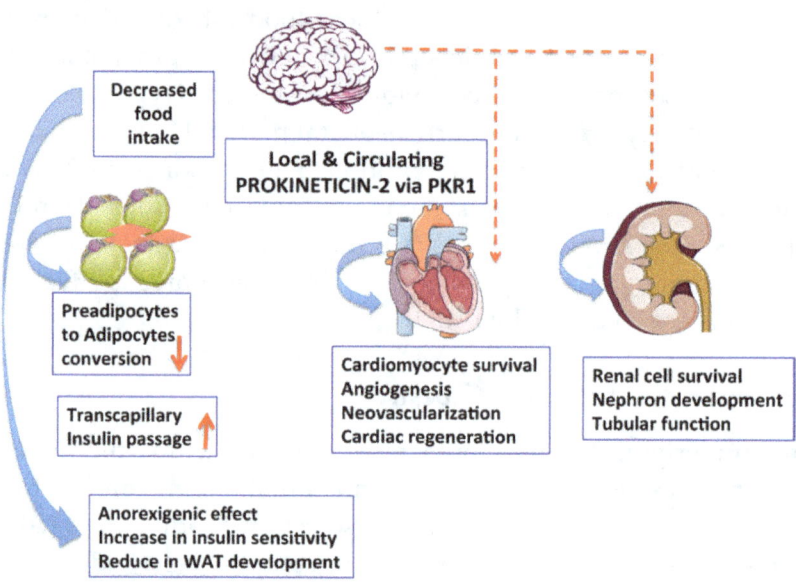

Figure 1. Prokineticin-2/PKR1 signaling may act as a new connector between development of obesity, diabetes and cardiovascular diseases. Prokineticin-2/PKR1 signaling in central nervous system (CNS) regulates food intake. Prokineticin-2 released from adipocytes controls preadipocyte conversion to adipocyte via PKR1 signaling. Prokineticin-2/PKR1 signaling promotes survival of cardiomyocytes and angiogenesis and involved in neovascularization by activating cardiac progenitor cells. Prokineticin-2/PKR1 signaling contributes to heart and kidney development as well as kidney function. Whether this signaling involves heart and kidney regulation through CNS remains to be studied.

2.3. Prokineticin in insulin resistance

The endothelium is essential for insulin transcapillary delivery to the skeletal muscle interstitium. This process is the rate-limiting step in insulin-stimulated glucose uptake. [24] The impairment of insulin delivery process contributes to insulin resistance [25]. On the other hand, insulin resistance leads to endothelial dysfunction [26]. Thus, the vascular endothelium is a potential therapeutic target for the prevention of insulin resistance and related complications [27].

Endothelium-specific PKR1-knockout mice (PKR1[ec-/-]) display impaired capillary formation and low transcapillary insulin uptake [23]. Impaired insulin delivery and signaling in endothelial cells (ECs) has been observed in cases of insulin resistance with type 2 diabetes and obesity. Endothelial cells overexpressing PKR1 promotes insulin transendothelial uptake [9] and angiogenesis [28]. PKR1[ec-/-] mice display lipodystrophy due to poor capillary formation in the AT. Lipodystrophies, involving a loss of WAT, cause hyperphagia and peripheral insulin resistance [29].

As a summary, prokineticin regulates appetite (effects in central nervous system (CNS)) and suppresses adipocyte expansion (direct effect on adipocyte tissue), promotes normal fat storage (endothelial-dependent effect) and increases insulin sensitivity. Therapeutic strategies targeting PKR1 could be important to treat obesity and obesity-associated insulin resistance.

2.4. Prokineticin in cardiovascular regulation

Obesity is both an independent risk factor and a risk marker for the development of asymptomatic and symptomatic coronary artery disease, heart failure and atrial fibrillation [2]. The relationship between obesity and cardiovascular diseases may be associated with hemodynamic and anatomic cardiovascular changes related to excess body mass [30]. However, the relationship can also be mediated by obesity-related metabolic, inflammatory and neurohormonal changes.

Altered expression of prokineticins and their receptors has been implicated in the development of a number of pathological cardiac conditions, including heart failure [31]. Prokineticins and their receptors have been identified as an important cardiovascular-signaling system especially cardiac cell commitment and cell-to-cell communications [32].

PKR1-mediated signaling contributes to cardiomyocyte survival and adult heart repair. PKR1 activates Akt in cardiomyocyte to protect these cells against hypoxia-mediated apoptosis [33]. Transgenic (TG) mice-overexpressing PKR1 in the cardiomyocytes (TG-PKR1) had an increased number of epicardial-derived progenitor cells (EPDCs), with an increase of capillary density and coronary arterioles. [32] The cardiac-PKR1 signaling up-regulates its own ligand prokineticin-2 to stimulate the EPDC differentiation into endothelial and smooth muscle cells to promote neovasculogenesis [32]. However, cardiomyocyte-PKR1 is essential for cardiomyocyte survival and contractility. PKR1^{null} mice displayed cardiomyocyte-contractile defects and apoptosis partially due to lack of PKR1 signaling in cardiomyocytes. [34]

In endothelial cells (ECs), PKR1 activates Akt and MAPK to promote proliferation, migration and angiogenesis. In agreement with the *in vitro* findings, the specific loss of PKR1 from mouse ECs resulted in defective angiogenesis, leading to necrosis/apoptosis in the surrounding tissues in several organs, including the heart and kidneys [23].

There was significantly less capillary formation in adult PKR1$^{ec-/-}$ hearts. The posterior walls of PKR1$^{ec-/-}$ hearts were thinner, which was due to the loss of capillary formation and a high level of apoptosis [23]. The remaining viable heart muscle is subject to greater biomechanical stress, triggering hypertrophy [23]. Shortening fractions (indicators of left ventricular contractility) were progressively reduced in mutant mice. PKR1$^{ec-/-}$ hearts displayed EC deregulation, capillary refraction, apoptosis, fibrosis and ectopic lipid deposition, abnormal insulin signaling in hearts resulting in impaired diastolic function.

The ECs of hearts exhibited severely decreased FICT-insulin uptake, indicating defective *transcapillary* transport of insulin in the vascular wall of these mice. Isolated ECs from the mutant cardiac and renal tissues exhibited very little insulin uptake, confirming that the loss of PKR1 from EC decreased insulin transport [23]. Overexpressing PKR1 in these ECs promoted fluorescein isothiocyanate (FITC)-insulin passage. Indeed, the primary defect linking insulin resistance and endothelial dysfunction is believed to be nitric oxide deficiency of endothelial origin [35]. In agreement, insulin uptake and insulin-mediated eNOS activation were impaired in all mutant ECs. Similarly, altered eNOS activation and low insulin action have recently been demonstrated in the endothelium of patients with diabetes mellitus [36]. Thus, impaired insulin delivery to ECs may lead to defective NOS and eNOS activation in PKR1[ec-/-] aortas, consequently impairing endothelium-dependent relaxation. These data highlight the role of PKR1 as a positive regulator of insulin uptake [37].

PKR1 signaling also contributes to heart development. In developing heart, PKR1 regulates epicardial-mesenchymal transition (EMT) to form epicardial-derived progenitor cell (EPDC) [38]. Genetic ablation of PKR1 in epicardium leads to ventricular hypoplasia and septal defects during embryogenesis. Impaired vasculogenesis in these mice is due to impaired EPDC proliferation as well as a defective EPDC differentiation into endothelial and smooth muscle cell type. PKR1 in EPDCS activates Akt signaling, changes cell morphology, actin cytoskeleton remodeling and EMT gene expression profile. Epicardial-PKR1 contributes to cardiomyocyte, proliferation and rhythmicity in a paracrine pathway.

2.5. Prokineticin in renal development and function

Global PKR1-knockout mice have peripheral obesity accompanied by a diabetes-like syndrome at the late ages (36 weeks old) [7], mainly due to endothelial dysfunction and impaired adipose tissue functions [37]. These mice also exhibited cardiomegaly, severe interstitial fibrosis and cardiac dysfunction under the stress conditions. These mice also displayed impaired renal tubular dilation, reduced glomerular capillaries, urinary phosphate excretion and proteinuria [34].

Similarly, endothelial-specific PKR1-knockout mice (PKR1[ec-/-]) also displayed dilatation of Bowman's spaces in most glomeruli, a compact glomerulus, fibrosis and enlarged tubular structures with a swollen necrotic nucleus, abnormal mitochondria and aberrant organization of podocytes. Abnormal tubular function with higher levels of absolute renal phosphate (Pi) excretion in the PKR1[ec-/-] mice is due to lower levels of sodium-calcium and sodium phosphate exchanger. The morphological changes in the PKR1[ec-/-] kidneys were associated with higher levels of apoptosis and impaired insulin signaling and lipid accumulation. Mutant mice displayed high levels of creatinine clearance and proteinuria. [34] Endothelial dysfunction resulted from loss of PKR1 signaling partially underlies the pathological features of heart and kidney.

PKR1 signaling in kidney is essential for nephron development during embryogenesis [38]. Recently, it has been shown that mutant mice with targeted PKR1 gene disruptions in nephron progenitors exhibited partial embryonic and postnatal lethality due to hypoplastic kidneys with premature glomeruli and necrotic nephrons. Kidney developmental defects in these mice are manifested in the adult stage as renal atrophy with glomerular defects, nephropathy and uremia. Thus, PKR1 is necessary for renal mesenchymal-epithelial transition (MET) that is involved in the formation of renal progenitors, regulating glomerulogenesis toward forming nephrons during kidney development. Indeed, PKR1 through NFATc3 modifies MET processing to the development of nephron.

3. Conclusion

PKR1 signaling has various beneficial effects, e.g., central regulation of appetite, the suppression of adipocyte mass and insulin-sensitizing effects on skeletal muscle and other tissues, cardiac regenerative effects and regulation of kidney function. This has attracted considerable interest in the possible use of this receptor as a target for treatments combating obesity, diabetes and cardiovascular diseases. Intracardiac PKR1 gene transfer improved survival rate and heart functions after myocardial infarction [33]. Since PKR2 has been found to contribute to vascular leakage and hypertrophic cardiomyopathy [39], several laboratories are focused on the discovery of PKR1 agonist. Recently, PKR1 non-peptide agonist has been identified [40]. PKR1 agonist prevents cardiac lesion formation and improved cardiac function after myocardial infarction in mice, promoting proliferation of cardiac progenitor cells and neovasculogenesis. PKR1 agonist in treatment strategies of metabolic disease remains to be studied.

How prokineticin-2 contributes to the AT remodeling [41], how it modulates the interaction between the adipocytes, macrophages and endothelial cells to regulate AT expansion [42] remains also to be determined. Circulating prokineticin levels in obese, diabetic and heart failure patients remain to be explored.

Acknowledgements

I wish to thank people involved in the studies described here, including Kyoji Urayama, Célia Guilini, Gulen Turkeri, Monia Boulberdaa, Mojdeh Dormishian, Rehana Qureshi, Himanshu Arora and Adeline Gasser. The publication was supported in part by grants from Fondation pour la Recherche Médicale (Equipe Labellisée), Centre National de la Recherche Scientifique and Université de Strasbourg. This work has also been published within the LABEX ANR-10-LABX- 0034_Medalis and received a financial support from the French government managed by Agence Nationale de la Recherche (ANR) under "Programme d'investissement d'avenir."

Author details

Canan Nebigil

Address all correspondence to: nebigil@unistra.fr

CNRS-University of Strasbourg, (UMR 7242), Illkirch, France

References

[1] Haslam DW and James WP. Obesity. *Lancet*. 2005;366:1197–209.

[2] Mandviwala T, Khalid U and Deswal A. Obesity and cardiovascular disease: a risk factor or a risk marker? *Curr Atheroscler Rep*. 2016;18:21.

[3] Valassi E, Scacchi M and Cavagnini F. Neuroendocrine control of food intake. *Nutr Metab Cardiovasc Dis*. 2008;18:158–68.

[4] Mikulaskova B, Maletinska L, Zicha J and Kunes J. The role of food intake regulating peptides in cardiovascular regulation. *Mol Cell Endocrinol*. 2016;436:78–92.

[5] Monnier J and Samson M. Cytokine properties of prokineticins. *FEBS J*. 2008;275:4014–21.

[6] Kaser A, Winklmayr M, Lepperdinger G and Kreil G. The AVIT protein family. Secreted cysteine-rich vertebrate proteins with diverse functions. *EMBO Rep*. 2003;4:469–73.

[7] Szatkowski C, Vallet J, Dormishian M, Messaddeq N, Valet P, Boulberdaa M, Metzger D, Chambon P and Nebigil CG. Prokineticin receptor 1 as a novel suppressor of preadipocyte proliferation and differentiation to control obesity. *PLoS One*. 2013;8:e81175.

[8] Li M, Bullock CM, Knauer DJ, Ehlert FJ and Zhou QY. Identification of two prokineticin cDNAs: recombinant proteins potently contract gastrointestinal smooth muscle. *Mol Pharmacol*. 2001;59:692–8.

[9] LeCouter J and Ferrara N. EG-VEGF and the concept of tissue-specific angiogenic growth factors. *Semin Cell Dev Biol*. 2002;13:3–8.

[10] Wechselberger C, Puglisi R, Engel E, Lepperdinger G, Boitani C and Kreil G. The mammalian homologues of frog Bv8 are mainly expressed in spermatocytes. *FEBS Lett*. 1999;462:177–81.

[11] Nebigil CG. Prokineticin receptors in cardiovascular function: foe or friend? *Trends Cardiovasc Med*. 2009;19:55–60.

[12] Ross MG and Desai M. Developmental programming of appetite/satiety. *Ann Nutr Metab*. 2014;64(Suppl 1):36–44.

[13] Coll AP, Farooqi IS, Challis BG, Yeo GS and O'Rahilly S. Proopiomelanocortin and energy balance: insights from human and murine genetics. *J Clin Endocrinol Metab*. 2004;89:2557–62.

[14] Sobrino Crespo C, Perianes Cachero A, Puebla Jimenez L, Barrios V and Arilla Ferreiro E. Peptides and food intake. *Front Endocrinol (Lausanne)*. 2014;5:58.

[15] Gardiner JV, Bataveljic A, Patel NA, Bewick GA, Roy D, Campbell D, Greenwood HC, Murphy KG, Hameed S, Jethwa PH, Ebling FJ, Vickers SP, Cheetham S, Ghatei MA,

Bloom SR and Dhillo WS. Prokineticin 2 is a hypothalamic neuropeptide that potently inhibits food intake. *Diabetes*. 2010;59:397–406.

[16] Chaly AL, Srisai D, Gardner EE and Sebag JA. The melanocortin receptor accessory protein 2 promotes food intake through inhibition of the prokineticin receptor-1. *Elife*. 2016;5. p ii: e12397.

[17] Beale K, Gardiner JV, Bewick GA, Hostomska K, Patel NA, Hussain SS, Jayasena CN, Ebling FJ, Jethwa PH, Prosser HM, Lattanzi R, Negri L, Ghatei MA, Bloom SR and Dhillo WS. Peripheral administration of prokineticin 2 potently reduces food intake and body weight in mice via the brainstem. *Br J Pharmacol*. 2013;168:403–10.

[18] Iwasa T, Matsuzaki T, Munkhzaya M, Tungalagsuvd A, Kawami T, Murakami M, Yamasaki M, Kato T, Kuwahara A, Yasui T and Irahara M. Changes in the responsiveness of hypothalamic prokineticin 2 mRNA expression to food deprivation in developing female rats. *Int J Dev Neurosci*. 2014;34:76–8.

[19] Sarfati J, Guiochon-Mantel A, Rondard P, Arnulf I, Garcia-Pinero A, Wolczynski S, Brailly-Tabard S, Bidet M, Ramos-Arroyo M, Mathieu M, Lienhardt-Roussie A, Morgan G, Turki Z, Bremont C, Lespinasse J, Du Boullay H, Chabbert-Buffet N, Jacquemont S, Reach G, De Talence N, Tonella P, Conrad B, Despert F, Delobel B, Brue T, Bouvattier C, Cabrol S, Pugeat M, Murat A, Bouchard P, Hardelin JP, Dode C and Young J. A comparative phenotypic study of Kallmann syndrome patients carrying monoallelic and biallelic mutations in the prokineticin 2 or prokineticin receptor 2 genes. *J Clin Endocrinol Metab*. 2010;95:659–69.

[20] Hill JO, Wyatt HR and Peters JC. Energy balance and obesity. *Circulation*. 2012;126:126–32.

[21] Ma X, Lee P, Chisholm DJ and James DE. Control of adipocyte differentiation in different fat depots; implications for pathophysiology or therapy. *Front Endocrinol (Lausanne)*. 2015;6:1.

[22] Lafontan M. Adipose tissue and adipocyte dysregulation. *Diabetes Metab*. 2014;40:16–28.

[23] Dormishian M, Turkeri G, Urayama K, Nguyen TL, Boulberdaa M, Messaddeq N, Renault G, Henrion D and Nebigil CG. Prokineticin receptor-1 is a new regulator of endothelial insulin uptake and capillary formation to control insulin sensitivity and cardiovascular and kidney functions. *J Am Heart Assoc*. 2013;2:e000411.

[24] Kubota T, Kubota N, Kumagai H, Yamaguchi S, Kozono H, Takahashi T, Inoue M, Itoh S, Takamoto I, Sasako T, Kumagai K, Kawai T, Hashimoto S, Kobayashi T, Sato M, Tokuyama K, Nishimura S, Tsunoda M, Ide T, Murakami K, Yamazaki T, Ezaki O, Kawamura K, Masuda H, Moroi M, Sugi K, Oike Y, Shimokawa H, Yanagihara N, Tsutsui M, Terauchi Y, Tobe K, Nagai R, Kamata K, Inoue K, Kodama T, Ueki K and Kadowaki T. Impaired insulin signaling in endothelial cells reduces insulin-induced glucose uptake by skeletal muscle. *Cell Metab*. 2011;13:294–307.

[25] Genders AJ, Frison V, Abramson SR and Barrett EJ. Endothelial cells actively concentrate insulin during its transendothelial transport. *Microcirculation*. 2013;20:434–9.

[26] Prieto D, Contreras C and Sanchez A. Endothelial dysfunction, obesity and insulin resistance. *Curr Vasc Pharmacol*. 2014;12:412–26.

[27] Cao Y. Angiogenesis as a therapeutic target for obesity and metabolic diseases. *Chem Immunol Allergy*. 2014;99:170–9.

[28] Guilini C, Urayama K, Turkeri G, Dedeoglu DB, Kurose H, Messaddeq N and Nebigil CG. Divergent roles of prokineticin receptors in the endothelial cells: angiogenesis and fenestration. *Am J Physiol Heart Circ Physiol*. 2010;298:H844–52.

[29] Guo T, Bond ND, Jou W, Gavrilova O, Portas J and McPherron AC. Myostatin inhibition prevents diabetes and hyperphagia in a mouse model of lipodystrophy. *Diabetes*. 2012;61:2414–23.

[30] von Bibra H, Paulus W and St John Sutton M. Cardiometabolic syndrome and increased risk of heart failure. *Curr Heart Fail Rep*. 2016;13 :4 ;1–11

[31] Urban JD, Clarke WP, von Zastrow M, Nichols DE, Kobilka B, Weinstein H, Javitch JA, Roth BL, Christopoulos A, Sexton PM, Miller KJ, Spedding M and Mailman RB. Functional selectivity and classical concepts of quantitative pharmacology. *J Pharmacol Exp Ther*. 2007;320:1–13.

[32] Urayama K, Guilini C, Turkeri G, Takir S, Kurose H, Messaddeq N, Dierich A and Nebigil CG. Prokineticin receptor-1 induces neovascularization and epicardial-derived progenitor cell differentiation. *Arterioscler Thromb Vasc Biol*. 2008;28:841–9.

[33] Urayama K, Guilini C, Messaddeq N, Hu K, Steenman M, Kurose H, Ert G and Nebigil CG. The prokineticin receptor-1 (GPR73) promotes cardiomyocyte survival and angiogenesis. *FASEB J*. 2007;21:2980–93.

[34] Boulberdaa M, Turkeri G, Urayama K, Dormishian M, Szatkowski C, Zimmer L, Messaddeq N, Laugel V, Dolle P and Nebigil CG. Genetic inactivation of prokineticin receptor-1 leads to heart and kidney disorders. *Arterioscler Thromb Vasc Biol*. 2011;31:842–50.

[35] Duncan ER, Crossey PA, Walker S, Anilkumar N, Poston L, Douglas G, Ezzat VA, Wheatcroft SB, Shah AM and Kearney MT. Effect of endothelium-specific insulin resistance on endothelial function in vivo. *Diabetes*. 2008;57:3307–14.

[36] Tabit CE, Shenouda SM, Holbrook M, Fetterman JL, Kiani S, Frame AA, Kluge MA, Held A, Dohadwala MM, Gokce N, Farb MG, Rosenzweig J, Ruderman N, Vita JA and Hamburg NM. Protein kinase C-beta contributes to impaired endothelial insulin signaling in humans with diabetes mellitus. *Circulation*. 2013;127:86–95.

[37] Von Hunolstein JJ and Nebigil CG. Can prokineticin prevent obesity and insulin resistance? *Curr Opin Endocrinol Diabetes Obes*. 2015;22:367–73.

[38] Arora H, Boulberdaa M, Qureshi R, Bitirim V, Gasser A, Messaddeq N, Dolle P and Nebigil CG. Prokineticin receptor-1 signaling promotes epicardial to mesenchymal transition during heart development. *Sci Rep*. 2016;6:25541.

[39] Urayama K, Dedeoglu DB, Guilini C, Frantz S, Ertl G, Messaddeq N and Nebigil CG. Transgenic myocardial overexpression of prokineticin receptor-2 (GPR73b) induces hypertrophy and capillary vessel leakage. *Cardiovasc Res*. 2009;81:28–37.

[40] Gasser A, Brogi S, Urayama K, Nishi T, Kurose H, Tafi A, Ribeiro N, Desaubry L and Nebigil CG. Discovery and cardioprotective effects of the first non-Peptide agonists of the G protein-coupled prokineticin receptor-1. *PLoS One*. 2015;10:e0121027.

[41] Sun K, Kusminski CM and Scherer PE. Adipose tissue remodeling and obesity. *J Clin Invest*. 2011;121:2094–101.

[42] Molgat AS, Gagnon A and Sorisky A. Macrophage-induced preadipocyte survival depends on signaling through Akt, ERK1/2 and reactive oxygen species. *Exp Cell Res*. 2011;317:521–30.

2

Obesity and Coronary Artery Disease

Ibrahim Akin, Uzair Ansari and

Christoph A. Nienaber

Abstract

The impact of obesity can be better understood by studying the growing medical and socioeconomic burden of this often neglected public health epidemic. Traditionally associated with cardiovascular risk factors like hypertension, hyperlipidemia, and diabetes mellitus, morbid obesity has increasingly contributed to mortality among Western as well as Third World populations. Contemporary evidence has also consistently linked this patient cohort with a greater risk to develop coronary artery disease. Recent population-based registries indicate that 43 and 24% of all cases of coronary revascularization were performed in overweight and obese patients, respectively. In this context, although popular thought has reaffirmed the positive correlation between obesity and increased cardiovascular morbidity, some authors have opined a better clinical outcome in overweight and obese patients, a phenomenon they termed "obesity paradoxon." Conflicting data and the possibility of confounding bias have festered an ongoing debate challenging this "obesity paradox." In this review article, we present updated evidence and discuss the validity of the "obesity paradoxon" in a variety of clinical settings.

Keywords: coronary stent, obesity paradox, mortality, BMI

1. Introduction

Obesity has traditionally been defined as a body mass index (BMI) value $>30 \, \text{kg/m}^2$, and its prevalence in the Western world, according to recent epidemiological data, could be as high as 36.5% [1]. Evidence of the growing prevalence of obesity can be inferred from the USA, where almost 70% of the population has been classified as obese; a significant increase from the 25% reported forty years ago [2]. The clinical relevance of obesity and its cluster of associated disorders, like arterial hypertension, dyslipidemia, diabetes mellitus, and sleep apnea syndrome, are demonstrated by its persistent link to an increased morbidity as well as mortality [3, 4]. It is for this reason that initiatives detailing the primary and secondary prevention of cardiovascular disease in overweight and obese patients have laid specific emphasis on the significance of weight loss so as to modify cardiovascular risk [5–7]. Obese patients have an increased preponderance to develop atherosclerotic disease, especially coronary artery disease, which is characterized by a reduced sensitivity to insulin, enhanced free fatty acid turnover, increased basal sympathetic tone, a hyper-coagulable state, and finally with promotion of systemic inflammation [8, 9]. Population-based data suggest that 43 and 24% of all coronary revascularization in recent years were carried out in overweight and obese patients, respectively [10]. It has been speculated that the obese patient cohort is somehow associated with a clinical outcome far worse than that of a normal weight patient, and this theory is further substantiated by the existence of evidence describing the causative association of morbid obesity in cardiovascular disease. Interestingly, contemporary studies have recently elucidated the role of an "obesity paradoxon," describing the protective effect of obesity (when considering postoperative morbidity and mortality) in patients receiving either surgical or minimally invasive coronary revascularization [11]. This observation suggesting a better clinical outcome for obese patients is not only restricted to the clinical setting of coronary revascularization, as similar data have also been reported in cases of an acute myocardial infarction and heart failure [12, 13].

In this review article, we attempt to present an overview and summarize the evidence documented on "obesity paradoxon" in coronary artery disease.

2. Stable coronary artery disease

The correlation of BMI with clinical endpoints in the setting of interventional coronary revascularization from a single-center experience in patients (n = 3571) receiving balloon angioplasty was first reported in 1996 [14]. A detailed study of the in-hospital outcomes suggested higher rates of mortality (2.8% vs. 0.9% vs. 3.7%; $p < 0.001$) in normal weight and obese patients as compared to overweight patients. This bias could also noted in the patients' need for blood transfusions (11.9% vs. 7.4% vs. 8.4%; $p = 0.003$) and their corresponding rise in creatinine value >1 mg/dl (3.6% vs. 1.8% vs. 1.8%; $p = 0.018$). Interestingly, the rates of myocardial infarction did not reflect any such patient group preference (3.5% vs. 3.4% vs. 4.7%; p = n.s.). The multicenter BARI registry evaluated the BMI of 3634 patients undergoing elective revascularization [2108 by interventional procedure (PCI) and 1526 by surgery (CABG)] at study entry between 1988 and 1991 [15]. Initial analyses of the results elicited a correlation between the body mass index and an increased risk of a major in-hospital event in the PCI arm. At the five-year follow-up interval, this correlation between BMI and mortality existed only in the CABG arm. The final results from the BARI registry suggested an inverse relationship between BMI and in-hospital outcome post-PCI without any major difference in long-term follow-up. Interestingly, although the study by Gruberg et al. [11] did indicate an inverse relationship in the 9633 patients evaluated between 1994 and 1999 at the 12-month follow-up for mortality (10.6% vs. 5.7% vs 4.9%:

$p < 0.0001$), rates of myocardial infarction (7.4% vs. 7.0% vs. 6.7%: $p = 0.66$) and target vessel revascularization (20.2% vs. 22.0% vs. 22.4%: $p = 0.16$) did not vary significantly. Certain post-procedural clinical events like arterial hypertension, pulmonary congestion, impairment of renal function, bleeding events, access site complications, as well as those leading to mortality were seen more often in underweight patients as compared to the overweight and obese patient cohort.

The Scottish Coronary Revascularization Register offers another perspective to this debate. In contrast to previous all-comers trials, this study included only those patients ($n = 4880$) undergoing elective PCI between 1997 and 2006, and without any known history of coronary artery disease. Patients evaluated to have a BMI in the range between 27 and 30 kg/m^2 were linked with lower all-cause mortality after 5 years of follow-up as compared to other weight groups. The introduction of a blanking time (<30 days) to exclude periprocedural events as well as an adjustment to different baseline data did not impact the outcome of their study [16]. These conclusions were reaffirmed in the APPROACH registry, where a collective of 310,121 patients were treated conservatively ($n = 7801$), by PCI ($n = 7017$), or by CABG ($n = 15,601$) [17]. Lower mortality rates were recorded among overweight and obese patients as compared to normal weight patients in the cohort treated conservatively. These findings were also consistent for the CABG as well as the PCI group. An interesting corollary to these results centered around the use of bare-metal stents (BMS) as well as a discussion on the meta-analysis of these single trials, suggesting an inverse relationship between BMI and the clinical outcome after stenting [18]. The results from studies of the balloon angioplasty and the BMS era are in stark contrast to other studies conducted in this timeframe, wherein patients receiving any of the two stents, DES or BMS, did not observe the "obesity paradoxon." An additional note in this context is summarized by the study of Poston et al. conducted in 1631 patients, suggesting that normal weight patients were older than obese or overweight patients at the time of hospital admission [18]. The 1-year follow-up mortality and risk for procedure revision were comparable in both groups.

In the TAXUS trials, of the 1307 patients stratified according to BMI and type of stent used (BMS versus DES) [20], higher rates of BMS in-stent restenoses were observed in obese and overweight patients than in normal-weight patients (29.2% vs. 30.5% vs. 9.3%; $p = 0.01$). The patients receiving DES had major cardiac event (MACE) rates skewing in favor of normal weight patients, and however, the clinical event rates in these different patient groups did not vary significantly. Subsequent results obtained from the German DES.DE registry would also validate these findings [21]. A total of 5806 patients assimilated from 98 sites in Germany were included in this registry for DES patients and followed up over a period of 12 months. The results would summarize suggestions made in previous trials, stating that the baseline comorbidity index was higher in obese patients as compared to overweight and normal weight patients, while the rates of in-hospital events were similar in all three groups. The follow-up after 1 year indicated no significant variability in mortality rates (3.3% vs. 2.4% vs. 2.4%; $p = 0.17$), myocardial infarction (2.8% vs. 2.3% vs. 2.3%; $p = 0.45$), target vessel revascularization (10.9% vs. 11.7% vs. 11.6%; $p = 0.56$), and major bleeding

Author	Year	n	Follow-up (months)	Mortality	Myocardial infarction	Target vessel revascularization	Renal insufficiency	Vascular complications
Ellis et al. [14]	1996	3571	12	+	−	−	+	+
Gurm et al. [15]	2002	3634	60	+	n.a.	n.a.	n.a.	−
Gruberg et al. [11]	2002	9633	12	+	−	−	+	−
Poston et al. [19]	2004	1631	12	−	n.a.	−	n.a.	n.a.
Nikolsky et al. [20]	2005	1301	12	−	−	−	n.a.	n.a.
Romero-Corral et al. [18]	2006	250, 152	45	+	n.a.	n.a.	n.a.	n.a.
Oreopoulos et al. [17]	2009	31, 021	46	+	n.a.	n.a.	n.a.	n.a.
Hastie et al. [16]	2010	4880	60	+	n.a.	n.a.	n.a.	n.a.
Akin et al. [21]	2012	5806	12	−	−	−	−	−

Table 1. Overview of literature addressing the "obesity paradox" in patients suffering from stable coronary artery disease undergoing coronary angiography and/or revascularization.

(2.5% vs. 2.1% vs. 2.8%; $p = 0.53$) between normal weight, overweight, and obese patients, respectively (**Table 1**).

3. Acute coronary syndrome

The essential difference between stable coronary artery disease and an acute myocardial infarction is the existence of a pro-inflammatory state with different forms of hemodynamic, rhythmogenic, and hemostatic disturbance in the latter. Although the "obesity paradoxon" phenomenon has been evaluated in the patient population, there is lack of homogenous data establishing a potential link between BMI and clinical events in patients with acute myocardial infarction. Data analyses of the 6359 acute coronary syndrome (ACS) patients included in the PREMIER and TRIUMPH registries drawn to establish a relationship between BMI and survival rate yielded novel results [22]. BMI and mortality rates shared an inverse relationship (9.2% vs. 6.1% vs. 4.7%; $p < 0.001$) irrespective of demographic age and sex distribution. The KAMIR registry yielded similar results in its 3824 ST-elevation myocardial infarction patient collective [23]. The baseline characteristics defined an older group of normal weight patients, with impairment of left ventricular ejection fraction and having a higher comorbidity index. The study eventually summarized that normal weight patients were associated with higher mortality rates.

An attempt to reaffirm this inverse relationship between BMI and clinical outcome in this scenario, however, was not possible in many other similarly conducted trials [24, 25]. Our research working group analyzed data from 890 patients diagnosed with ST-elevated myocardial infarction and followed them up for a duration of 12 months. This group also constituted patients diagnosed with cardiogenic shock. Interestingly, results indicated that clinical events did not vary significantly between all three weight groups, thus challenging the premise of the "obesity paradox" [26] (**Table 2**).

Author	Year	N	Follow-up (months)	Mortality	Myocardial infarction	Target vessel revascularization	Renal insufficiency	Vascular complications
Kosuge et al. [25]	2008	3076	hospital	–	n.a.	n.a.	n.a.	n.a.
Kang et al. [23]	2010	3824	12	+	–	–	n.a.	n.a.
Camprubi et al. [24]	2012	824	hospital	–	n.a.	n.a.	n.a.	n.a.
Bucholz et al. [22]	2012	6359	12	+	n.a.	n.a.	n.a.	n.a.
Li et al. [27]	2013	1429	12	–	–	–	n.a.	n.a.
Shehab et al. [28]	2014	4379	1	–	–	–	n.a.	n.a.
Akin et al. [26]	2015	890	12	–	–	–	–	–

Table 2. Overview of literature addressing the "obesity paradox" in patients suffering from acute coronary syndrome, including cardiogenic shock, undergoing coronary revascularization.

4. Rationale for the "obesity paradox"

The growing incidence of obesity can be construed from data suggesting an increase of 37% from 13.6 to 18.6%, in the cases of self-reported obesity, among men aged 35–49 since 1970. Epidemiological factors attributed to the development of obesity and cardiovascular disease like arterial hypertension and diabetes mellitus are also on the rise [29, 30]. Recent efforts directed to reducing cholesterol levels and prevention of damaging smoking habits have helped sustain a decline in mortality from an acute coronary event. Frequent vessel revascularization has also possibly played a role in this positive development [31–33]. This, however, does not discount the influence of the metabolic syndrome and its link to various cardiovascular risk factors. Overweight and obese patients are derivatives of this syndrome, and the continual process of endothelial dysfunction and inflammation is often associated with the risk of developing atherosclerosis.

Evidence of this correlation constitutes an interesting paradox where better survival rates in an acute coronary event are real despite an increased incidence of obesity. This pertinent question has festered an ongoing debate as to the existence of the "obesity paradoxon" phenomenon in the spectrum of coronary artery disease [10–26].

An examination of current literature indicates that certain published data, essentially that comprising retrospective information, have claimed a U-shaped nonsignificant trend to suggest lower survival among underweight patients as compared to normal or mildly overweight patients. This, however, could be the result of a technical bias, which unfortunately cannot be fully corrected by statistical means.

A detailed analysis of these patient groups has suggested that up to 2% of patients who are underweight are likely to suffer from comorbid conditions, including malignancies, heart failure, malnutrition, and multi-organ dysfunction (MODS). This patient group also happens to constitute a significantly older age group demographic as compared to normal and obese patients [10, 11, 15], and clear evidence has linked elderly and frail patients to significantly poorer clinical outcomes regardless of management or reperfusion strategy [34, 35].

An interesting highlight in this respect is the influence of increasing age with its concomitant comorbidities on weight change [36–38]. The possibility of chronic disease leading to gradual weight loss had not been factored into presented trials. Another important confounding observation was the increased tendency of obese patients receiving diagnosis and treatment at an earlier stage in comparison with lean patients.

A recent survey of >130,000 patients suggested that patients with higher BMI adhere more sincerely to guidelines with regard to the use of standard drugs such as aspirin, beta-blockers, acetylcholinesterase inhibitors, angiotensin II receptor blockers, as well as lipid-lowering drugs and are increasingly likely to undergo invasive diagnostic and therapeutic interventions [15, 18, 21]. Additionally, overweight and obese subjects tended to be more stable at presentation, with the general constellation describing a patient lacking hemodynamic compromise, having a lower Killip class and also a preserved or less impaired ventricular function, which in turn proffers a better prognosis to the existing clinical scenario. These preliminary results present a clear challenge to the "obesity parodoxon" phenomenon.

Novel theories explaining the post-PCI "obesity paradoxon" hypothesize that obese patients have "larger vessels" somehow instituting a beneficial effect. A further consolidation of this hypothesis naturally suggests that post-PCI outcome is significantly worse in patients with smaller vessels [39, 40]. The pharmacology of antithrombotic drugs is another interesting topic of discussion in this regard. The use of a standard dose rather than weight-adjusted dosages precludes accurate measurement of the pharmacokinetic and pharmacodynamic effects of these medications in each patient. For example, the standard dose could very well be too high for an underweight patient (as calculated by BMI) resulting in significant bleeding events and is associated with a higher mortality rate [41]. Similarly, the sheath-to-artery size ratio varies in different BMI groups, and this could influence the rates of vascular complications [15]. These superficial differences observed in the context of a periprocedural event can reflect on the perceived improved survival noted among overweight patients [11, 42].

An absolute limiting factor in most studies centers around the use of BMI as a measure of obesity. The inadequate documentation of obesity distribution questions the plausibility of several results as this vital information has a significant impact in the clinical scenario. For example, central obesity has been associated with a poorer clinical outcome [43]. Other parameters such as waist circumference, waist-to-hip ratio, and weight change have not found mention in several of these trials [44–47]. Additionally, the inherent limitation of all these trials hypothesizing the "obesity paradoxon" is that they are an observational retrospective registry.

The failure to analyze potentially confounding variables such as physical inactivity, unintended weight loss, the influence of socioeconomic factors, as well as the short follow-up of these registries may have contributed to additional bias. Any existing relationship between obesity and in-hospital and short-term survival may have been lost, and the longer patients were followed. The possible buildup of the detrimental effects of obesity overtime could also have been studied in an extended follow-up period, perhaps establishing a link to increased late mortality [48, 49].

The "obesity paradoxon" hypothesis hinges on certain questionable data. The proponents of this theory claim that replete adipose tissue plays the role of an endocrine organ [50] producing soluble tissue necrosis factor receptor and hence ensues the protective effect [51].

Conversely, higher levels of thrombotic factors as well as elevated plasminogen activator inhibitor-I in patients who are morbidly obese (BMI > 40 Kg/m^2) probably contribute to the higher adjusted rates of post-PCI mortality seen in this patient group [52].

The suggestion, in early studies, that there exists an inverse relationship between underweight patients and outcomes in heart failure is what heralded the concept of "obesity paradoxon." However, an in-depth analysis of recently published data questions any such claim in the setting of coronary artery disease and modern coronary intervention. In fact, there is insufficient evidence or even proof of concept to veer away from the classic relationship between risk factors, confounding variables and prognostic outcomes. These association studies are limited not only by the lack of pathophysiological underpinnings, but also hindered by the use of descriptive notions and confounding variables with unknown impact to substantiate their results. While analyzing the neutralizing results of the German DES.DE Registry [21], the perception of obesity demonstrating a protective effect on outcomes post-PCI is seriously held in doubt and the provocative construct of an "obesity paradoxon" debased, as this hypothesis was never really substantiated in the clinical setting of coronary artery disease and PCI.

Finally, the support expressed by associative studies (in light of little or no statistical and biological evidence) leading to the hypothesis of an "obesity paradox" has been effectively debunked by the interpretation of recent clinical data. A contrarian concept would only hold traction if supported by plausible pathophysiology. In the context of coronary artery disease and PCI, there are hardly any convincing explanation and certainly no clinical data to justify an "obesity paradoxon."

Author details

Ibrahim Akin[1,*], Uzair Ansari[1] and Christoph A. Nienaber[2]

*Address all correspondence to: ibrahim.akin@umm.de

1 University Mannheim, Mannheim, Germany

2 Royal Brompton Hospital and Harefield Trust, London, UK

References

[1] Berghöfer A, Pischon T, Reinhold T, Apovian CM, Sharma AM, Willich SN. Obesity prevalence from a European perspective: a systematic review. BMC Public Health 2008; 8: 200. [PMID:18533989 doi:10.1186/1471-2458-8-200]

[2] Ogden CL, Carroll MD, Curtin LR, McDowell MA, Tabak CJ, Flegal KM. Prevalence of overweight and obesity in the United States, 1999–2004. JAMA 2006; 295: 1549–1555. [PMID:16595758 doi:10.1001/jama.295.13.1549]

[3] Garrison RJ, Higgins MW, Kannel WB. Obesity and coronary heart disease. Curr Opin Lipidol 1996; 4: 199–202. [PMID:8883494]

[4] Lakka HM, Laaksonen DE, Lakka TA, et al. The metabolic syndrome and total and cardiovascular disease mortality in middle-aged men. JAMA 2002; 288: 2709–2716. [PMID:12460094 doi:10.1001/jama.288.21.2709]

[5] Smith SC Jr, Blair SN, Bonow RO, Brass LM, Cerqueira MD, Dracup K, Fuster V, Gotto A, Grundy SM, Miller NH, Jacobs A, Jones D, Krauss RM, Mosca L, Ockene I, Pasternak RC, Pearson T, Pfeffer MA, Starke RD, Taubert KA. AHA/ACC guidelines for preventing heart attack and death in patients with atherosclerotic Cardiovascular Disease: 2001 update-a statement for healthcare professionals from the American Association and the American College of Cardiology. J Am Coll Cardiol 2001; 38: 1581–1583. [PMID:11691544 doi:10.1016/S0735-1097(01)01682-5]

[6] De Backer G, Ambrosioni E, Borch-Johnsen K, Brotons C, Cifkova R, Dallongeville J, Ebrahim S, Faergeman O, Graham I, Mancia G, Cats VM, Orth-Gomér K, Perk J, Pyörälä K, Rodicio JL, Sans S, Sansoy V, Sechtem U, Silber S, Thomsen T, Wood D; European Society of Cardiology Committee for Practice Guidelines. European guidelines on cardiovascular disease prevention in clinical practice: third joint task force of Eurpean and other societies on cardiovascular disease prevention in clinical practice (constituted by representatives of eight societies and by invited experts). Eur J Cardiovasc Prev Rehab 2003; 10: S1–S10. [PMID:1455889 doi:10.1097/01.hjr.0000087913.96265.e2]

[7] Willett WC, Dietz WH, Colditz GA. Guidelines for health weight. N Engl J Med 1999; 341: 427–434. [PMID:10432328 doi:10.1056/NEJM199908053410607]

[8] Hubert HB, Feinleib M, McNamara PM, Castelli WP. Obesity as an independent risk factor for cardiovascular disease: a 26-year follow-up of participiants in the Framingham Heart Study. Circulation 1983; 67: 968–977. [PMID:6219830 doi:10.1161/01.CIR.67.5.968]

[9] Whitlock G, Lewington S, Sherliker P, Clarke R, Emberson J, Halsey J, Qizilbash N, Collins R, Peto R. Body-mass index and cause-specific mortality in 900,000 adults: collaborative analyses of 57 prospective studies. Lancet 2009; 373: 1083–1096. [PMID:19299006 doi:10.1016/S0140-6736(09)60318-4]

[10] Minutello RM, Chou ET, Hong MK, Bergman G, Parikh M, Iacovone F, Wong SC. Impact of body mass index on in-hospital outcomes following percutaneous coronary intervention (report from the New York State Angioplasty Registry). Am J Cardiol 2004; 93: 1229–1232. [PMID:15135694 doi:10.1016/j.amjcard.2004.01.065]

[11] Gruberg L, Weissman NJ, Waksman R, Fuchs S, Deible R, Pinnow EE, Ahmed LM, Kent KM, Pichard AD, Suddath WO, Satler LF, Lindsay J Jr. The impact of obesity

on the short-term and long-term outcomes after percutaneous coronary intervention: the obesity paradox? J Am Coll Cardiol 2002; 39: 578–584. [PMID:11849854 doi:10.1016/S0735-1097(01)01802-2]

[12] Califf RM, Pieper KS, Lee KL, Van De Werf F, Simes RJ, Armstrong PW, Topol EJ. Prediction of 1-year survival after thrombolysis for acute myocardial infarction in the global utilization of streptokinase and TPA for occluded coronary arteries trial. Circulation 2000; 101: 2231–2238. [PMID:10811588 doi:10.1161/01.CIR.101.19.2231]

[13] Fonarow GC, Srikanthan P, Costanzo MR, Cintron GB, Lopatin M; ADHERE Scientific Advisory Committee and Investigators. An obesity paradox in acute heart failure: analysis of body mass index and in hospital mortality for 108,927 patients in the Acute Decompensated Heart Failure National Registry. Am Heart J 2007; 153: 74–81. [PMID:17174642 doi:10.1016/j.ahj.2006.09.007]

[14] Ellis SG, Elliott J, Horrigan M, Raymond RE, Howell G. Low-normal or excessive body mass index: newly identified and powerful risk factors for death and other complications with percutaneous coronary intervention. Am J Cardiol 1996; 78: 642–646. [PMID:8831397 doi:10.1016/S0002-9149(96)00386-4]

[15] Gurm HS, Whitlow PL, Kip KE, et al. The impact of body mass index on short- and long-term outcomes in patients undergoing coronary revascularization. Insight from the Bypass Angioplasty Revascularization Investigations (BARI). J Am Coll Cardiol 2002; 39: 834–840. [PMID:11869849 doi:10.1016/S0735-1097(02)01687-X]

[16] Hastie CE, Padmanabhan S, Slack R, Pell AC, Oldroyd KG, Flapan AD, Jennings KP, Irving J, Eteiba H, Dominiczak AF, Pell JP. Obesity paradox in a cohort of 4880 consecutive patients undergoing percutaneous coronary intervention. Eur Heart J 2010; 31: 222–226. [PMID:19687163 doi:10.1093/eurheartj/ehp317]

[17] Oreopoulos A, Mc Allister FA, Kalantar-Zadeh K, Padwal R, Ezekowitz JA, Sharma AM, Kovesdy CP, Fonarow GC, Norris CM. The relationship between body mass index, treatment, and mortality in patients with established coronary artery disease: a report from APPROACH. Eur Heart J 2009; 30: 2584–2592. [PMID:19617221 doi:10.1093/eurheartj/ehp288]

[18] Romero-Corral A, Montori VM, Somers VK, Korinek J, Thomas RJ, Allison TG, Mookadam F, Lopez-Jimenez F. Association of bodyweight with total mortality and with cardiovascular events in coronary artery disease: a systematic review of cohort studies. Lancet 2006; 368: 666–678. [PMID:16920472 doi:10.1016/S0140-6736(06)69251-9]

[19] Poston WS, Haddock CK, Conard M, Spertus JA. Impact of obesity on disease-specific health status after percutaneous coronary intervention in coronary disease patients. Int J Obes Relat Metab Disord 2004; 28: 1011–1017. [PMID:15211370 doi:10.1038/sj.ijo.0802703]

[20] Nikolsky E, Kosinski E, Mishkel GJ, Kimmelstiel C, McGarry TF Jr, Mehran R, Leon MB, Russell ME, Ellis SG, Stone GW. Impact of obesity on revascularization and restenosis

rates after bare-metal and drug-eluting stent implantation (from the TAXUS-IV trial). Am J Cardiol 2005; 95: 709–715. [PMID:15757595 doi:10.1016/j.amjcard.2004.11.020]

[21] Akin I, Tölg R, Hochadel M, Khattab AA, Schneider S, Senges J, Kuck KH, Richardt G, Nienaber CA; DES.DE (German Drug-Eluting Stent) Study Group. No evidence of "obesity paradox" after treatment with drug-eluting stents in a routine clinical practice: results from the prospective multicenter German DES.DE (German Drug-Eluting Stent) registry. JACC Cardiovasc Interv 2012; 5: 162–169. [PMID:22361600 doi:10.1016/j. jcin.2011.09.021]

[22] Bucholz EM, Rathore SS, Reid KJ, Jones PG, Chan PS, Rich MW, Spertus JA, Krumholz HM. Body mass index and mortality in acute myocardial infarction patients. Am J Med 2012; 125: 796–803. [PMID:22483510 doi:10.1016/j.amjmed.2012.01.018]

[23] Kang WY, Jeong MH, Ahn YK, Kim JH, Chae SC, Kim YJ, Hur SH, Seong IW, Hong TJ, Choi DH, Cho MC, Kim CJ, Seung KB, Chung WS, Jang YS, Rha SW, Bae JH, Cho JG, Park SJ; Korea Acute Myocardial Infarction Registry Investigators. Obesity paradox in Korean patients undergoing primary percutaneous coronary intervention in ST-segment elevation myocardial infarction. J Cardiol 2010; 55: 84–91. [PMID:20122553 doi:10.1016/j. jjcc.2009.10.004]

[24] Camprubi M, Cabrera S, Sans J, et al. Body mass index and hospital mortality in patients with acute coronary syndrome receiving care in a university hospital. J Obes 2012;2012:287939. [PMID:22900151 doi:10.1155/2012/287939]

[25] Kosuge M, Kimura K, Kojima S, Sakamoto T, Ishihara M, Asada Y, Tei C, Miyazaki S, Sonoda M, Tsuchihashi K, Yamagishi M, Shirai M, Hiraoka H, Honda T, Ogata Y, Ogawa H; Japanese Acute Coronary Syndrome Study (JACSS) Investigators. Impact of body mass index on in-hospital outcomes after percutaneous coronary intervention for ST segment elevation acute myocardial infarction. Circ J 2008; 72: 521–525. [PMID:18362419 doi:JST.JSTAGE/circj/72.521]

[26] Akin I, Schneider H, Nienaber CA, Jung W, Lübke M, Rillig A, Ansari U, Wunderlich N, Birkemeyer R. Lack of "obesity paradox" in patients presenting with ST-segment elevation myocardial infarction including cardiogenic shock-a multicenter German network registry analysis. BMC Cardiovasc Disord 2015; 15: 67. [PMID: 26162888 doi:10.1186/ s12872-015-0065-6]

[27] Li Y, Wu C, Sun Y, Jiang D, Zhang B, Ren L, Gao Y, Yu H, Yang G, Guan Q, Tian W, Zhang H, Guo L, Qi G. Obesity paradox: clinical benefits not observed in obese patients with ST-segment elevation myocardial infarction: a multivcenter, prospective, cohort study of the northern region of China. Int J Cardiol 2013; 168: 2949–2950. [PMID:23642605 doi:10.1016/j.ijcard.2013.03.169]

[28] Shehab A, Al-Dabbagh B, AlHabib K, Alsheikh-Ali A, Almahmeed W, Sulaiman K, Al-Motarreb A, Suwaidi JA, Hersi A, AlFaleh H, Asaad N, AlSaif S, Amin H, Alanbaei M, Nagelkerke N, Abdulle A. The obesity paradox in patients with acute coronary syndrome:

results from the Gulf RACE-2 study. Angiology 2014; 65: 585–589. [PMID:23921507 doi:10.1177/0003319713497087]

[29] Ford ES, Capewell S. Coronary heart disease mortality among young adults in the U.S. from 1980 through 2002: concealed leveling of mortality rates. J Am Coll Cardiol 2007; 50: 2128–2132. [PMID:18036449 doi:10.1016/j.jacc.2007.05.056]

[30] O'Flaherty M, Ford E, Allender S, Scarborough P, Capewell S. Coronary heart disease trends in England and Wales from 1984 to 2004: concealed levelling of mortality rates among young adults. Heart 2007; 94: 178–181. [PMID: 17641070 doi:10.1136/hrt.2007.118323]

[31] Unal B, Critchley JA, Capewell S. Explaining the decline in coronary heart disease mortality in England and Wales between 1981 and 2000. Circulation 2004; 109: 1101–1107. [PMID:14993137 doi:10.1161/01.CIR.0000118498.35499.B2]

[32] Ford ES, Ajani UA, Croft JB, Critchley JA, Labarthe DR, Kottke TE, Giles WH, Capewell S. Explaining the decrease in US deaths from coronary disease, 1980–2000. N Engl J Med 2007; 356: 2388–2398. [PMID:17554120 doi:10.1056/NEJMsa053935]

[33] Gregg EW, Cheng YJ, Cadwell BL, Imperatore G, Williams DE, Flegal KM, Narayan KM, Williamson DF. Secular trends in cardiovascular disease risk factors according to body mass index in US adults. JAMA 2005; 293: 1868–1874. [PMID:15840861 doi:10.1001/jama.293.15.1868]

[34] Holmes DR Jr, White HD, Pieper KS, Ellis SG, Califf RM, Topol EJ. Effect of age on outcome with primary angioplasty versus thrombolysis. J Am Coll Cardiol 1999; 33: 412–419. [PMID:9973021 doi:10.1016/S0735-1097(98)00579-8]

[35] Halkin A, Singh M, Nikolsky E, Grines CL, Tcheng JE, Garcia E, Cox DA, Turco M, Stuckey TD, Na Y, Lansky AJ, Gersh BJ, O'Neill WW, Mehran R, Stone GW. Prediction of mortality after primary percutaneous coronary intervention for acute myocardial infarction. The CADILLAC risk score. J Am Coll Cardiol 2005; 45: 1397–1405. [PMID:15862409 doi:10.1016/j.jacc.2005.01.041]

[36] Strandberg TE, Strandberg AY, Salomaa VV, Pitkälä KH, Tilvis RS, Sirola J, Miettinen TA. Explaining the obesity paradox: cardiovascular risk, weight change, and mortality during long-term follow-up in men. Eur Heart J 2009; 30: 1720–1727. [PMID:19429917 doi:10.1093/eurheartj/ehp162]

[37] Calle EE, Thun MJ, Petrelli JM, Rodriguez C, Heatzh CW Jr. Body-mass index and mortality in a prospective cohort of U.S. adults. N Engl J Med 1999; 341: 1097–1105. [PMID:10511607 doi:10.1056/NEJM199910073411501]

[38] O'Donovan G, Owen A, Kearney EM, Jones DW, Nevill AM, Woolf-May K, Bird SR. Cardiovascular disease risk factors in habitual exercisers, lean sedentary men and abdominal obese sedentary men. Int J Obes (Lond) 2005; 29: 1063–1069. [PMID:15925958 doi:10.1038/sj.ijo.0803004]

[39] Schunkert H, Harrell L, Palacios IF. Implications of small reference vessel diameter in patients undergoing percutaneous coronary revascularization. J Am Coll Cardiol 1999; 34: 40–48. [PMID:10399990 doi:10.1016/S0735-1097(99)00181-3]

[40] Foley DP, Melkert R, Serruys PW. Influence of coronary vessel size on renarrowing process and late angiographic outcome after successful balloon angioplasty. Circulation 1994; 90: 1239–1251. [PMID:8087933 doi:10.1161/01.CIR.90.3.1239]

[41] Powell BD, Lennon RJ, Lerman A, Bell MR, Berger PB, Higano ST, Holmes DR Jr, Rihal CS. Association of body mass index with outcome after percutaneous coronary inetrvention. Am J Cardiol 2003; 91: 472–476. [PMID:12586271 doi:10.1016/S0002-9149(02)03252-6]

[42] Manson JE, Stampfer MJ, Henneckens CH, Williett WC. Body weight and longevity: a reassessment. JAMA 1987; 257: 353–358. [PMID:3795418 doi:10.1001/jama.1987.03390030083026]

[43] Folsom AR, Kushi LH, Anderson KE, Mink PJ, Olson JE, Hong CP, Sellers TA, Lazovich D, Prineas RJ. Association of general and abdominal obesity with multiple health outcomes in older women: the Iowa Women's Health study. Arch Intern Med 2000; 160: 2117–2128. [PMID:10904454 doi:10.1001/archinte.160.14.2117]

[44] Yusuf S, Hawken S, Ounpunn S, Bautista L, Franzosi MG, Commerford P, Lang CC, Rumboldt Z, Onen CL, Lisheng L, Tanomsup S, Wangai P Jr, Razak F, Sharma AM, Anand SS; INTERHEART Study Investigators. Obesity and the risk of myocardial infarction in 27,000 participants from 52 countries: a case-control study. Lancet 2005; 366: 1640–1649. [PMID:16271645 doi:10.1016/S0140-6736(05)67663-5]

[45] Dagenais GR, Yi Q, Mann JF, Bosch J, Pogue J, Yusuf S. Prognostic impact of body weight and abdominal obesity in women and men with cardiovascular disease. Am Heart J 2005; 149: 54–60. [PMID:15660034 doi:10.1016/j.ahj.2004.07.009]

[46] Pischon T, Boeing H, Hoffmann K, Bergmann M, Schulze MB, Overvad K, van der Schouw YT, Spencer E, Moons KG, Tjønneland A, Halkjaer J, Jensen MK, Stegger J, Clavel-Chapelon F, Boutron-Ruault MC, Chajes V, Linseisen J, Kaaks R, Trichopoulou A, Trichopoulos D, Bamia C, Sieri S, Palli D, Tumino R, Vineis P, Panico S, Peeters PH, May AM, Bueno-de-Mesquita HB, van Duijnhoven FJ, Hallmans G, Weinehall L, Manjer J, Hedblad B, Lund E, Agudo A, Arriola L, Barricarte A, Navarro C, Martinez C, Quirós JR, Key T, Bingham S, Khaw KT, Boffetta P, Jenab M, Ferrari P, Riboli E. General and abdominal adiposity and risk of death in Europe. N Engl J Med 2008; 358: 2105–2120. [PMID:19005195 doi:10.1056/NEJMoa0801891]

[47] Lavie CJ, Milani RV, Ventura HO. Obesity and cardiovascular disease. Risk factor, paradox, and impact of weight loss. J Am Coll Cardiol 2009; 53: 1925–1932. [PMID:19460605 doi:10.1016/j.jacc.2008.12.068]

[48] Rhoads GG, Kagan A. The relation of coronary disease, stroke and mortality to weight in youth and middle age. Lancet 1983; 1: 492–495. [PMID:6131209 doi:S0140-6736(83)92189-X]

[49] Allison DB, Faith MS, Heo M, Kotler DP. Hypothesis concerning the U-shaped rela-
      tion between body mass index and mortality. Am J Epidemiol 1997; 146: 339–349.
      [PMID:9270413]

[50] Kerhaw EE, Flier JS. Adipose tissue as an endocrine organ. J Clin Endocrinol Metab 2004;
      89: 2548–2556. [PMID:15181022 doi:10.1210/jc.2004-0395]

[51] Mohamed-Ali V, Goodrick S, Bulmer K, Holly JM, Yudkin JS, Coppack SW. Production
      of soluble tumor necrosis factor receptors by human subcutanoeus adipose tissue *in vivo*.
      Am J Physiol 1999; 277: E971–E975. [PMID:10600783]

[52] De Pergola G, Pannacciulli N. Coagulation and fibrinolysis abnormalities in obesity.
      J Endocrinol Invest 2002; 25: 899–904. [PMID:12508953 doi:10.1007/BF03344054]

3

Vitamin D Status in Obesity: Relation with Expression of Vitamin D Receptor and Vitamin D Hydroxylation Enzymes in Subcutaneous and Visceral Adipose Tissue

Adryana Cordeiro and Andrea Ramalho

Abstract

Currently and worldwide, a high prevalence of obesity, obesity-associated metabolic dysfunction, and vitamin D (VD) deficiency occurs. Besides participating in bone mineralization and calcium homeostasis, VD has other major functional roles. The vitamin D receptor (VDR) signaling pathway is crucial for the proper functioning of adipose tissue (AT). AT is a reservoir for VD and can activate/inactivate VD by hydroxylation. Subcutaneous and visceral AT (SAT, VAT) have different and prime roles in metabolic regulation/dysfunction. A search was done on PubMed/Medline, Web of Science, and Scopus databases using the following keywords: vitamin D, vitamin D receptor, hydroxylases, subcutaneous adipose tissue, visceral adipose tissue, obesity, and metabolic dysfunction. Our chapter focuses on human studies on VD status and expression of VDR and VD activation/inactivation enzymes in SAT and VAT in an obese environment.

Keywords: obesity, adiposity measures, visceral adipose tissue, subcutaneous adipose tissue, vitamin D, vitamin D receptor, vitamin D hydroxylation

1. Introduction

Obesity is defined as an excess amount of body fat that may impair health [1] and has been strongly associated with chronic low-grade or metabolic inflammation characterized by the activation of inflammatory signaling pathways and abnormal secretion of a large set of immune response mediators and several bioactive proteins [2, 3] known as adipokines [4] and a deficit of mediators responsible for the resolution of this process [5]. Within the adipose tissue (AT), other cells are also present including preadipocytes, mast cells, and macrophages, which also contribute to this inflammatory environment. Currently and worldwide, obesity is the fifth greatest risk factor for mortality [6], and it is associated with vitamin D deficiency (VDD) [7].

Vitamin D (VD) is essential for the development and maintenance of bone tissue, as well as for normal homeostasis of calcium and phosphorus [8]. Moreover, VD has other major functional roles; it is related to differentiation, cell proliferation, and hormone secretion. It is an important nutrient with crucial role in obesity onset (AT) and in the comorbidities associated with the chronic inflammation [9].

An estimated 80–90% of VD from the human body originates from skin synthesis, with sunlight activation, while the rest is supplied through supplements or food [10]. VD status is measured by means of the plasma levels of 25-hydroxyvitamin D [25(OH)D] or calcidiol, the dominant circulating form and the best indicator of VD status [11]. The action of $1,25(OH)_2D$, active form of VD [12], is mediated through the vitamin D receptor (VDR), a member of the nuclear receptor superfamily, which regulates the transcription of many target genes [13].

The VDR signaling pathway is crucial for the proper functioning of AT that is called an active endocrine organ, which plays an important role in fat storage and in the production and secretion of adipokines [14, 15]; is a reservoir for VD; and, besides, can activate/inactivate it by hydroxylation. VD and VDR are implicated in preadipocyte differentiation into adipocytes [16].

Major differences between subcutaneous adipose tissue (SAT) and visceral adipose tissue (VAT) were shown in the expression of VD-metabolizing enzymes. The expression of the VDR, 25-hydroxyvitamin D 1α-hydroxylase (CYP27B1) genes, and 24-hydroxylase enzymes has been shown in human adipocytes [17].

In line, our chapter will focus on VD status and expression of VDR and VD hydroxylase enzymes in SAT and VAT in an obese environment.

2. Vitamin D, VDR, and hydroxylase enzymes on adipose tissue

2.1. Vitamin D

VD is a hormone mainly described for its role as a regulator of phosphate and calcium homeostasis [18, 19], therefore playing an important part in bone metabolism, and seems to have some anti-inflammatory and immune-modulating properties. This micronutrient can be obtained through animal (VD_3, cholecalciferol) or plant (VD_2, ergocalciferol) food sources. However, vitamin D_3 is the only form that is found naturally in human subjects and other animals. Although the main source of vitamin D_3 is through endogenous synthesis in the skin, the vitamin can also be obtained from the diet, and this is important for those who have limited exposure to the sun [20].

VD_3 is produced endogenously in the skin after UVB irradiation, between 290 and 315 nm, present for limited number of hours also varying with respect to latitude and reason. VD_3 is formed from the precursor 7-dehydrocholesterol to give pre-VD_3 and further is released into the circulation [21]. Vitamin D_3, whether derived from sunlight or the diet, enters the circulation bound to vitamin D–binding protein (DBP) and is transported to the liver. VD_3 is hydroxylated in the liver to 25(OH)D, the major circulating vitamin D metabolite; it has a relatively long half-life (15 days) but, however, is an inactive form. The Institute of Medicine proposed that serum 25(OH)D concentrations below 50 nmol/l or 20 ng/ml should be considered to represent the deficiency of this nutrient [22]. 25(OH)D is then further hydroxylated by 1α-hydroxylase enzyme (gene: CYP27B1), and this occurs primarily in the kidney to produce $1,25(OH)_2D$, the biologically active form of VD [23, 24].

In relation of signaling of VD in AT, 25(OH)D can promote the differentiation of human adipocytes, most likely via its activation to $1,25(OH)_2D$ [25]. The local metabolism of VD in AT may regulate the conversion of preadipocytes to adipocytes and later support the healthy remodeling of human AT. Also, $1,25(OH)_2D$ may promote the differentiation of human preadipocytes by maintaining a high expression level of key adipogenic transcription factors, like C/EBPα and PPARγ gene expression, the two master regulators of adipogenesis that were increased during the late phase of differentiation [26]. Besides, 1,25-dihydroxyvitamin D modulates adipogenesis through VDR-dependent inhibition of critical molecular components of it such as PPARγ [27].

The emerging role of VD in immune regulation suggests that this endocrine factor can modulate the inflammatory responses in AT. $1,25(OH)_2D$ displayed an anti-inflammatory effect and its ability to improve the insulin-stimulated uptake of glucose, as well as enhance and improve the function of pancreatic β-cell [28]. To strongly support the anti-inflammatory effect of $1,25(OH)_2D$ in adipocytes, the improvement of pro-inflammatory status and glucose uptake in adipocytes under $1,25(OH)_2D$ effect suggest that low-grade inflammation could be linked to VDD [29].

The $1,25(OH)_2D$ significantly reduced the basal release of MCP-1, IL-8, and IL-6 from preadipocytes (MCP-1 is produced by macrophages which increase further macrophage infiltration into AT [30], and circulating levels of IL-8 are increased in obesity). It should also be pointed out that since adipocytes store VD, adipocytes and monocytes/macrophages are able to locally convert 25(OH)D to $1,25(OH)_2D$ [31, 32], and the concentrations of VD within AT could be higher than implied by the plasma levels. Vitamin D_3 may protect against AT inflammation in obesity by disrupting the deleterious cycle of macrophage recruitment [33].

Lower 25(OH)D is associated with greater regional adiposity; this is stronger in VAT than SAT and significant across the spectrum of body size [34]. VD has been reported to act as an acute phase reactant as a consequence of such an inflammatory response occurs in obesity, which can suppress the concentration of 25(OH)D [35].

2.2. Vitamin D receptor

The human VDR is a 50- to 60-kDa molecule, a member of the nuclear receptor superfamily that is the only nuclear receptor that binds to $1,25(OH)_2D$ with high affinity and specificity. VDR forms a heterodimer with the retinoid X receptor acting as a transcription factor that binds to VD response elements in the promoter region of target genes [36]. VDR expression has been identified in most human tissues, including in osteoblasts, skin keratinocytes, macrophages, smooth muscle, pancreatic β-cells and epithelial cells [37, 38], and it is also highly expressed in adipocytes.

The action of 1,25(OH)$_2$D is mediated through the VDR, which regulates the transcription of many target genes [13]. There are more than 1000 genes that are directly or indirectly regulated by 1,25(OH)$_2$D and involved in various physiological processes such as cell proliferation, differentiation, apoptosis, and angiogenesis [38].

VDR expression is increased in obese, which has more VAT than lean subjects, but the physiological relevance of this upregulation has not yet been elucidated. VAT *VDR* gene expression correlated positively with body mass index (BMI) [39]. The ubiquitous expression of VDR may underlie the diverse effects of VD and provide a mechanistic basis for the link between VDD and a number of disorders that are linked with obesity like certain types of cancer, inflammatory bowel disease, cardiovascular diseases (CVD), diabetes (type 1 and type 2), and the metabolic syndrome [40–42].

Expanding to another approach, there are associations of VDR variants with the more metabolically active fat, VAT, which is more closely tied to the metabolic consequences of adiposity. Association of VDR SNP rs4,328,262 with VAT supports the notion that the VDR gene is likely to be related to the development of obesity and obesity-related outcomes [43]. Polymorphisms in the VDR gene might play a role in regulating AT activity body fatness and susceptibility to adiposity among African Americans, albeit genetic factors that contribute to adiposity are certainly more complex than to be explained totally by variations in a single gene.

2.3. Hydroxylase enzymes

The formation, activation, and catabolism of 25(OH)D are complex processes, which involve mitochondrial and microsomal cytochrome P450 enzymes. In humans, four cytochrome P450 enzymes, CYP2R1, CYP3A4, CYP27A1, and CYP2J2, [44–47] possess 25-hydroxylase activity, with CYP2R1 being the most specific. Hydroxylation in the 1α-position is effected by the mitochondrial CYP27B1. This process was classically located to the kidney, but recently, extrarenal 1α-hydroxylase activity has been described in several other tissues [48]. 1,25(OH)$_2$D stimulates its own degradation by induction of the 24-hydroxylase (CYP24A1), which catabolizes 25(OH)D and 1,25(OH)$_2$D to calcitroic acid and other inactive metabolites [49].

2.3.1. 25-Hydroxylation

Various enzymes may be associated with the first hydroxylation of 25(OH)D, but CYP2R1 seems to be the key to this hydroxylation [50]. In humans, other cytochromes P450 such as CYP3A4, CYP27A1, and CYP2J2 show activity of 25-hydroxylase to vitamin D molecules but less efficient. CYP2J3, CYP2D25, and CYP2C11 also show activity of 25-hydroxylase but are only expressed in male pigs and rats, respectively [51]. 25-Hydroxylation appears to be functional in AT. Interestingly, in human AT, biopsies have confirmed the expression of

CYP27A1, CYP2R1, and CYP2J2, suggesting that human AT and adipocytes are able to convert vitamin D_3 into 25(OH)D.

2.3.2. 1α-Hydroxylation

25(OH)D is then secreted into the circulation or directed to 1α-hydroxylase CYP27B1 mitochondria to be metabolized to 1,25(OH)$_2$D. CYP27B1 is the key enzyme 1α-hydroxylation, and its activity is regulated by the parathyroid hormone (PTH), fibroblast growth factor 23 (FGF23), calcium, and phosphorus and self-regulated by 1,25(OH)$_2$D via negative feedback mechanism [18]. CYP27B1 mRNA, which encodes the 1α-hydroxylase that converts 25(OH)D to the biologically active 1,25(OH)$_2$D, was present at significant levels in SAT and VAT. This gene was mainly expressed in the stromal vascular fraction of human AT that contains preadipocytes, macrophages, and endothelial cells. The expression of CYP27B1 has also been detected in adipocytes of murine [17] and human AT biopsies [52].

2.3.3. 24-Hydroxylation

Vitamin D 24-hydroxylase (CYP24A1) is responsible for the inactivation of 1,25(OH)$_2$D. This inactivation is self-regulated, from 1,25(OH)$_2$D induces the expression of CYP24A1 which converts 25(OH)D in 1,25(OH)$_2$D within the less active metabolites (24,25(OH)$_2$D and 1,24,25(OH)$_3$D), which are later catabolized into inactive calcitroic acid [53]. In AT, the expression of CYP24A1 has been detected in murine and human adipocytes. Additionally, levels of CYP24A1 mRNA are strongly induced by incubation of 1,25(OH)$_2$D.

The expression of 25-hydroxyvitamin D 1α-hydroxylase (CYP27B1) genes and 24-hydroxylase enzyme has been shown in human adipocytes [17]. The CYP24 gene, which encodes the enzyme catalyzing 1,25(OH)$_2$D, was also found to be expressed by human adipocytes and preadipocytes [31, 54]. Recently, a low expression of CYP27B1 gene in SAT of obese individuals has been shown [52]; this finding corroborates the ability of AT to metabolize VD locally. One of the main mechanisms by which this vitamin may act in human AT is via the expression of VD-metabolizing enzymes such as 25-hydroxylase CYP2J2, CYP27B1, and CYP24 [55]. This capacity to metabolize VD locally was demonstrated when, after weight loss in obese subjects, plasma 25(OH)D increased and expression levels of 25-hydroxylase CYP2J2 and 1α-hydroxylase CYP27B1 declined in the SAT of these subjects. So, a dynamic alteration may occur in AT during weight loss and obesity.

In the SAT of the obese individuals have a lower expression of one of the enzymes responsible for 25-hydroxylation of VD (CYP2J2), as well as a tendency toward a decreased expression of the 1α-hydroxylase, 25-hydroxylation and the 1α-hydroxylation in SAT are impaired in obesity AT expresses the enzymes for both the formation of 25(OH)D and of 1,25(OH)$_2$D, and for degradation of VD. To explain an altered VD metabolism in obesity, major differences between SAT and VAT in the expression of VD-metabolizing enzymes occur with difference in spreading between lean and obese subjects [52]. The expression of CYP27A1 is more pronounced in VAT than in SAT, without differences between lean and obese women, while the expression of

CYP2J2 is more prominent in SAT than in VAT in lean women. So, these findings lead to a compromised of 25-hydroxylation in SAT in obese, taken by a lower expression of the CYP2J2.

3. Mechanisms suggested for VDD in obesity

Several studies have shown the relationship between obesity and inadequacy of VD [56–58]. Evidence suggests that one of the VDDs in subjects with obesity may be connected to storage of VD in the adipocytes, reducing its bioavailability and activating the hypothalamus to develop a cascade of reactions that result in increased feelings of hunger and decreased energy expenditure [59]. Low serum of 25(OH)D concentrations is found to be inversely correlated with measures of obesity, including body mass index (BMI) ($\geq$30kg/m^2), fat mass, and WC [60, 61]. A bidirectional genetic study has suggested that higher BMI chiefs to lower 25(OH)D; each unit increase in BMI is being associated with 1.15% lower concentration of 25(OH)D, after adjusting for age, sex, laboratory collection, and month of measurement [62]. The relationship between obesity and 1,25(OH)$_2$D is less clear, and this is probably due to the dynamic nature of the production and regulation of the active hormone. However, the study in vitro showed that 1,25(OH)$_2$D acts as a potent inhibitor of leptin secretion in a culture of human adipocytes [63].

Extensive evidence has demonstrated that adipocytes become enlarged and dysregulated the following weight gain, which subsequently produces an imbalance in the inflammatory profile of AT. So, obesity is commonly linked to an upregulation of pro-inflammatory molecules and downregulation of anti-inflammatory molecules [64]. Individuals with both high SAT and high VAT have an approximately threefold prevalence of VDD compared with those with both low SAT and low VAT [34]. A predominant effect of VD on macrophages could explain the differences observed in relations of VD response in VAT versus SAT. Is observed a greater macrophage infiltration of VAT when compared with SAT in individuals with obesity. In contrast, inflammatory markers in AT strongly correlate with macrophage infiltration [65], and many metabolic differences could potentially explain the different VD-induced anti-inflammatory response observed between these two types of AT, including the number of cells expressing the VDR [52]. Because ATs of obese are infiltrated with macrophages, it seems likely that macrophages also contribute to the local activation of VD. Because SAT and BMI are closely correlated, it is possible that most of the association between SAT and 25(OH)D is attributable to the difference in body size that is seized by BMI. It is observed that lower 25(OH)D was associated with greater regional adiposity.

In fact, the basis of low concentration in subjects with obesity is not totally known but could be the result of various mechanisms. There are five suggested mechanisms that are most commonly cited within the literature which may explain a low VD status in obesity:

- *Obese individuals have reduced sun exposure compared with lean subjects.*

- *Low 1.25(OH)$_2$D inhibits adipogenesis.*

- *Negative feedback control.*

- *Vitamin D is sequestered within adipose tissue.*

- *Lower 25(OH)D concentration is just due to volumetric dilution.*

3.1. Reduced sun exposure

Obese individuals reduce their exposure to sunlight, reportedly have a limited mobility, avoid performing outdoor activities, and/or use clothes that cover more of the body [56], which limit exposure to the sun and, consequently, cutaneous VD synthesis. However, in a study based on the Framingham cohort, which evaluated the association between obesity and VD, it was reported that after adjustments for practicing outdoor physical activities, this theory was insufficient to explain the relationship between obesity and VDD [34]. In addition, the study indicates that daily exposure to 0.5 standard erythemal dose (SED) between 11:00 and 13:00h, using typical summer clothing, was not enough to achieve the state suitable of VD in the late summer [66]. Until now, it is still unclear which VD supplementation dose corresponds to the amount of UVB radiation exposed, in regard to efficiency to increase serum concentrations of 25(OH)D and as little establishing a standard exposure solar time daily necessary to achieve an adequate state of VD [67].

3.2. Low 1.25(OH)$_2$D inhibits adipogenesis

Some experimental data have suggested that VDD can favor greater adiposity by promoting increased PTH hormone levels and greater inflow of calcium into adipocytes, so increasing lipogenesis [68]. Evidence suggests that low 1.25(OH)$_2$D inhibits adipogenesis through actions modulated by vitamin D-dependent receptors [69]. Thus, depletion of vitamin D can lead to excessive differentiation of preadipocytes to adipocytes.

3.3. Negative feedback control

Excess AT impairs the VD status from activating energy expenditure. In this mechanism, the leptin stimulates osteocytic FGF23, inhibits renal synthesis of 1α-hydroxylase, and consequently impairs the production of 1,25 (OH)$_2$D, creating a negative feedback mechanism [70].

3.4. Sequestration in adipose tissue

Wortsman et al. [71] published the first study to provide strong convincing evidence that VD (as a fat-soluble vitamin) may become sequestered within AT. In their study, the concentration of circulating cholecalciferol was similar between obese and lean groups at baseline, but the obese group had a significantly reduced response to the UVB intervention, resulting in a 57% lower serum cholecalciferol concentration postintervention, compared with the control group (lean). This suggested that the limitation in the obese group was the bioavailability of the synthesized cholecalciferol in circulation [71]. This sequestration theory is probably the most supported in the literature.

3.5. Volumetric dilution

Most recently, Drincic et al. [72] showed that body weight and body fat are inversely correlated with 25(OH)D levels across the spectrum of body weight ranging from normal to obese. This inverse association is related to the greater volume of distribution for both VD_3 and 25(OH)D in tissue mass. They suggested that simple volumetric dilution is the most thrifty explanation for the low VD status in obesity. A hyperbolic model best explains the lower 25(OH)D values in obesity, and when serum 25(OH)D values was adjusted for body weight, difference between obese and normal subjects disappeared. These authors went on to recommend that the VD dosing for treatment of VDD in obesity should be based on body weight, for example, "one size does not fit all" [72].

Overall, although these are the five most commonly suggested mechanisms, the latter two theories have more robust evidences available. The strong evidence presented for the sequestration and volumetric dilution hypotheses, and more importantly, a lack of contradictory evidence for either, suggest that they are the most probable, independently or in combination, to explain the low VD status widely reported in obesity.

4. Conclusions

The prevalence of obesity and VDD is growing exponentially in recent decades, and several studies have been conducted worldwide, particularly, the signs of VDR and hydroxylase enzymes in AT (SAT and VAT). VD is a nutrient with important role in the genesis of obesity and also in diseases associated with chronic inflammation. It features an anti-inflammatory effect in AT, anti-adipogenic activity, exerts immunoregulatory effect, and has the capacity to limit the expression of inflammatory markers in AT. Scientific evidences suggest that AT is a target for VD action, as CYP27B1 and VDR genes that are expressed by adipocytes. All evidence suggests that 25(OH)D, 1,25(OH)$_2$D, and VDR are involved in the AT, through the endocrine system as well as autocrine/paracrine actions of VD.

Based on news researches, there is a hypothesis that AT is not only a stock of VD but also has a dynamic ability to activation and deactivation of this vitamin in obesity. Low VD status in obesity may have implications for AT biology based on recent data from different research groups which are converging to highlight the impacts of VD on AT/adipocyte biology. Therefore, some key points have yet to be elucidated in relation to VD metabolism and its regulation on AT, especially in obese environment.

Acknowledgements

The authors acknowledge the contribution of Coordenação de Aperfeiçoamento de Pessoal de Nível Superior (CAPES) that provided the payment of publication this book's chapter.

Author details

Adryana Cordeiro[1,3]* and Andrea Ramalho[1,2,3]

*Address all correspondence to: adrynutri@yahoo.com.br

1 Micronutrients Research Center (NPqM), Institute of Nutrition Josué de Castro (INJC) of the Federal University of Rio de Janeiro (UFRJ), Rio de Janeiro, Brazil

2 Social Applied Nutrition Department, Institute of Nutrition Josué de Castro (INJC) of the Federal University of Rio de Janeiro (UFRJ), Rio de Janeiro, Brazil

3 Medical Clinic Program, Faculty of Medicine, UFRJ, Rio de Janeiro, Brazil

References

[1] World Health Organization (WHO). Fact Sheet Obesity and Overweight [Internet]. 2013 [Updated: 2016]. Available from: http://www.who.int/mediacentre/factsheets/fs311/en/ [Accessed: July 2016.]

[2] Gregor MF, Hotamisligil GS. Inflammatory mechanisms in obesity. Annu Rev Immunol. 2011;29:415–445.

[3] Olefsky JM, Glass CK. Macrophages, inflammation, and insulin resistance. Annu Rev Physiol. 2010;72:219–246.

[4] Antuna-Puente B, Feve B, Fellahi S, Bastard JP. Adipokines: the missing link between insulin resistance and obesity. Diabetes Metab. 2008;34:2–11.

[5] Olatz Izaola, Daniel de Luis, Ignacio Sajoux, Joan Carles Domingo y Montserrat Vidal. Inflamation and obesity. Nutr Hosp. 2015;31(6):2352–2358.

[6] World Health Organization (WHO). Fact Sheet Obesity and Overweight [Internet]. 2013 [Updated: 2016]. Available from: http://www.who.int/mediacentre/factsheets/fs311/en/ [Accessed: May 2016]

[7] Afzal S, Brøndum-Jacobsen P, Bojesen SE, Nordestgaard BG. Vitamin D concentration, obesity, and risk of diabetes: a Mendelian randomisation study. Lancet Diabetes Endocrinol. 2014;2:298–306.

[8] Reid IR, Bolland MJ, Grey A. Effects of vitamin D supplements on bone mineral density: a systematic review and meta-analysis. Lancet. 2014;383:146–155.

[9] de Souza WN, Martini LA. The role of vitamin D in obesity and inflammation at adipose tissue. J Obes Metab Res. 2015;2:161–166.

[10] Holick MF. Sunlight and vitamin D for bone health and prevention of autoimmune diseases, cancers, and cardiovascular disease. Am J Clin Nutr. 2004;80:1678s–1688s.

[11] Holick MF, Binkley NC, Bischoff-Ferrari HA, Gordon CM, Hanley DA, Heaney RP et al. Evaluation, treatment, and prevention of vitamin D deficiency: an endocrine society clinical practice guideline. J Clin Endocrinol Metab. 2011;96:1911–1930.

[12] Daniel D. Bikle. Vitamin D and bone. Curr Osteoporos Rep. 2012;10(2):151–159.

[13] Demay MB. Mechanism of vitamin D receptor action. Ann N Y Acad Sci. 2006;1068:204–213.

[14] Vaidya A, Pojoga L, Underwood PC, et al. The association of plasma resistin with dietary sodium manipulation, the renin-angiotensin-aldosterone system, and 25-hydroxyvitamin D3 in human hypertension. Clin Endocrinol. 2011;74:294–299.

[15] Ultutas O, Taskapan H, Taskapan MT, Temel I. Vitamin D deficiency, insulin resistance, serum adipokine and leptin levels in peritoneal dialysis patients. Int Urol Nephrol. 2013;45:879–884.

[16] Ding C, Gao D, Wilding J, et al. Vitamin D signaling in adipose tissue. Br J Nutr. 2012;108:1915–1923.

[17] Li J, Byrne ME, Chang E, Jiang Y, Donkin SS, Buhman KK, Burgess JR, Teegarden D. 1α,25-Dihydroxyvitamin D hydroxylase in adipocytes. J Steroid Biochem Molecular Biol. 2008;112(1–3):122–126.

[18] Holick MF. Vitamin D deficiency. N Engl J Med. 2007;357:266–281.

[19] Allina Leal Bringel; Kalliasmin Francielle Sacerdote Andrade; Nadson Duarte Silva Júnior; George Gonçalves dos Santos. Nutritional supplementation of calcium and vitamin D for bone health and prevention of osteoporotic fractures. Revista Brasileira de Ciências da Saúde. 2014;18(4):353–358.

[20] Fuleihan Gel-H, Bouillon R, Clarke B, Chakhtoura M, Cooper C, McClung M, Singh RJ. Serum 25-hydroxyvitamin D levels: variability, knowledge gaps, and the concept of a desirable range. J Bone Miner Res. 2015;30(7):1119–1133.

[21] Holick MF. Vitamin D: a D-lightful solution for health. J Invest Med. 2011;59:872–880.

[22] Ross AC, Manson JE, Abrams SA, et al. The 2011 report on dietary reference intakes for calcium and vitamin D from the institute of medicine: what clinicians need to know. J Clin Endocrinol Metab. 2011;96:53–58.

[23] Masuda S, Byford V, Arabian A, et al. Altered pharmacokinetics of 1alpha,25-dihydroxyvitamin D3 and 25-hydroxyvitamin D3 in the blood and tissues of the 25-hydroxyvitamin D-24-hydroxylase (Cyp24a1) null mouse. Endocrinology. 2005;146:825–834.

[24] Xu Y, Hashizume T, Shuhart MC, et al. Intestinal and hepatic CYP3A4 catalyze hydroxylation of 1alpha,25-dihydroxyvitamin D(3): implications for drug-induced osteomalacia. Mol Pharmacol. 2006;69:56–65.

[25] Nimitphong H, Holick MF, Fried SK, Lee MJ. 25-hydroxyvitamin D_3 and 1,25-dihydroxyvitamin D_3 promote the differentiation of human subcutaneous preadipocytes. PLoS One. 2012;7(12):e52171.

[26] White UA, Stephens JM. Transcriptional factors that promote formation of white adipose tissue. Mol Cell Endocrinol. 2010;318(1–2):10–14.

[27] Vinh quốc Lu'o'ng K, Hoàng Nguyễn LT. The beneficial role of vitamin D in obesity: possible genetic and cell signaling mechanisms. Nutr J. 2013;12:89.

[28] Sung CC, Liao MT, Lu KC, Wu CC. Role of vitamin D in insulin resistance. J Biomed Biotechnol. 2012;2012:634195.

[29] Marcotorchino J, Gouranton E, Romier B, Tourniaire F, Astier J, Malezet C, Amiot MJ, Landrier JF. Vitamin D reduces the inflammatory response and restores glucose uptake in adipocytes and its ability to improve the insulin-stimulated uptake of glucose. Mol Nutr Food Res. 2012;56(12):1771–1782.

[30] Gao D, Trayhurn P, Bing C. Macrophage-secreted factors inhibit ZAG expression and secretion by human adipocytes. Mol Cell Endocrinol. 2010;325:135–142. .

[31] Ching S, Kashinkunti S, Niehaus MD, Zinser GM. Mammary adipocytes bioactivate 25-hydroxyvitamin D_3 and signal via vitamin D_3 receptor, modulating mammary epithelial cell growth. J Cell Biochem. 2011;112:3393–3405.

[32] Hewison M. Antibacterial effects of vitamin D. Nat Rev Endocrinol. 2011;7:337–345.

[33] Gao D, Trayhurn P, Bing C. 1,25-dihydroxyvitamin D3 inhibits the cytokine-induced secretion of MCP-1 and reduces monocyte recruitment by human preadipocytes. Int J Obes (Lond). 2013;37(3):357–365.

[34] Cheng S, Massaro JM, Fox CS, et al. Adiposity, cardiometabolic risk, and vitamin D status: the Framingham heart study. Diabetes. 2010;59:242–248.

[35] Waldron JL, Ashby HL, Cornes MP, et al. Vitamin D: a negative acute phase reactant. J Clin Pathol. 2013;66:620–622.

[36] Bikle D. Nonclassic actions of vitamin D. J Clin Endocrinol Metabol. 2009;94(1):26–34.

[37] Norman AW. Minireview: vitamin D receptor: new assignments for an already busy receptor. Endocrinology. 2006;147:5542–5548.

[38] Plum LA & DeLuca HF. Vitamin D, disease and therapeutic opportunities. Nat Rev Drug Discov. 2010;9:941–955.

[39] Clemente-Postigo M, Munoz-Garach A, Serrano M et al. Serum 25-hydroxyvitamin d and adipose tissue vitamin D receptor gene expression: relationship with obesity and type 2 diabetes. J Clin Endocrinol Metab. 2015;100:E591–E595.

[40] Osei K. 25-OH vitamin D: is it the universal panacea for metabolic syndrome and type 2 diabetes?. J Clin Endocrinol Metab. 2010;95:4220–4222.

[41] Dretakis OE, Tsatsanis C, Fyrgadis A, et al. Correlation between serum 25-hydroxyvitamin D levels and quadriceps muscle strength in elderly Cretans. J Int Med Res. 2010;38:1824–1834.

[42] Yiu YF, Chan YH, Yiu KH, et al. Vitamin D deficiency is associated with depletion of circulating endothelial progenitor cells and endothelial dysfunction in patients with type 2 diabetes. J Clin Endocrinol Metab 2011;96:E830–E835.

[43] Khan RJ, Riestra P, Gebreab SY, Wilson JG, Gaye A, Xu R, Davis SK. Vitamin D receptor gene polymorphisms are associated with abdominal visceral adipose tissue volume and serum adipokine concentrations but not with body mass index or waist circumference in African Americans: the jackson heart study. J Nutr. 2016;146(8):1476–1482.

[44] Cheng JB, Levine MA, Bell NH, Mangelsdorf DJ, Russell DW. Genetic evidence that the human CYP2R1 enzyme is a key vitamin D 25-hydroxylase. Proc Natl Acad Sci U S A. 2004;101:7711–7715.

[45] Shinkyo R, Sakaki T, Kamakura M, Ohta M, Inouye K. Metabolism of vitamin D by human microsomal CYP2R1. Biochem Biophys Res Commun. 324:451–457.

[46] Gupta RP, Hollis BW, Patel SB, Patrick KS, Bell NH. CYP3A4 is a human microsomal vitamin D 25-hydroxylase. J Bone Miner Res. 2004;19:680–688.

[47] Aiba I, Yamasaki T, Shinki T, Izumi S, Yamamoto K, Yamada S et al. Characterization of rat and human CYP2J enzymes as vitamin D 25-hydroxylases. Steroids. 2006; 71:849–856.

[48] Zehnder D, Bland R, Williams MC, McNinch RW, Howie AJ, Stewart PM et al. Extrarenal expression of 25-hydroxyvitamin d(3)-1 alpha-hydroxylase. J Clin Endocrinol Metab. 2001;86: 888–894.

[49] Jones G, Prosser DE, Kaufmann M. 25-Hydroxyvitamin D-24-hydroxylase (CYP24A1): its important role in the degradation of vitamin D. Arch Biochem Biophys 2011;523:9–18.

[50] Schuster I. Cytochromes P450 are essential players in the vitamin D signaling system. Biochim Biophys Acta. 2011;1814:186–199.

[51] Rahmaniyan M, Patrick K & Bell NH. Characterization of recombinant CYP2C11: a vitamin D 25-hydroxylase and 24-hydroxylase. Am J Physiol Endocrinol Metab. 2005;288:E753–E760.

[52] Wamberg L, Christiansen T, Paulsen SK, Fisker S, Rask P, Rejnmark L, Richelsen B, Pedersen SB. Expression of vitamin D-metabolizing enzymes in human adipose tissue

—the effect of obesity and diet-induced weight loss. Int J Obes (Lond). 2013;37(5):651–657.

[53] Dusso AS, Brown AJ, Slatopolsky E. Vitamin D. Am J Physiol Renal Physiol. 2005;289: F8–F28.

[54] Trayhurn P, O'Hara A, Bing C. Interrogation of microarray datasets indicates that macrophage-secreted factors stimulate the expression of genes associated with Vitamin D metabolism (VDR and CYP27B1) in human adipocytes. Adipobiology. 2011;3:29–34.

[55] Ding C, Wilding JP, Bing C. 1,25-dihydroxyvitamin D_3 protects against macrophage-induced activation of NFkB and MAPK signalling and chemokine release in human adipocytes. PLoS One. 2013;8:e61707.

[56] Vanlint S. Vitamin D and obesity. Nutrients 2013;5:949–956.

[57] I. González-Molero, G. Rojo-Martínez, S. Morcillo et al. Hypovitaminosis D and incidence of obesity: a prospective study. Eur J Clin Nutr. 2013;67 (6):680–682.

[58] Cordeiro A, Pereira SE, Saboya CJ, Ramalho A. Association between 25(OH) D concentrations and metabolic syndrome components in class III obese subjects. Int J Med Med Sci. 2015;48(1):1597–1603.

[59] Sun X; Zemel MB. 1 Alpha, 25-dihydroxyvitamin D and corticosteroid regulate adipocyte nuclear vitamin D receptor. Int J Obes (Lond). 2008;32(8):1305–1311.

[60] Jorde R, Sneve M, Emaus N, et al. Cross-sectional and longitudinal relation between serum 25-hydroxyvitamin D and body mass index: the tromso study. Eur J Nutr. 2010;49:401–407.

[61] Rajakumar K, de las Heras J, Chen TC, et al. Vitamin D status, adiposity, and lipids in black American and Caucasian children. J Clin Endocrinol Metab. 2011;96:1560–1567.

[62] Vimaleswaran KS, Berry DJ, Lu C, et al. Causal relationship between obesity and vitamin D status: bi-directional Mendelian randomization analysis of multiple cohorts. PLoS Med. 2013;10(2):e1001383.

[63] Menendez C, Lage M, Peino R. Retinoic acid and vitamin D_3 powerfully inhibit in vitro leptin secretion by human adipose tissue. J Endocrinol 2011;170:425–431.

[64] Galic S, Oakhill JS, Steinberg GR. Adipose tissue as an endocrine organ. Mol Cell Endocrinol. 2010;316(2):129–139.

[65] Weisberg SP, McCann D, Desai M, Rosenbaum M, Leibel RL, Ferrante AW. Obesity is associated with macrophage accumulation in adipose tissue. J Clin Invest. 2003;112(2): 1796–1808.

[66] Lagunova Z, Porojnicu, AC, Aksnes, L et al. Effect of vitamin D supplementation and ultraviolet B exposure on serum 25-hydroxyvitamin D concentrations in healthy volunteers: a randomized, crossover clinical trial. Br J Dermatol. 2013;169(2):434–440.

[67] Wacker M, Holick MF. Vitamin D—effects on skeletal and extraskeletal health and the need for supplementation. Nutrients 2013;5:111–148.

[68] Wood RJ. Vitamin D and adipogenesis: new molecular insights. Nutr Rev. 2008;66:40–46.

[69] Martini LA, Wood RJ. Vitamin D status and the metabolic syndrome. Nutr Rev. 2006;64:479–486.

[70] Bouillon R, Carmeliet G, Lieben L, Watanabe M, Perino A, Auwerx J, et al. Vitamin D and energy homeostasis: of mice and men. Nat Rev Endocrinol. 2014;10:79–87.

[71] Wortsman J, Matsuoka LY, Chen TC, et al. Decreased bioavailability of vitamin D in obesity. Am J Clin Nutr. 2000;72:690–693.

[72] Drincic AT, Armas LA, Van Diest EE, et al. Volumetric dilution, rather than sequestration best explains the low vitamin D status of obesity. Obesity (Silver Spring). 2012;20: 1444–1448.

Adiponectin, Inflammation and Cardiometabolic Risk Factors in Paediatric Obese Patients: Impact of Interventional Studies

Henrique Nascimento, Susana Coimbra, Carla Rêgo,

Alice Santos-Silva and Luís Belo

Abstract

Paediatric obesity has significant physic, social and psychological implications. Childhood obesity is usually associated in adulthood with increased risk of type 2 diabetes, metabolic syndrome and cardiovascular diseases. Aggregation of cardiometabolic risk factors is already observed at young ages, with a nonlinear association with enhancement of adiposity. Adiponectin is an adipokine that inhibits inflammation, oxidative stress and metabolic syndrome components, namely dyslipidaemia, high blood pressure and insulin resistance. Obesity has been associated with hypoadiponectinaemia in both adult and paediatric patients, which may contribute to co-morbidities observed in these patients. Interventional studies that aim to tackle obesity reported controversial results. Although the general positive effect on weight loss, inflammatory and cardiometabolic markers has been studied, the impact of these interventional studies on adiponectin remains unclear. Some studies reported that the improvement in adiponectin might only occur in paediatric obese patients with great weight loss or intensive physical exercise; the magnitude of the changes in body composition appears to be of particular importance. A revision about the knowledge on the relation between adiponectin, inflammation and cardiometabolic risk factors in paediatric patients is performed; the impact of interventional studies on adiponectin levels and markers of cardiometabolic risk is also addressed.

Keywords: adiponectin, inflammation, obesity, paediatric age, cardiometabolic risk factors

1. Introduction

The worldwide increase in obesity at paediatric ages has been accompanied by the appearance of diseases that were considered exclusive of adults, namely type 2 diabetes (T2D), dyslipidaemia and hypertension. These pathologies are commonly associated with central obesity, and this association is related with increased cardiometabolic risk [1, 2].

Obesity is closely associated with hypoadiponectinaemia, and low levels of circulating adiponectin are a potential predictor of some obesity-related co-morbidities. Therefore, adiponectin has been studied as a possible link between these conditions. Furthermore, growing evidence supports a relationship between obesity in childhood and low levels of adiponectin, and increased cardiometabolic risk factors in adulthood [3, 4].

2. Adiponectin and its isoforms

Adiponectin is important as a mediator of inflammatory factors and as an anti-atherogenic, anti-dyslipidaemic and insulin sensitiser factor. Adiponectin has particular characteristics, different from most of the other mediators: each one of its three circulating isoforms (high- (HMW), medium- (MMW) and low-molecular weight (LMW)) appears to be linked with different, sometimes opposite, actions in the organism. High-molecular weight (HMW) isoform has been considered a better metabolic marker than total adiponectin [5, 6].

Total and HMW adiponectin concentration were reported to be lower in obese (OB) children and adolescents, when compared to lean controls (CT) [6, 7]. Besides, the relative percentages of the isoforms are, usually, altered: HMW% adiponectin decreases, while low-molecular weight (LMW)% adiponectin increases. In children, HMW adiponectin multimer is usually linked to an improvement in insulin resistance (IR) and lipid profile [6], and it has been negatively associated with cardiometabolic complications [8]. The negative associations of HMW adiponectin with IR and adiposity appear to be present even in pre-pubertal (PP) individuals [9, 10]. Zimmet et al. reported that in PP children, HMW adiponectin was negatively associated with body mass index (BMI) z-score, IR, triglycerides (TG), leptin and soluble intracellular adhesion molecule (sICAM); however, after adjustment for age and sex, only BMI z-score and TG maintained their negative association with HMW adiponectin [11]. These authors did not detect correlations between HMW adiponectin and proinflammatory mediators, such as resistin, interleukin (IL)-8 and IL-18 [11]. This lack of correlation with inflammatory mediators suggests that the levels of adiponectin multimers might be more linked to changes in glucose and lipid metabolisms at young ages.

Figure 1 resumes the reported associations between total, HMW and LMW adiponectin with inflammatory mediators, hormones and other factors [12–31].

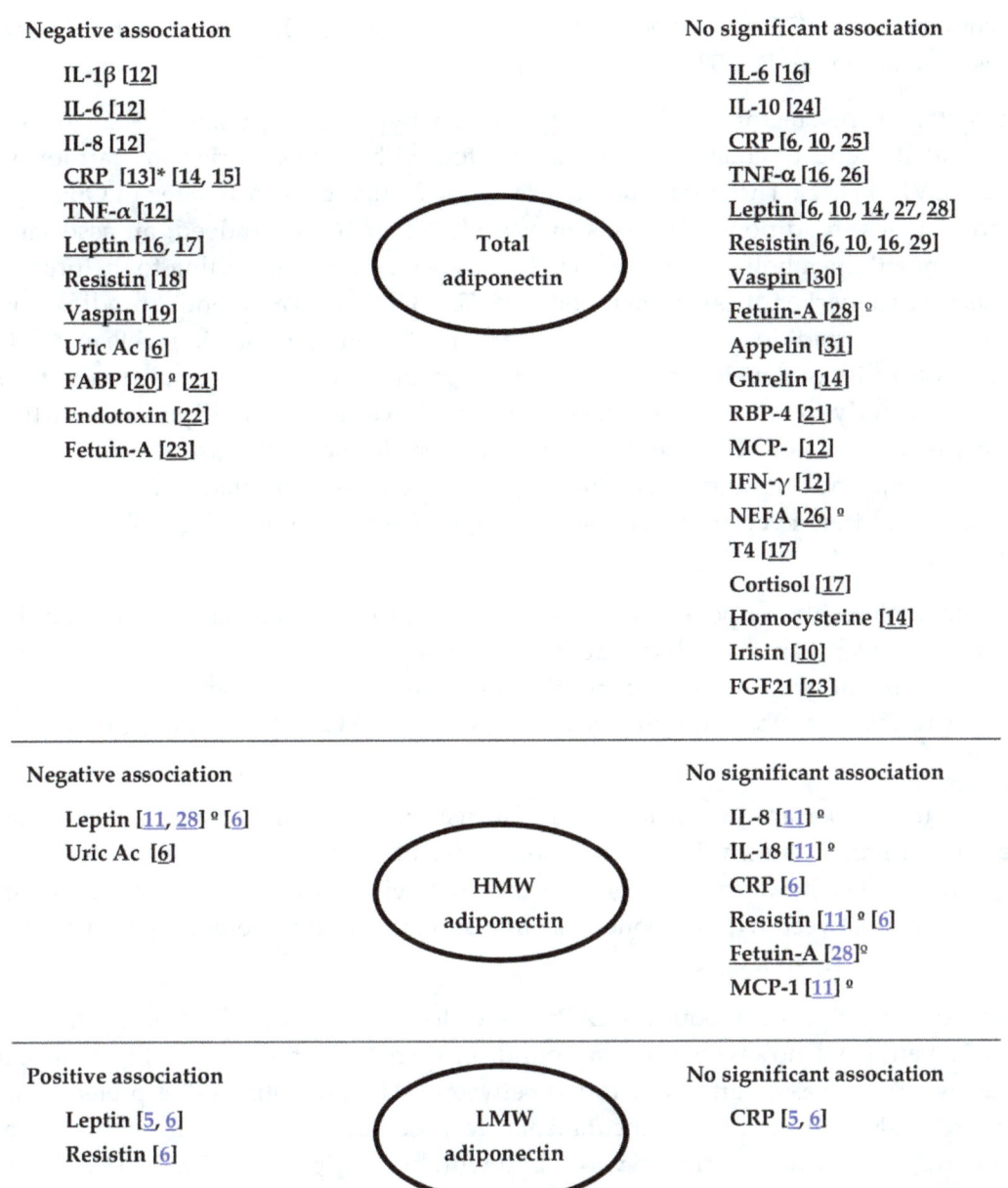

Negative association

IL-1β [12]
IL-6 [12]
IL-8 [12]
CRP [13]* [14, 15]
TNF-α [12]
Leptin [16, 17]
Resistin [18]
Vaspin [19]
Uric Ac [6]
FABP [20] º [21]
Endotoxin [22]
Fetuin-A [23]

Total adiponectin

No significant association

IL-6 [16]
IL-10 [24]
CRP [6, 10, 25]
TNF-α [16, 26]
Leptin [6, 10, 14, 27, 28]
Resistin [6, 10, 16, 29]
Vaspin [30]
Fetuin-A [28] º
Appelin [31]
Ghrelin [14]
RBP-4 [21]
MCP- [12]
IFN-γ [12]
NEFA [26] º
T4 [17]
Cortisol [17]
Homocysteine [14]
Irisin [10]
FGF21 [23]

Negative association

Leptin [11, 28] º [6]
Uric Ac [6]

HMW adiponectin

No significant association

IL-8 [11] º
IL-18 [11] º
CRP [6]
Resistin [11] º [6]
Fetuin-A [28]º
MCP-1 [11] º

Positive association

Leptin [5, 6]
Resistin [6]

LMW adiponectin

No significant association

CRP [5, 6]

Figure 1. Studies reporting associations between inflammatory markers and total, high-molecular weight (HMW) and low-molecular weight (LMW) adiponectin. Underlined are the inflammatory factors that appear in both columns (ambiguous results). º, pre-pubertal; *, post-pubertal; Ac, acid; CRP, C-reactive protein; FABP, fat acid-binding protein; FGF, fibroblast growth factor; IL, interleukin; IFN, interferon; MCP, monocyte chemoattractant protein; NEFA, non-esterified fatty acid; RBP, retinol-binding protein; T4, thyroxine; TNF, tumour necrosis factor.

3. Adiponectin and the risk of developing co-morbidities

Some contradiction exists in literature regarding adiponectin levels in young OB patients. Total adiponectin levels are generally accepted to be lower in OB children and adolescents when compared with CT and overweight (OW) subjects [25, 32]. However, contradictory data have also been reported [12, 33].

Cardiometabolic risk factors, such as dyslipidaemia, hyperglycaemia, hypertension, central obesity and IR, tend to cluster and are associated with increased risk for cardiovascular diseases (CVDs) [1, 2]. These risk factors are already altered in early ages in OB individuals, and changes in adiponectin levels may underlie such risk. Indeed, an association of adiponectin with metabolic risk factors [1, 34] has been reported, leading to the proposal of adiponectin as a marker of cardiometabolic risk [24, 35], and as a potential predictor of obesity-related co-morbidities [36, 37]. An association between adiponectin levels in childhood and the probability of developing co-morbidities in the future has been also raised [21]. In agreement, a study by Morrison et al. showed that lower levels of adiponectin in 16-year-old females were related with the development of cardiometabolic risk features at the age of 23 years [38]. Another study also showed adiponectin as a predictor of cardiometabolic risk, in OW children, even when adjusted for age, gender, Tanner stage, BMI, visceral fat and IR [34].

In T2D OB adolescents, adiponectin levels were found to be lower than in normal individuals, and even lower than in OB individuals without T2D. In this population, IR appeared as a main determinant of adiponectin concentrations, more than BMI itself [2]. There are, however, controversial data about the changes in adiponectin, in OB adolescents with and without T2D [23].

In obesity, it is important to consider body fat distribution, besides weight excess. Indeed, increased abdominal obesity has been associated with lower levels of adiponectin [1, 25, 39, 40] and adiponectin was negatively associated with visceral-to-subcutaneous fat ratio [41]. The association between hypoadiponectinaemia and increased visceral adipose tissue (VAT) seems to appear early in life [33].

Younger age of adiposity rebound (AAR) associates with increased adiposity later in life [42, 43]. Nevertheless, no association was found between AAR and adiponectin in 10-year-old children, whereas an association was found between AAR and leptin [44]. A preferential relationship of AAR with increased subcutaneous adipose tissue, rather than with VAT, might partially explain why no association was found with hypoadiponectinaemia [43].

In adolescents, the increased abdominal obesity and reduced adiponectin levels are accompanied by enhanced TG and decreased levels of high-density lipoprotein cholesterol (HDLc) [1], suggesting that central body fat distribution is also associated with a worse control on lipid metabolism.

The inverse relation of adiponectin with cardiometabolic risk appears to be accepted, especially in pubertal subjects. It is important to highlight that the diagnosis of metabolic syndrome (MS) in young children (under 10 years) should be avoided, as recommended by the International Diabetes Federation, considering the lack of age- and gender-adjusted cut-offs for MS components and the ambiguous causality evidence in such young ages relating MS and increased risk of CVD later in life [45].

4. Adiponectin and cardiometabolic risk factors

4.1. Lipid profile

The effect of adiponectin on lipid metabolism has been widely studied. Adiponectin is known to lower the synthesis of free fatty acids and to stimulate β-oxidation [46]. Furthermore, HMW adiponectin seems to lower the release of apolipoprotein (apo) B and apo E from the liver, decreasing the release of lipoproteins rich in TG (e.g. very-low-density lipoprotein (VLDL)) and increasing HDLc levels [47].

The positive association between adiponectin and an improved lipid profile has been confirmed by several data. The most consensual effects for adiponectin are a positive association with HDLc and a negative correlation with TG [1, 13, 27, 29, 48, 49]. These associations are present even in PP ages [26, 50] (**Table 1**). Through its effect on lipid metabolism, adiponectin might even modulate the influence of genetics. Lower levels of apo B/apo A1 ratios and total cholesterol/HDLc were found for individuals with higher adiponectin levels despite presenting an apo E genotype associated with a worse lipid profile [51]. In adolescent OB girls, adiponectin levels were positively associated with HDLc measured 7 years later, highlighting that adiponectin might modulate lipid metabolism even for a long term. However, no correlation was found between adiponectin and TG or low-density lipoprotein cholesterol (LDLc) [38]. Oppositely, no relation between lipid profile and adiponectin was reported in other paediatric studies [14, 21].

Reference	Country	n (f%)	Age (years)	Cohort	Adiposity	IR	Dyslip
Martos-Moreno et al. [9]	Spain	70 (31.4)	8.92 ± 1.80	OB (61 lean CT)	NS	(-)	
Bansal et al. [50]	UK	138 (35.5) European; 77 South Asian (35.1)	3	Global population	(-)		(-)^z
Gajewska et al. [7]	Poland	30 (40.0)	7.8 ± 1.3	OB (35 lean CT)	NS		
Gil-Campos et al. [26]	Spain	34 (32.4)	9.4 ± 0.4	OB (20 lean CT)	(-)*	(-)	(-)
Medina-Bravo et al. [33]	Mexico	33 (45.4)	9.0 ± 1.6	OB (13 lean CT)	(-)		
Murdolo et al. [11]	Italy	305 (52.8)	5–13	Global population	NS		
Gajewska et al. [71]	Poland	100 (54.0)	8.3 (7.0–9.3)	OB (70 lean CT)	(-)		
Nascimento et al. [72]	Portugal	13 (46.2)	7.9 ± 1.4	OB (10 lean CT)	NS		
Murdolo et al. [28]	Italy	200 (55.5)	5–13	Global population	(-)	NS	(-)^z

*, Correlation with total and central adiposity; ^{z}, positive correlation with HDL. CT, control; Dyslip, Dyslipidaemia; f, female; IR, insulin resistance; (-), negative association; NS, not significant; OB, obese; OW, overweight.

Table 1. Studies assessing the relation between total adiponectin levels and cardiometabolic risk factors in pre-pubertal children.

Concerning adiponectin multimers, while LMW adiponectin seems to be linked with a worse lipid profile, through a positive association with TG [5], HMW adiponectin has shown opposite effects [6], even in PP individuals [11].

4.2. Blood vessels and blood pressure (BP)

Adiponectin-positive effects on blood vessels are, apparently, independent of its effect on IR [52]. Adiponectin improves vessel status and reduces atherogenesis by inducing nitrous oxide production by endothelial cells that promotes vasodilatation and reduces platelet adhesion/aggregation. It also reduces vascular smooth muscle cells proliferation [53, 54] and avoids macrophage activation, preventing, therefore, vascular wall remodelling and foam cells formation [55]. Through these effects, adiponectin prevents the development of atherosclerosis while still in early stages. Adiponectin association with vascular changes appears since paediatric ages, as its levels are positively correlated with brachial artery distensibility [52], and inversely correlated with the internal media thickness (IMT) of carotid arteries (cIMT) [56–59]. However, some intervention programmes did not find any correlation between adiponectin improvement and cIMT [13], cIMT variation [60], or retinal vessel diameter [61].

Adiponectin presents anti-oxidant activity reducing the production of reactive oxygen species (ROS) that are deleterious to endothelial cells. Actually, the enhanced production of ROS favours the development of oxidative stress, which is a predictive factor for cardiovascular events (e.g. coronary artery disease) [62, 63]. In OB children, increased markers of oxidative stress have been found together with lower adiponectin levels [64]. The lower anti-oxidant status [65] leads to increased HDL and LDL oxidation in OB children [66]. Increased oxidised LDL (oxLDL) is linked to the formation of foam cells, a key step in atherosclerosis initiation. The anti-oxidant enzyme paraoxonase (PON)1 presents a reduced activity in OB subjects, being adiponectin positively correlated with PON1 arylesterase activity in OB children [66].

Decreased adiponectin levels are negatively associated with other oxidative stress markers, as adipocyte fatty acid-binding protein (A-FABP) and lipocalin-2 [21, 67]. In a 3-year longitudinal study, higher concentrations of A-FABP and lower levels of adiponectin were reported as predictors for the development of CVD risk factors [21]. The improvement of adiponectin levels after an exercise-based intervention programme has been associated with improvements in the oxidant status in paediatric populations [68].

Similar to their opposite biological effects in lipid metabolism, LMW and HMW adiponectin multimers present contrasting activity regarding oxidative stress and vascular changes. An increase in systolic BP (SBP), cIMT and oxidative stress (higher-circulating oxLDL) was positively associated with LMW% adiponectin [6], while HMW adiponectin correlated inversely with a marker of oxidative stress that is increased in OB children—isoprostane [69].

Conflicting results exist in literature regarding the association of adiponectin with BP. Some data reported a negative association between adiponectin and both SBP and diastolic BP (DBP) [13, 16, 36], or with SBP alone [25, 29, 34, 37, 70]. Fewer studies describe the absence of association between adiponectin and BP [14, 27, 49].

Longitudinal studies usually show no association between fluctuations of adiponectin and changes in BP. Choi et al. found in 9-year-old children a positive correlation between baseline adiponectin and BP changes, during a 3-year follow-up study; however, the significances were lost when adjusted for Tanner stage [21]. Another study [38] reported no association between adiponectin concentration in OB 16-year-old girls and the values of BP 7 years later.

4.3. Insulin resistance

IR plays a central role in the pathophysiology of obesity-related co-morbidities such as dyslipidaemia, nonalcoholic fatty liver disease (NAFLD), hypertension and inflammation.

Apart from PP individuals (**Table 1**), the relation between adiponectin, obesity and IR appears to be clear. Total adiponectin levels are negatively correlated with IR, and the increase in adiponectin, following a lifestyle intervention, leadvvvs to a decrease in IR [29, 73]. However, there is still some controversy concerning this association [10].

Hepatic IR is particularly important for the metabolic changes observed in obesity, as it modifies the profile of lipoproteins released by the liver, towards a more atherogenic profile [47, 74]. IR also leads to TG accumulation in hepatocytes, leading to the development of NAFLD. The structural and metabolic changes in hepatocytes induce macrophage activation, increasing the hepatic production of inflammatory mediators and transaminases [74]. Adiponectin is reduced in OB children and adolescents with NAFLD [75–77], and, when adiponectin increases, IR and NAFLD are also improved [75]. Adipose tissue-specific IR also accounts for important metabolic and inflammatory changes in OB individuals, as insulin-resistant adipocytes release more free fatty acids and proinflammatory adipokines [78].

In OB children [6], including PP subjects [12], total adiponectin, and HMW in particular, has a more close relation with IR markers, namely with homeostatic model assessment (HOMA), than with BMI or body fat. On the contrary, a positive association between LMW% adiponectin and HOMA has been reported [6].

The negative association of adiponectin with IR might not be present from birth. Insulin levels increase until 1 year of age, which is accompanied by a reduction in adiponectin; however, those changes are not associated with HOMA [79]. The inverse association between total and HMW adiponectin with IR seems to appear only after 2–6 years of age [11, 14, 26, 80, 81].

The insulin-sensitiser effect of adiponectin is likely to explain, in part, why individuals with two clinical conditions associated with hyperadiponectinaemia, such as Prader-Willi syndrome (PWS) (associated with cognitive impairment) [82] and Laron syndrome (associated with dwarfism) [83], present decreased markers of IR despite severe obesity when compared to BMI-matched CT. HMW% adiponectin is found to be particularly increased in PWS. These two syndromes also have in common a diminished level or activity of the growth hormone (GH). Changes in this hormone might partially explain their paradoxical hyperadiponectinaemia, increased insulin sensitivity and lower percentage of visceral fat.

Adiponectin and leptin are closely related, presenting, however, an inverse association with adiposity and IR. A study by Schiper et al. showed that an increased inflammatory profile increased leptin and leukocyte activation, and IR, in childhood obesity, while lean children presented increased adiponectin, insulin sensitivity and lower leukocyte activation [84]. Adiponectin-to-leptin ratio appears as a relevant marker of IR, with a strong negative association with HOMA and insulin. In fact, it might be a better marker than HOMA to predict IR, as was shown in OB adolescent cohorts [18, 85]. A cross-sectional study in Chinese children proposed leptin as the best predictor of IR, once adiponectin predicted IR only in OB and OW boys and girls, and had no predictive value for lean individuals [32].

The association of adiponectin with IR, adiposity and other CVD markers might be different in paediatric populations, with different/special characteristics. The mechanisms underlying IR in subjects with type 1 diabetes (T1D) are different from those leading to T2D [86, 87]. In adult cohorts of T1D patients, adiponectin is increased, when compared to the general population, and is associated with cardiovascular and all-cause mortality [87]. The exact mechanisms underlying this paradoxal association are still uncertain.

The relation between adiponectin and other metabolic parameters is influenced by the population background. Some ethnic groups, as South Asians (sub-continental India), showed reduced adiponectin levels in infants, despite the normal values of insulin or lipid profile [50]. Lower adiponectin is also present in both adult [88] and adolescent black individuals [38, 89]. Even though presenting lower adiponectin levels, increased prevalence of IR in black adolescents is less clear [38, 89]. It must be highlighted, once again, that the association between adiponectin and other metabolic parameters should always be considered regarding the ethnicity.

4.4. Adiponectin and markers of inflammation

In paediatric ages, as in adults, obesity is a low-grade inflammatory state, usually accompanied by a rise in proinflammatory mediators, and by a decrease in anti-inflammatory molecules, especially adiponectin. In accordance, adiponectin, in paediatrics, is negatively associated with proinflammatory mediators, such as IL-1β, IL-6, IL-8 and tumour necrosis factor (TNF)-α [12]. Different mediators are known to influence adiponectin levels, including other adipokines, hormones (e.g. insulin, insulin-like growth factor 1 (IGF-1), GH), and different types of molecules, produced within the adipose tissue or in other organs and tissues.

Inflammatory status appears to vary according to the degree of obesity, as severely OB children and adolescents, when compared with individuals presenting a moderate type of obesity, present reduced adiponectin and increased C-reactive protein (CRP), leptin, IL-6 and resistin [90]. However, this relation between adiponectin, inflammation and the severity of obesity is still controversial [51].

Adiponectin reduces TNF-α secretion by macrophages [88], and both TNF-α and IL-6 reduce adiponectin mRNA expression, explaining, at least in part, the relations of these cytokines with IR [88, 91]. Actually, TNF-α is known to inhibit insulin signalling [92]. In agreement, Lopez-Alarcon et al. reported that OB and OW adolescents with IR who participated in a

1-month n3 fatty acids supplementation protocol presented an improvement in the inflammatory status (higher-circulating levels of adiponectin and lower TNF-α and leptin), and of IR [93].

In PP individuals, the association between TNF-α and adiponectin might be less obvious, as the studies in this population failed to find any correlation between those adipokines [16, 26]. Another study in OB and OW adolescents, presenting a decrease in TNF-α, IL-10 and IL-8 after weight and body fat loss, following a physical exercise (PE) programme, did not present changes in adiponectin [94].

Leptin is one of the adipokines more closely associated to adiposity, presenting a negative correlation with adiponectin and a positive correlation with BMI. A 3-year longitudinal study showed that children with the highest increase in BMI presented lower adiponectin and increased leptin [3]. Likewise, adiponectin levels were negatively associated with leptin in female adolescents [17]. In OB Romanian children, a worse adipokine profile was observed, when compared to lean CT, with increased IL-6, leptin and resistin, and decreased adiponectin, which correlated, negatively, with leptin; this correlation with leptin disappeared when corrected for waist circumference (WC) and BMI z-score. Actually, WC has been proposed as a good predictor of adiponectin levels, highlighting the influence of adiposity distribution in adipokines [16].

As referred, adiponectin-to-leptin ratio might be a better marker of IR than adiponectin and leptin separated, or even HOMA [18, 85]. Due to the opposite association of adiponectin and leptin with adiposity, this ratio could be also used as an indicator of the anti- or proinflammatory adipokine balance in obesity [95].

The adiponectin multimers are also associated with leptin; the HMW adiponectin is negatively correlated, while LMW and LMW% adiponectin present positive associations [5, 6]. By contrast, other authors did not find any correlation between adiponectin and leptin [10, 14, 96] in OW and OB children, despite the association of both adipokines with IR and adiposity.

CRP is a well-recognised marker of CVD risk in adults. Although it has been associated with the increased inflammation in paediatric obesity patients [48], its association with adiponectin is not so clear in these ages [5, 6, 10, 13, 14, 37, 48, 51]. Nevertheless, there are strong evidence that both are related to obesity and IR [48, 51].

IL-6 is a proinflammatory mediator, usually increased in obesity. In lean individuals, IL-6 controls energy intake but, in OB individuals, a state of resistance to IL-6 appears to develop.

In animal models, resistin was found to associate positively with IR. In human studies, especially in children, the results are not conclusive. No associations between resistin and total adiponectin in children [6, 10, 16, 29], or in PP OB patients [11], as well as with HMW and LMW adiponectin [6], were found.

The anti-inflammatory effect of adiponectin is partially related with IL-10, an anti-inflammatory and anti-atherogenic interleukin, once adiponectin induces the synthesis of

IL-10 by macrophages. Considering that in obesity adiponectin is reduced and an increased infiltration of macrophages occurs in the adipose tissue, hypoadiponectinaemia would lead to diminished IL-10 levels. Despite that, increased circulating IL-10 was reported in OB adults. This increase is probably linked to a state of IL-10 resistance in OB individuals, as observed for IL-6, leptin and insulin. It could be also a response to the obese-related increase in inflammation, as IL-10 is an anti-inflammatory mediator [24, 97]. Conversely, Calcaterra et al. did not find in OB children, the correlation between adiponectin and IL-10 reported in adults [24].

4.5. Interventional studies and adiponectin levels

Longitudinal studies are crucial to obtain causal associations between adiponectin and other factors. **Table 2** presents a summary of interventional studies involving PE and/or nutritional counselling/supplementation programmes and their impact on adiponectinaemia.

Improvements in adiponectin levels may be obtained by energy restriction and PE, and the combination of both approaches appears to have a greater impact, as was observed in OB adolescent boys [18]. According to this study, the magnitude of the weight loss does not seem to be a confounding factor, as the group practicing only exercise had no significant weight loss, but, even so, the adiponectin levels increased. These data raise the hypothesis that variations in adiponectin levels are closely associated with changes in body composition [18]. In fact, even when the weight loss is not significant, changes in plasmatic adiponectin are negatively correlated with the variations in body fat percentage, in children [73]. Similarly, another interventional study for OB adolescents found that increases in adiponectin levels were associated with weight loss, and improvements were kept if the adiposity reduction was sustained [98].

Other factors, such as genetics, PE, inflammation and nutritional habits could influence adiponectin levels. For instance, when considering an intervention programme, involving diet and PE, performed on OB females with eating disorders (nervous bulimia or binge eating) and on BMI-matched controls, both groups benefited from the intervention, as both presented improvements in adiponectin. Nevertheless, changes in adiponectin correlated negatively with changes in HOMA and body fat percentage, only in the CT, and baseline and post-intervention adiponectin levels did not differ between them [99]. The independent role of PE, besides anthropometric improvements, in raising adiponectin levels has also been highlighted [100].

Despite the recognised influence of other factors, studies in children and adolescents have proposed that significant changes in adiponectin require a marked improvement in adiposity [25, 29]. A cut-off value of BMI z-score of 0.5 has been proposed as a target for achieving such changes [12, 101, 102].

The need for a considerable adiposity reduction in paediatric ages, even when compared to adults, in order to obtain significant results regarding adiponectin, is partially linked to the age-related decrease in this adipokine levels that occur during this period of life; this decrease is more enhanced during puberty and in boys. In fact, a BMI z-score reduction of 0.3 in OB

Intervention programme	Reference	Country	n ($f\%$)	Age (years)	Cohort	Duration	Adiposity	IR	Effect
EP	Shultz et al. [114]	New Zealand	14 (57.1%)	16.1 ± 1.6	OB	16 months			(+) Programme
	Lopes et al. [115]	Brazil	17 (100%)	14.6 ± 1.15	OW (17 OW CT)	12 weeks			NS Programme
ENCP	Lazzer et al. [98]	France	26 (53.8%)	12–16	Severely OB	9 months	(-)		(+) Programme
	Reinehr et al. [116]	Germany	37 (64.9%)	8–12	OB	12 months			(+) Programme (D-BMIzsc > 0.5)
	Elloumi et al. [18]	Tunisia	21 (0%)		OB	2 months$^¥$			(+) Programme (> combined energy restriction + exercise)
	Lee et al. [30]	Korea	50 (50.0%)	12.0 ± 0.9	OW + OB	7 days			(+) Programme
	Roth et al. [12]	Germany	62 (54.8%)	11 ± 0.5	OB	12 months	(-)	(-)	(+) Programme (D-BMIzsc>0.5)
	Romeo et al. [94]	Spain	25 (48.0%)	13–16	OW + OB	13 months	NS		NS Programme
	Reinehr et al. [31]	Germany	80 (52.5%)	10.9 ± 0.3	OB	12 months	(-)		(+) Programme
	Carnier et al. [99]	Brazil	83 (66.3%)	15–19	OB*	12 months	(-)	(-)	(+) Programme
	Leao da Silva et al. [95] [22, 41, 59, 60, 75, 117]*	Brazil	84 (59.5%)	15–19	OB	12 months		(-)	(+) Programme
	Siegrist et al. [96]	Germany	402 (59.2%)	13.9 ± 2.3	OW + OB	4–6 weeks			(+) Programme
	Nemet et al. [100]	Israel	21 (47.6%)	10.41 ± 1.96	OB (20 OB CT)	3 months	(-)		(+) Programme
	Racil et al. [118]	Tunisia	34 (100%)	15.9 ± 0.3	OB	12 weeks	(-)		(+) Programme
	Bluher et al. [10]	Germany	65 (46.1%)	12.6 (11.6–13.9)	OW + OB	12 months	NS		NS Programme
	Bocca et al. [104]	Netherlands	75 (72.0%)	4.6 ± 0.8	PP OW + OB	16 weeks	NS	NS	NS Programme
	Inoue et al. [119][106, 120, 121]*	Brazil	45 (62.2%)	16.28 ± 1.34	OB	12 months (AT or AET)	(-)	(-)	(+) Programme (AET)NS (AT)
	Nascimento et al. [15]	Portugal	80 (46.3%)	10.0 ± 2.7	OW + OB (37 OW + OB CT)	8 months	(-)		(+) Programme
	Seabra et al. [107]	Portugal	58 (0%)	8–12	OB (30 OB CT)	6 months			NS Programme
	Nunes et al. [68]	Brazil	17 (52.9%)	16.18 ± 1.51	OB (8 OB CT)	6 months			(+) Programme^a

Intervention programme	Reference	Country	n (f %)	Age (years)	Cohort	Duration	Adiposity	IR	Effect
MENCP	Cambuli et al. [73]	Italy	48 (45.8%)	10.7 ± 3.2	OW + OB	12 months	(-) (D-%fat mass)NS (D-weight)		(+) Programme
	Martos-Moreno et al. [9]	Spain	70 (31.4%)	8.92 ± 1.80	OB	18 months	(-) (T, HMW)		(+) Programme
	Gajewska et al. [7]	Poland	30 (40.0%)	7.8 ± 1.3	PP OB	3 months			(+) Programme (T, HMW, HMW%, and MMW) (-) Programme (LMW%)
	Vos et al. [25]	Netherlands	40 (55.0%)	13.3 ± 2.0	OB (39 OB CT)	3, 12 and 24 months			NS Programme
	Nascimento et al. [48]	Portugal	60 (48.3%)	11.0 ± 2.4	OB	12 months	(-)		NS Programme
	Gajewska et al. [71]	Poland	100 (54.0%)	8.3 (7.0–9.3)	PP OB	3 months	NS		(+) Programme
	Huang et al. [29]	Mexico	54 (40.7%)	13. 6 ± 1.3	OB	6 months	(-) (WC) NS (BMI and BMI z-sc)	NS	(+) Programme
	Rambhojan et al. [111]	Guadalupe Island, France	55	11–15	OW + OB (28 lean CT)	12 months	NS		(+) Programme
NCP	Pedrosa et al. [14]	Portugal	61 (55.7%)	7–9	OW + OB	12 months		NS	NS
	Saneei et al. [105]	Iran	49 (100%)	11–18	MS	6 weeks	(-)	NS	(+) Programme
	Jensen et al. [122]	Australia	74 (74.3%)	13.3 ± 2.0	OB	12 weeks	(-)	NS	(+) Programme
	Rouhani et al. [123]	Iran	25 (100%)	12–18	OW + OB (25 OW + OB CT)	10 weeks			NS Programme
NSupp	Janczyk et al. [124]	Poland	76 (14.5%)	13 (11.5-15.2)	NAFLD OW + OB	6 months (Ω3 fatty-acids)			(+) Programme
	Machado et al. [125]	Brazil	75 (56.0%)	13.7 ± 2.1	OW	11 weeks (flaxseed)			NS Programme

Intervention programme	Reference	Country	n (f%)	Age (years)	Cohort	Duration	Adiposity	IR	Effect
PI	Clarson et al. [126]	Canada	11 (63.6%)	10–16	IR OB (14 OB CT)	6 months φ			(+) Programme
	Kendall et al. [127]	UK	74 (66.2%)	13.68 ± 2.3	IR OB (77 OB CT)	6 months φ			(+) Programme

*, Different studies from the same group with similar results; +, increase of adiponectin with intervention programme; -, negative association; ¥, exercise and energy restriction, separately or combined; #, 28 with binge eating or bulimia nervous; a, no increase in intervention group versus reduction control group; φ, 1.5 g of metformin daily.

AET, aerobic and endurance training; AT, aerobic training; BMI, body mass index; CT, control; ENCP, Exercise and Nutritional Counselling Programme; EP, Exercise Programme; f, female; HMW, high-molecular weight adiponectin; IR, insulin resistance; LMW, low-molecular weight adiponectin; MENCP, Motivation to Exercise and Nutritional Counselling Programme; MS, metabolic syndrome; NAFLD, nonalcoholic fatty liver disease; NCP, Nutritional Counselling Programme; NS, not significant; NSupp, nutritional supplementation; PI, pharmacological intervention; PP, pre-puberty; T, total adiponectin; WC, waist circumference.

Table 2. Interventional studies evaluating the effect on adiponectin levels in overweight (OW) and obese (OB) children and adolescents and the relation between changes in adiponectin and the variation of adiposity and insulin resistance (IR).

children, although already associated with improvements in HOMA and lipid profile, only prevents the age/puberty-associated reduction in adiponectin, observed in the group that did not reach that cut-off [48].

Different strategies have been used in interventional studies; those that appear to achieve changes in body composition, necessary to obtain improvements in adiponectin, are usually short-term/high-intensity programmes that are able to produce in a smaller period of time a greater adiposity reduction [48]. In agreement, adiponectin increased, while BMI reduced, in high-intensity short-term intervention protocols lasting 7 days [30] and 4–6 weeks, in OB children [96].

Strengthening the importance of weight-loss magnitude, Lira et al. found that only the OB adolescents that reduced more than 5% of their fat mass, following PE and dietary intervention, had an increase in adiponectin levels [22]. Nevertheless, the participants in this study were all post-pubertal (Tanner stage 5) and, thus, the improvement in adiponectin might have been facilitated by the absence of the counteracting physiologic reduction. Following a similar intervention, by the same group, decreased IR and increased adiponectin levels were associated with improvements in NAFLD in an OB paediatric population [75].

Regarding the influence of lifestyle interventions on multimeric distribution of adiponectin, a study in PP children found that total and HMW adiponectin were lower in OB children when compared to lean CT. Variation in multimers, in OB children, is probably associated with changes in the multimerisation process that occurs inside the adipocyte, before secretion. In OB individuals, there is a reduction in the percentage of MMW and HMW adiponectin, while LMW% adiponectin increases [7]. Following a lifestyle intervention in OB PP children, a decrease in BMI of 10% was associated with an increase in total adiponectin, along with a decrease in LMW% adiponectin and an increase in the percentage of the other multimers (HMW% and MMW%), despite no association was observed at baseline, between BMI and the multimers or total adiponectin [7]. In a similar way to total adiponectin, changes in multimers concentrations might only be evident if there is a change in body composition, namely a reduction in adiposity, as studies that did not achieve significant reductions also did not have impact on adiponectin multimer levels [103].

Concerning interventional programmes, not only in adolescents but also (and particularly) in children, controversial results are found (**Table 2**). Indeed, some authors report no association with anthropometric changes in PP individuals, as well as no correlation with changes in lipid profile and in IR [104].

Adiponectin did not improve after a lifestyle intervention only with nutritional counselling (without PE programme), despite BMI z-score reduction and lipid profile improvement being achieved [14]. Likewise, in another study involving PE and diet, even though improvements in body fat and BMI were obtained, adiponectin did not increase [94]. Changes in adiponectin levels might be harder to obtain even when compared to other inflammation markers. For example, a decrease in CRP was present following a nutritional intervention programme, despite no significant changes in adiponectin levels and adiposity [105].

The type of PE chosen, namely the training routines and intensity used, will influence the results obtained regarding the body composition and cardiorespiratory fitness and, consequently, adiponectin levels [94, 106, 107]. For instance, although improvements in visceral fat, BMI and dyslipidaemia were obtained by both aerobic training (AT) and aerobic combined with endurance training (AET), these changes were greater with AET, which also presented a significant increase in adiponectin and reduction of IR. It was hypothesised that the greater improvement in dyslipidaemia and IR observed in the AET group was partially caused by the increase found for adiponectin in these individuals, but absent in the AT group [106].

Differences in baseline body composition and physical fitness might also influence the impact of intervention protocols on inflammation mediators, namely on adiponectin. Studies involving non-OB subjects or a mixed population can present different results from those found when only OB individuals are included. Ballet, for instance, is characterised by intense physical activity (PA), associating with an increase in lean mass. Girls practicing ballet have increased adiponectinaemia, when compared to lean CT. Moreover, their adiponectin levels increased during pubertal years (contrarily to CT), despite the trend towards central fat distribution following an increase in BMI z-score in this group [108].

A school-based study in Denmark did not find changes in adiponectin after a 6-week-day camp intervention (involving PA and health classes), although reduction in CRP and leptin and beneficial changes in body composition were achieved [109]. Contrarily, a 12-week exercise intervention study with lean adolescents males found an increase in adiponectin, IL-6 and CRP, although none of these changes were associated with variations in body fat composition [110]. Similar results were found in other studies [111]. It is known that PE, particular high-intensity PE, increases oxidative stress and inflammation markers [112]. As the metabolic profile, the inflammatory balance also differs between lean and OB individuals, with the last presenting a turn towards a more proinflammatory profile. Thus, it is likely that their response to interventional studies also vary, suggesting that comparisons should be done carefully.

A longitudinal study involving only PP lean individuals reported a negative association between adiponectin and the level of PA. Also, the traditional negative association between adiponectin and IR was influenced by the PA levels in this cohort, being stronger for the less-active groups. A mechanism of negative feedback might be present, as children with increased levels of PA would present greater insulin sensitivity (consequence of the PE), making the insulin-sensitiser agent adiponectin less 'necessary'. The opposite effect would occur in the less-active individuals [113]. This postulated negative feedback could also occur in OB individuals participating in interventional programmes, and cause a reduction in adiponectin, following the initial increase, as the intervention continued, due to the increased insulin sensitivity [30]. Actually, in T1D children the increase in IR is accompanied by higher levels of circulating adiponectin [128, 129].

Pharmacological strategies to tackle obesity and obesity-related co-morbidities have been explored. Metformin associates with a small, but consistent, BMI reduction, and increases adiponectin and adiponectin-to-leptin ratio in OB children and adolescents, without noticeable side effects. Still, the effect of long-term maintenance of metformin on adiponectin levels in children and adolescents is still unknown, particularly in children; thus, its use should be carefully considered [126, 127].

In conclusion, adiponectin association with obesity-related cardiometabolic risk factors, such as IR, dyslipidaemia, atherosclerosis and NAFLD, have been well demonstrated. Interventional studies are good options to tackle obesity and the referred co-morbidities, pharmacological adjuvants being an option to be considered. The variety of interventional approaches, with different study designs, populations and PE protocol makes the impact of these interventions on inflammatory mediators, and particularly on adiponectin, less clear; however, a positive effect is almost consistently found.

5. Conclusions and final remarks

The relation between adiponectin and cardiometabolic risk in children and adolescents is still under research.

Considering the different adiponectin multimers, HMW adiponectin has been associated with a better metabolic control, improving IR, while the LMW multimer presents an opposite effect. The concentrations and the relative percentage of the multimers should be considered as potential markers of CVD risk.

Obesity, and particularly abdominal obesity, is closely associated with lower adiponectin values in paediatric ages. Adiponectin acts as an insulin sensitiser, decreasing as the IR rises. Nevertheless, there might be a negative feedback mechanism, causing a relative decrease in adiponectin as insulin sensitivity improves. Higher adiponectin levels are associated with an improvement in lipid profile, with decreased TG and increased HDLc, being the influence on LDLc more limited. Besides the contribution to a less atherogenic lipid profile, adiponectin further prevents atherosclerosis by a direct positive effect on blood vessels. It reduces the formation of foam cells, macrophage infiltration and activation, and the vascular wall remodelling. Adiponectin is also associated with smaller arterial IMT and increased vessel elasticity, in children. Likewise, increased adiponectin is linked to reduced, healthier, BP.

Combining the specific effects of adiponectin in lipid profile, BP and IR, a decrease in this adipokine will induce clustering of several cardiovascular risk factors in OB children and adolescents that predicts cardiometabolic diseases in the future.

HMW adiponectin seems to be a better predictor of cardiometabolic risk factors than total adiponectin. An increase in total and HMW adiponectin is achieved following interventional programmes, particularly those involving exercise and diet interventions. Changes in body composition, with reduction of total and central body fat, more than changes in body weight, appear to be the key for therapeutic success.

The positive effects of adiponectin on general metabolism are not so clear in PP individuals, particularly the improvement in IR. No significant differences are usually observed between genders in PP individuals. After puberty, and possibly through a mechanism involving sexual hormones, adiponectin decreases with age in both genders, more markedly in boys [72, 130]. Several studies have reported similar adiponectin levels for both genders, even in OB paediatric populations involving post-pubertal subjects [10, 29, 61, 111, 131].

The controversial data on adiponectin following interventional programmes are, probably, related to different study designs and strategies used, including age, nutritional/body composition characterisation and pubertal stage of the studied subjects, PE or PA practice and type (e.g. aerobic, endurance, strength), group or individual therapy, among others; the population background should also be considered, as genetics plays an important part on adiponectin-circulating levels and, thus, might affect the results. Different populations also have different diets, and nutritional influence on adiponectin levels deserves further studies. Thus, although it is hard to control all variables, a good characterisation of the interventional studies is crucial for future comparisons.

Adiponectin, obesity and IR are so closely associated that it is hard to establish which are causes and which are consequences. The clarification of adiponectin physiological role, the evolution of its normal values throughout life and its relation with other metabolic markers and diseases need well-designed and objective longitudinal studies. These studies should focus on increased follow-up periods, including PP and CT individuals, and evaluate adiponectin isoforms, considering the lack of information on individual multimer levels and function. Further studies would help to better understand the metabolic changes in obesity, and to find new therapeutic targets to obesity itself and obesity-related complications.

Author details

Henrique Nascimento[1], Susana Coimbra[1, 2]*, Carla Rêgo[3], Alice Santos-Silva[1] and Luís Belo[1]

*Address all correspondence to: ssn.coimbra@gmail.com

1 UCIBIO\REQUIMTE, Department of Biological Sciences, Laboratory of Biochemistry, Faculty of Pharmacy, University of Porto, Porto, Portugal

2 CESPU, Institute of Research and Advanced Training in Health Sciences and Technologies (IINFACTS), Gandra-PRD, Portugal

3 Children and Adolescent Centre, CUF Hospital, Center for Health Technology and Services Research (CINTESIS), Faculty of Medicine, University of Porto, Porto, Portugal

References

[1] Yoshinaga M, Takahashi H, Shinomiya M, Miyazaki A, Kuribayashi N, Ichida F. Impact of having one cardiovascular risk factor on other cardiovascular risk factor levels in adolescents. *J Atheroscler Thromb* 2010;17:1167–75.

[2] Nadeau KJ, Zeitler PS, Bauer TA, Brown MS, Dorosz JL, Draznin B, Reusch JE, Regensteiner JG. Insulin resistance in adolescents with type 2 diabetes is associated with impaired exercise capacity. *J Clin Endocrinol Metab* 2009;94:3687–95.

[3] Nishimura R, Sano H, Matsudaira T, Morimoto A, Miyashita Y, Shirasawa T, Kokaze A, Tajima N. Changes in body mass index, leptin and adiponectin in Japanese children during a three-year follow-up period: a population-based cohort study. *Cardiovasc Diabetol* 2009;8:30.

[4] Toprak D, Toprak A, Chen W, Xu JH, Srinivasan S, Berenson GS. Adiposity in childhood is related to C-reactive protein and adiponectin in young adulthood: from the Bogalusa Heart Study. *Obesity (Silver Spring)* 2011;19:185–90.

[5] Mangge H, Almer G, Haj-Yahya S, Grandits N, Gasser R, Pilz S, Moller R, Horejsi R. Nuchal thickness of subcutaneous adipose tissue is tightly associated with an increased LMW/total adiponectin ratio in obese juveniles. *Atherosclerosis* 2009;203:277–83.

[6] Mangge H, Almer G, Haj-Yahya S, Pilz S, Gasser R, Moller R, Horejsi R. Preatherosclerosis and adiponectin subfractions in obese adolescents. *Obesity (Silver Spring)* 2008;16:2578–84.

[7] Gajewska J, Weker H, Ambroszkiewicz J, Chelchowska M, Wiech M, Laskowska-Klita T. Changes in concentration of serum adiponectin multimeric forms following weight reduction programme in prepubertal obese children. *Med Wieku Rozwoj* 2011;15:298–305.

[8] Araki S, Dobashi K, Kubo K, Asayama K, Shirahata A. High molecular weight, rather than total, adiponectin levels better reflect metabolic abnormalities associated with childhood obesity. *J Clin Endocrinol Metab* 2006;91:5113–6.

[9] Martos-Moreno GA, Barrios V, Martinez G, Hawkins F, Argente J. Effect of weight loss on high-molecular weight adiponectin in obese children. *Obesity (Silver Spring)* 2010;18:2288–94.

[10] Bluher S, Panagiotou G, Petroff D, Markert J, Wagner A, Klemm T, Filippaios A, Keller A, Mantzoros CS. Effects of a 1-year exercise and lifestyle intervention on irisin, adipokines, and inflammatory markers in obese children. *Obesity (Silver Spring)* 2014;22:1701–8.

[11] Murdolo G, Nowotny B, Celi F, Donati M, Bini V, Papi F, Gornitzka G, Castellani S, Roden M, Falorni A, Herder C, Falorni A. Inflammatory adipokines, high molecular weight adiponectin, and insulin resistance: a population-based survey in prepubertal schoolchildren. *PLoS One* 2011;6:e17264.

[12] Roth CL, Kratz M, Ralston MM, Reinehr T. Changes in adipose-derived inflammatory cytokines and chemokines after successful lifestyle intervention in obese children. *Metabolism* 2011;60:445–52.

[13] Arnaiz P, Acevedo M, Barja S, Aglony M, Guzman B, Cassis B, Carvajal J, Moreno M, Navarrete C, Berrios X. Adiponectin levels, cardiometabolic risk factors and markers of subclinical atherosclerosis in children. *Int J Cardiol* 2010;138:138–44.

[14] Pedrosa C, Oliveira BM, Albuquerque I, Simoes-Pereira C, Vaz-de-Almeida MD, Correia F. Metabolic syndrome, adipokines and ghrelin in overweight and obese schoolchildren: results of a 1-year lifestyle intervention programme. *Eur J Pediatr* 2011;170:483–92.

[15] Nascimento H, Alves AI, Medeiros AF, Coimbra S, Catarino C, Bronze-da-Rocha E, Costa E, Rocha-Pereira P, Silva G, Aires L, Seabra A, Mota J, Ferreira Mansilha H, Rego C, Santos-Silva A, Belo L. Impact of a school-based intervention protocol—ACORDA project—on adipokines in an overweight and obese pediatric population. *Pediatr Exerc Sci* 2016;28:407–16.

[16] Gherlan I, Vladoiu S, Alexiu F, Giurcaneanu M, Oros S, Brehar A, Procopiuc C, Dumitrache C. Adipocytokine profile and insulin resistance in childhood obesity. *Maedica (Buchar)* 2012;7:205–13.

[17] Modan-Moses D, Stein D, Pariente C, Yaroslavsky A, Ram A, Faigin M, Loewenthal R, Yissachar E, Hemi R, Kanety H. Modulation of adiponectin and leptin during refeeding of female anorexia nervosa patients. *J Clin Endocrinol Metab* 2007;92:1843–7.

[18] Elloumi M, Ben Ounis O, Makni E, Van Praagh E, Tabka Z, Lac G. Effect of individualized weight-loss programmes on adiponectin, leptin and resistin levels in obese adolescent boys. *Acta Paediatr* 2009;98:1487–93.

[19] Suleymanoglu S, Tascilar E, Pirgon O, Tapan S, Meral C, Abaci A. Vaspin and its correlation with insulin sensitivity indices in obese children. *Diabetes Res Clin Pract* 2009;84:325–8.

[20] Canas JA, Damaso L, Hossain J, Balagopal PB. Fatty acid binding proteins 4 and 5 in overweight prepubertal boys: effect of nutritional counselling and supplementation with an encapsulated fruit and vegetable juice concentrate. *J Nutr Sci* 2015;4:e39.

[21] Choi KM, Yannakoulia M, Park MS, Cho GJ, Kim JH, Lee SH, Hwang TG, Yang SJ, Kim TN, Yoo HJ, Baik SH, Kim SM, Mantzoros CS. Serum adipocyte fatty acid-binding protein, retinol-binding protein 4, and adiponectin concentrations in relation to the development of the metabolic syndrome in Korean boys: a 3-y prospective cohort study. *Am J Clin Nutr* 2011;93:19–26.

[22] Lira FS, Rosa JC, Pimentel GD, Santos RV, Carnier J, Sanches PL, de Piano A, de Souza CT, Tock L, Tufik S, de Mello MT, Seelaender M, Oller do Nascimento CM, Oyama LM, Damaso AR. Long-term interdisciplinary therapy reduces endotoxin level and insulin resistance in obese adolescents. *Nutr J* 2012;11:74.

[23] Reinehr T, Karges B, Meissner T, Wiegand S, Fritsch M, Holl RW, Woelfle J. Fibroblast growth factor 21 and fetuin-A in obese adolescents with and without type 2 diabetes. *J Clin Endocrinol Metab* 2015;100:3004–10.

[24] Calcaterra V, De Amici M, Klersy C, Torre C, Brizzi V, Scaglia F, Albanesi M, Albertini R, Allais B, Larizza D. Adiponectin, IL-10 and metabolic syndrome in obese children and adolescents. *Acta Biomed* 2009;80:117–23.

[25] Vos RC, Wit JM, Pijl H, Houdijk EC. Long-term effect of lifestyle intervention on adiposity, metabolic parameters, inflammation and physical fitness in obese children: a randomized controlled trial. *Nutr Diabetes* 2011;1:e9.

[26] Gil-Campos M, Ramirez Tortosa MC, Aguilera CM, Canete R, Gil A. Fasting and postprandial adiponectin alterations anticipate NEFA and TNF-alpha changes in prepubertal obese children. *Nutr Metab Cardiovasc Dis* 2011;21:62–8.

[27] Papoutsakis C, Yannakoulia M, Ntalla I, Dedoussis GV. Metabolic syndrome in a Mediterranean pediatric cohort: prevalence using International Diabetes Federation-derived criteria and associations with adiponectin and leptin. *Metabolism* 2012;61:140–5.

[28] Murdolo G, Tortoioli C, Celi F, Bini V, Papi F, Brozzetti A, Falorni A. Fetuin-A, adiposity-linked insulin resistance and responsiveness to an educational-based weight excess reduction program: a population-based survey in prepubertal schoolchildren. *Endocrine* 2016.

[29] Huang F, Del-Rio-Navarro BE, Perez-Ontiveros JA, Ruiz-Bedolla E, Saucedo-Ramirez OJ, Villafana S, Bravo G, Mailloux-Salinas P, Hong E. Effect of six-month lifestyle intervention on adiponectin, resistin and soluble tumor necrosis factor-alpha receptors in obese adolescents. *Endocr J* 2014;61:921–31.

[30] Lee MK, Jekal Y, Im JA, Kim E, Lee SH, Park JH, Chu SH, Chung KM, Lee HC, Oh EG, Kim SH, Jeon JY. Reduced serum vaspin concentrations in obese children following short-term intensive lifestyle modification. *Clin Chim Acta* 2010;411:381–5.

[31] Reinehr T, Woelfle J, Roth CL. Lack of association between apelin, insulin resistance, cardiovascular risk factors, and obesity in children: a longitudinal analysis. *Metabolism* 2011;60:1349–54.

[32] Xu L, Li M, Yin J, Cheng H, Yu M, Zhao X, Xiao X, Mi J. Change of body composition and adipokines and their relationship with insulin resistance across pubertal development in obese and nonobese Chinese children: the BCAMS study. *Int J Endocrinol* 2012;2012:389108.

[33] Medina-Bravo P, Meza-Santibanez R, Rosas-Fernandez P, Galvan-Duarte R, Saucedo-Garcia R, Velazquez-Lopez L, Torres-Tamayo M. Decrease in serum adiponectin levels associated with visceral fat accumulation independent of pubertal stage in children and adolescents. *Arch Med Res* 2011;42:115–21.

[34] Shaibi GQ, Cruz ML, Weigensberg MJ, Toledo-Corral CM, Lane CJ, Kelly LA, Davis JN, Koebnick C, Ventura EE, Roberts CK, Goran MI. Adiponectin independently predicts metabolic syndrome in overweight Latino youth. *J Clin Endocrinol Metab* 2007;92:1809–13.

[35] Alikasifoglu A, Gonc N, Ozon ZA, Sen Y, Kandemir N. The relationship between serum adiponectin, tumor necrosis factor-alpha, leptin levels and insulin sensitivity in childhood and adolescent obesity: adiponectin is a marker of metabolic syndrome. *J Clin Res Pediatr Endocrinol* 2009;1:233–9.

[36] Klunder-Klunder M, Flores-Huerta S, Garcia-Macedo R, Peralta-Romero J, Cruz M. Adiponectin in eutrophic and obese children as a biomarker to predict metabolic syndrome and each of its components. *BMC Public Health* 2013;13:88.

[37] Gilardini L, McTernan PG, Girola A, da Silva NF, Alberti L, Kumar S, Invitti C. Adiponectin is a candidate marker of metabolic syndrome in obese children and adolescents. *Atherosclerosis* 2006;189:401–7.

[38] Morrison JA, Glueck CJ, Daniels S, Wang P, Stroop D. Paradoxically high adiponectin in obese 16-year-old girls protects against appearance of the metabolic syndrome and its components seven years later. *J Pediatr* 2011;158:208–14 e1.

[39] Cnop M, Havel PJ, Utzschneider KM, Carr DB, Sinha MK, Boyko EJ, Retzlaff BM, Knopp RH, Brunzell JD, Kahn SE. Relationship of adiponectin to body fat distribution, insulin sensitivity and plasma lipoproteins: evidence for independent roles of age and sex. *Diabetologia* 2003;46:459–69.

[40] Ogawa Y, Kikuchi T, Nagasaki K, Hiura M, Tanaka Y, Uchiyama M. Usefulness of serum adiponectin level as a diagnostic marker of metabolic syndrome in obese Japanese children. *Hypertens Res* 2005;28:51–7.

[41] Lira FS, Rosa JC, Dos Santos RV, Venancio DP, Carnier J, Sanches Pde L, do Nascimento CM, de Piano A, Tock L, Tufik S, de Mello MT, Damaso AR, Oyama LM. Visceral fat decreased by long-term interdisciplinary lifestyle therapy correlated positively with interleukin-6 and tumor necrosis factor-alpha and negatively with adiponectin levels in obese adolescents. *Metabolism* 2011;60:359–65.

[42] Williams SM, Goulding A. Patterns of growth associated with the timing of adiposity rebound. *Obesity (Silver Spring)* 2009;17:335–41.

[43] Ohlsson C, Lorentzon M, Norjavaara E, Kindblom JM. Age at adiposity rebound is associated with fat mass in young adult males-the GOOD study. *PLoS One* 2012;7:e49404.

[44] Flexeder C, Thiering E, Kratzsch J, Klumper C, Koletzko B, Muller MJ, Koletzko S, Heinrich J. Is a child's growth pattern early in life related to serum adipokines at the age of 10 years? *Eur J Clin Nutr* 2014;68:25–31.

[45] Zimmet P, Alberti G, Kaufman F, Tajima N, Silink M, Arslanian S, Wong G, Bennett P, Shaw J, Caprio S. The metabolic syndrome in children and adolescents. *Lancet* 2007;369:2059–61.

[46] Xu A, Wang Y, Keshaw H, Xu LY, Lam KS, Cooper GJ. The fat-derived hormone adiponectin alleviates alcoholic and nonalcoholic fatty liver diseases in mice. *J Clin Invest* 2003;112:91–100.

[47] Neumeier M, Sigruener A, Eggenhofer E, Weigert J, Weiss TS, Schaeffler A, Schlitt HJ, Aslanidis C, Piso P, Langmann T, Schmitz G, Scholmerich J, Buechler C. High molecular weight adiponectin reduces apolipoprotein B and E release in human hepatocytes. *Biochem Biophys Res Commun* 2007;352:543–8.

[48] Nascimento H, Costa E, Rocha-Pereira P, Rego C, Mansilha HF, Quintanilha A, Santos-Silva A, Belo L. Cardiovascular risk factors in Portuguese obese children and adolescents: impact of small reductions in body mass index imposed by lifestyle modifications. *Open Biochem J* 2012;6:43–50.

[49] Snehalatha C, Yamuna A, Ramachandran A. Plasma adiponectin does not correlate with insulin resistance and cardiometabolic variables in nondiabetic Asian Indian teenagers. *Diabetes Care* 2008;31:2374–9.

[50] Bansal N, Anderson SG, Vyas A, Gemmell I, Charlton-Menys V, Oldroyd J, Pemberton P, Durrington PN, Clayton PE, Cruickshank JK. Adiponectin and lipid profiles compared with insulins in relation to early growth of British South Asian and European children: the Manchester children's growth and vascular health study. *J Clin Endocrinol Metab* 2011;96:2567–74.

[51] Nascimento H, Silva L, Lourenco P, Weinfurterova R, Castro E, Rego C, Ferreira H, Guerra A, Quintanilha A, Santos-Silva A, Belo L. Lipid profile in Portuguese obese children and adolescents: interaction of apolipoprotein E polymorphism with adiponectin levels. *Arch Pediatr Adolesc Med* 2009;163:1030–6.

[52] Urbina EM, Khoury P, Martin LJ, D'Alessio D, Dolan LM. Gender differences in the relationships among obesity, adiponectin and brachial artery distensibility in adolescents and young adults. *Int J Obes (Lond)* 2009;33:1118–25.

[53] Kato H, Kashiwagi H, Shiraga M, Tadokoro S, Kamae T, Ujiie H, Honda S, Miyata S, Ijiri Y, Yamamoto J, Maeda N, Funahashi T, Kurata Y, Shimomura I, Tomiyama Y, Kanakura Y. Adiponectin acts as an endogenous antithrombotic factor. *Arterioscler Thromb Vasc Biol* 2006;26:224–30.

[54] Arita Y, Kihara S, Ouchi N, Maeda K, Kuriyama H, Okamoto Y, Kumada M, Hotta K, Nishida M, Takahashi M, Nakamura T, Shimomura I, Muraguchi M, Ohmoto Y, Funahashi T, Matsuzawa Y. Adipocyte-derived plasma protein adiponectin acts as a platelet-derived growth factor-BB-binding protein and regulates growth factor-induced common postreceptor signal in vascular smooth muscle cell. *Circulation* 2002;105:2893–8.

[55] Wang Y, Lam KS, Xu JY, Lu G, Xu LY, Cooper GJ, Xu A. Adiponectin inhibits cell proliferation by interacting with several growth factors in an oligomerization-dependent manner. *J Biol Chem* 2005;280:18341–7.

[56] Pilz S, Horejsi R, Moller R, Almer G, Scharnagl H, Stojakovic T, Dimitrova R, Weihrauch G, Borkenstein M, Maerz W, Schauenstein K, Mangge H. Early atherosclerosis in obese juveniles is associated with low serum levels of adiponectin. *J Clin Endocrinol Metab* 2005;90:4792–6.

[57] Litwin M, Michalkiewicz J, Niemirska A, Gackowska L, Kubiszewska I, Wierzbicka A, Wawer ZT, Janas R. Inflammatory activation in children with primary hypertension. *Pediatr Nephrol* 2010;25:1711–8.

[58] Jaakkola JM, Pahkala K, Viitala M, Ronnemaa T, Viikari J, Niinikoski H, Lagstrom H, Jula A, Simell O, Raitakari O. Association of adiponectin with adolescent cardiovascular health in a dietary intervention study. *J Pediatr* 2015;167:353–60 e1.

[59] Masquio DC, de Piano A, Campos RM, Sanches PL, Carnier J, Corgosinho FC, Netto BD, Carvalho-Ferreira JP, Oyama LM, Oller do Nascimento CM, Tock L, de Mello MT, Tufik S, Damaso AR. Reduction in saturated fat intake improves cardiovascular risks in obese adolescents during interdisciplinary therapy. *Int J Clin Pract* 2015;69:560–70.

[60] Sanches Pde L, Mello MT, Fonseca FA, Elias N, Piano A, Carnier J, Tock L, Oyama LM, Tufik S, Damaso A. Insulin resistance can impair reduction on carotid intima-media thickness in obese adolescents. *Arq Bras Cardiol* 2012;99:892–8.

[61] Siegrist M, Hanssen H, Neidig M, Fuchs M, Lechner F, Stetten M, Blume K, Lammel C, Haller B, Vogeser M, Parhofer KG, Halle M. Association of leptin and insulin with childhood obesity and retinal vessel diameters. *Int J Obes (Lond)* 2014;38:1241–7.

[62] Szmitko PE, Teoh H, Stewart DJ, Verma S. Adiponectin and cardiovascular disease: state of the art? *Am J Physiol Heart Circ Physiol* 2007;292:H1655–63.

[63] Ouedraogo R, Wu X, Xu SQ, Fuchsel L, Motoshima H, Mahadev K, Hough K, Scalia R, Goldstein BJ. Adiponectin suppression of high-glucose-induced reactive oxygen species in vascular endothelial cells: evidence for involvement of a cAMP signaling pathway. *Diabetes* 2006;55:1840–6.

[64] Kelly AS, Steinberger J, Kaiser DR, Olson TP, Bank AJ, Dengel DR. Oxidative stress and adverse adipokine profile characterize the metabolic syndrome in children. *J Cardiometab Syndr* 2006;1:248–52.

[65] Sumegova K, Nagyova Z, Waczulikova I, Zitnanova I, Durackova Z. Activity of paraoxonase 1 and lipid profile in healthy children. *Physiol Res* 2007;56:351–7.

[66] Koncsos P, Seres I, Harangi M, Illyes I, Jozsa L, Gonczi F, Bajnok L, Paragh G. Human paraoxonase-1 activity in childhood obesity and its relation to leptin and adiponectin levels. *Pediatr Res* 2010;67:309–13.

[67] Matarese G, Mantzoros C, La Cava A. Leptin and adipocytokines: bridging the gap between immunity and atherosclerosis. *Curr Pharm Des* 2007;13:3676–80.

[68] Nunes JE, Cunha HS, Freitas ZR, Nogueira AM, Damaso AR, Espindola FS, Cheik NC. Interdisciplinary therapy changes superoxide dismutase activity and adiponectin in obese adolescents: a randomised controlled trial. *J Sports Sci* 2016;34:945–50.

[69] Araki S, Dobashi K, Yamamoto Y, Asayama K, Kusuhara K. Increased plasma isoprostane is associated with visceral fat, high molecular weight adiponectin, and metabolic complications in obese children. *Eur J Pediatr* 2010;169:965–70.

[70] Kynde I, Heitmann BL, Bygbjerg IC, Andersen LB, Helge JW. Hypoadiponectinemia in overweight children contributes to a negative metabolic risk profile 6 years later. *Metabolism* 2009;58:1817–24.

[71] Gajewska J, Weker H, Ambroszkiewicz J, Szamotulska K, Chelchowska M, Franek E, Laskowska-Klita T. Alterations in markers of bone metabolism and adipokines following a 3-month lifestyle intervention induced weight loss in obese prepubertal children. *Exp Clin Endocrinol Diabetes* 2013;121:498–504.

[72] Nascimento H, Costa E, Rocha S, Lucena C, Rocha-Pereira P, Rego C, Mansilha HF, Quintanilha A, Aires L, Mota J, Santos-Silva A, Belo L. Adiponectin and markers of metabolic syndrome in obese children and adolescents: impact of 8-mo regular physical exercise program. *Pediatr Res* 2014;76:159–65.

[73] Cambuli VM, Musiu MC, Incani M, Paderi M, Serpe R, Marras V, Cossu E, Cavallo MG, Mariotti S, Loche S, Baroni MG. Assessment of adiponectin and leptin as biomarkers of positive metabolic outcomes after lifestyle intervention in overweight and obese children. *J Clin Endocrinol Metab* 2008;93:3051–7.

[74] Wang Y, Zhou M, Lam KS, Xu A. Protective roles of adiponectin in obesity-related fatty liver diseases: mechanisms and therapeutic implications. *Arq Bras Endocrinol Metabol* 2009;53:201–12.

[75] Sanches PL, de Piano A, Campos RM, Carnier J, de Mello MT, Elias N, Fonseca FA, Masquio DC, da Silva PL, Corgosinho FC, Tock L, Oyama LM, Tufik S, Damaso AR. Association of nonalcoholic fatty liver disease with cardiovascular risk factors in obese adolescents: the role of interdisciplinary therapy. *J Clin Lipidol* 2014;8:265–72.

[76] Tadokoro N, Shinomiya M, Yoshinaga M, Takahashi H, Matsuoka K, Miyashita Y, Nakamura M, Kuribayashi N. Visceral fat accumulation in Japanese high school students and related atherosclerotic risk factors. *J Atheroscler Thromb* 2010;17:546–57.

[77] Ozkol M, Ersoy B, Kasirga E, Taneli F, Bostanci IE, Ozhan B. Metabolic predictors for early identification of fatty liver using Doppler and B-mode ultrasonography in overweight and obese adolescents. *Eur J Pediatr* 2010;169:1345–52.

[78] Hershkop K, Besor O, Santoro N, Pierpont B, Caprio S, Weiss R. Adipose insulin resistance in obese adolescents across the spectrum of glucose tolerance. *J Clin Endocrinol Metab* 2016;101:2423–31.

[79] Bozzola E, Meazza C, Arvigo M, Travaglino P, Pagani S, Stronati M, Gasparoni A, Bianco C, Bozzola M. Role of adiponectin and leptin on body development in infants during the first year of life. *Ital J Pediatr* 2010;36:26.

[80] Ibanez L, Lopez-Bermejo A, Diaz M, Angulo M, Sebastiani G, de Zegher F. High-molecular-weight adiponectin in children born small- or appropriate-for-gestational-age. *J Pediatr* 2009;155:740–2.

[81] Nascimento H, Alves AI, Coimbras S, Catarino C, Gomes D, Bronze-da-Rocha E, Costa E, Rocha-Pereira P, Aires L, Mota J, Ferreira Mansilha H, Rêgo C, Santos-Silva A, Belo L. Bilirubin is independently associated with oxidized LDL levels in young obese patients. *Diabetology & Metabolic Syndrome* 2015;7:4.

[82] Haqq AM, Muehlbauer M, Svetkey LP, Newgard CB, Purnell JQ, Grambow SC, Freemark MS. Altered distribution of adiponectin isoforms in children with Prader-Willi syndrome (PWS): association with insulin sensitivity and circulating satiety peptide hormones. *Clin Endocrinol (Oxf)* 2007;67:944–51.

[83] Kanety H, Hemi R, Ginsberg S, Pariente C, Yissachar E, Barhod E, Funahashi T, Laron Z. Total and high molecular weight adiponectin are elevated in patients with Laron syndrome despite marked obesity. *Eur J Endocrinol* 2009;161:837–44.

[84] Schipper HS, Nuboer R, Prop S, van den Ham HJ, de Boer FK, Kesmir C, Mombers IM, van Bekkum KA, Woudstra J, Kieft JH, Hoefer IE, de Jager W, Prakken B, van Summeren M, Kalkhoven E. Systemic inflammation in childhood obesity: circulating inflammatory mediators and activated CD14++ monocytes. *Diabetologia* 2012;55:2800–10.

[85] Inoue M, Maehata E, Yano M, Taniyama M, Suzuki S. Correlation between the adiponectin-leptin ratio and parameters of insulin resistance in patients with type 2 diabetes. *Metabolism* 2005;54:281–6.

[86] Lipsky LM, Gee B, Liu A, Nansel TR. Body mass index and adiposity indicators associated with cardiovascular biomarkers in youth with type 1 diabetes followed prospectively. *Pediatr Obes* 2016.

[87] Forsblom C, Thomas MC, Moran J, Saraheimo M, Thorn L, Waden J, Gordin D, Frystyk J, Flyvbjerg A, Groop PH, FinnDiane Study G. Serum adiponectin concentration is a positive predictor of all-cause and cardiovascular mortality in type 1 diabetes. *J Intern Med* 2011;270:346–55.

[88] Bruun JM, Lihn AS, Verdich C, Pedersen SB, Toubro S, Astrup A, Richelsen B. Regulation of adiponectin by adipose tissue-derived cytokines: in vivo and in vitro investigations in humans. *Am J Physiol Endocrinol Metab* 2003;285:E527–33.

[89] Butani L, Dharmar M, Devaraj S, Jialal I. Preliminary report of inflammatory markers, oxidative stress, and insulin resistance in adolescents of different ethnicities. *Metab Syndr Relat Disord* 2016;14:182–6.

[90] Rank M, Siegrist M, Wilks DC, Langhof H, Wolfarth B, Haller B, Koenig W, Halle M. The Cardio-Metabolic Risk of Moderate and Severe Obesity in Children and Adolescents. *J Pediatr* 2013; 163(1):137–42.

[91] Ouchi N, Kihara S, Funahashi T, Nakamura T, Nishida M, Kumada M, Okamoto Y, Ohashi K, Nagaretani H, Kishida K, Nishizawa H, Maeda N, Kobayashi H, Hiraoka H, Matsuzawa Y. Reciprocal association of C-reactive protein with adiponectin in blood stream and adipose tissue. *Circulation* 2003;107:671–4.

[92] Maeda N, Takahashi M, Funahashi T, Kihara S, Nishizawa H, Kishida K, Nagaretani H, Matsuda M, Komuro R, Ouchi N, Kuriyama H, Hotta K, Nakamura T, Shimomura I, Matsuzawa Y. PPARgamma ligands increase expression and plasma concentrations of adiponectin, an adipose-derived protein. *Diabetes* 2001;50:2094–9.

[93] Lopez-Alarcon M, Martinez-Coronado A, Velarde-Castro O, Rendon-Macias E, Fernandez J. Supplementation of n3 long-chain polyunsaturated fatty acid synergistically decreases insulin resistance with weight loss of obese prepubertal and pubertal children. *Arch Med Res* 2011;42:502–8.

[94] Romeo J, Martinez-Gomez D, Diaz LE, Gomez-Martinez S, Marti A, Martin-Matillas M, Puertollano MA, Veiga OL, Martinez JA, Warnberg J, Zapatera B, Garagorri JM, Morande G, Campoy C, Moreno LA, Marcos A, Group ES. Changes in cardiometabolic risk factors, appetite-controlling hormones and cytokines after a treatment program in overweight adolescents: preliminary findings from the EVASYON study. *Pediatr Diabetes* 2011;12:372–80.

[95] Leao da Silva P, de Mello MT, Cheik NC, Sanches PL, Munhoz da Silveira Campos R, Carnier J, Inoue D, do Nascimento CM, Oyama LM, Tock L, Tufik S, Damaso AR. Reduction in the leptin concentration as a predictor of improvement in lung function in obese adolescents. *Obes Facts* 2012;5:806–20.

[96] Siegrist M, Rank M, Wolfarth B, Langhof H, Haller B, Koenig W, Halle M. Leptin, adiponectin, and short-term and long-term weight loss after a lifestyle intervention in obese children. *Nutrition* 2013; 29(6):851–7.

[97] Esposito K, Pontillo A, Giugliano F, Giugliano G, Marfella R, Nicoletti G, Giugliano D. Association of low interleukin-10 levels with the metabolic syndrome in obese women. *J Clin Endocrinol Metab* 2003;88:1055–8.

[98] Lazzer S, Vermorel M, Montaurier C, Meyer M, Boirie Y. Changes in adipocyte hormones and lipid oxidation associated with weight loss and regain in severely obese adolescents. *Int J Obes (Lond)* 2005;29:1184–91.

[99] Carnier J, Sanches Pde L, da Silva PL, de Piano A, Tock L, Campos RM, Corgosinho FC, Correa FA, Masquio D, do Nascimento CM, Oyama LM, Ernandes RH, de Mello MT, Tufik S, Damaso AR. Obese adolescents with eating disorders: analysis of metabolic and inflammatory states. *Physiol Behav* 2012;105:175–80.

[100] Nemet D, Oren S, Pantanowitz M, Eliakim A. Effects of a multidisciplinary childhood obesity treatment intervention on adipocytokines, inflammatory and growth mediators. *Horm Res Paediatr* 2013;79:325–32.

[101] Reinehr T, Stoffel-Wagner B, Roth CL. Adipocyte fatty acid-binding protein in obese children before and after weight loss. *Metabolism* 2007;56:1735–41.

[102] Reinehr T, Stoffel-Wagner B, Roth CL, Andler W. High-sensitive C-reactive protein, tumor necrosis factor alpha, and cardiovascular risk factors before and after weight loss in obese children. *Metabolism* 2005;54:1155–61.

[103] Knox GJ, Baker JS, Davies B, Rees A, Morgan K, Cooper SM, Brophy S, Thomas NE. Effects of a novel school-based cross-curricular physical activity intervention on cardiovascular disease risk factors in 11- to 14-year-olds: the activity knowledge circuit. *Am J Health Promot* 2012;27:75–83.

[104]   Bocca G, Corpeleijn E, Stolk RP, Wolffenbuttel BH, Sauer PJ. Effect of obesity intervention programs on adipokines, insulin resistance, lipid profile, and low-grade inflammation in 3- to 5-y-old children. *Pediatr Res* 2014;75:352–7.

[105]   Saneei P, Hashemipour M, Kelishadi R, Esmaillzadeh A. The Dietary Approaches to Stop Hypertension (DASH) diet affects inflammation in childhood metabolic syndrome: a randomized cross-over clinical trial. *Ann Nutr Metab* 2014;64:20–7.

[106]   de Mello MT, de Piano A, Carnier J, Sanches Pde L, Correa FA, Tock L, Ernandes RM, Tufik S, Damaso AR. Long-term effects of aerobic plus resistance training on the metabolic syndrome and adiponectinemia in obese adolescents. *J Clin Hypertens (Greenwich)* 2011;13:343–50.

[107]   Seabra A, Katzmarzyk P, Carvalho MJ, Coelho ESM, Abreu S, Vale S, Povoas S, Nascimento H, Belo L, Torres S, Oliveira J, Mota J, Santos-Silva A, Rego C, Malina RM. Effects of 6-month soccer and traditional physical activity programmes on body composition, cardiometabolic risk factors, inflammatory, oxidative stress markers and cardiorespiratory fitness in obese boys. *J Sports Sci* 2016;34:1822–9.

[108]   Donoso MA, Munoz-Calvo MT, Barrios V, Garrido G, Hawkins F, Argente J. Increased circulating adiponectin levels and decreased leptin/soluble leptin receptor ratio throughout puberty in female ballet dancers: association with body composition and the delay in puberty. *Eur J Endocrinol* 2010;162:905–11.

[109]   Huang CJ, Kwok CF, Chou CH, Chou YC, Ho LT, Shih KC. The effect of exercise on lipid profiles and inflammatory markers in lean male adolescents: a prospective interventional study. *J Investig Med* 2015;63:29–34.

[110]   Huang T, Larsen KT, Moller NC, Ried-Larsen M, Frandsen U, Andersen LB. Effects of a multi-component camp-based intervention on inflammatory markers and adipokines in children: A randomized controlled trial. *Prev Med* 2015;81:367–72.

[111]   Rambhojan C, Bouaziz-Amar E, Larifla L, Deloumeaux J, Clepier J, Plumasseau J, Lacorte JM, Foucan L. Ghrelin, adipokines, metabolic factors in relation with weight status in school-children and results of a 1-year lifestyle intervention program. *Nutr Metab (Lond)* 2015;12:43.

[112]   Santos-Silva A, Rebelo MI, Castro EM, Belo L, Guerra A, Rego C, Quintanilha A. Leukocyte activation, erythrocyte damage, lipid profile and oxidative stress imposed by high competition physical exercise in adolescents. *Clin Chim Acta* 2001;306:119–26.

[113]   Metcalf BS, Jeffery AN, Hosking J, Voss LD, Sattar N, Wilkin TJ. Objectively measured physical activity and its association with adiponectin and other novel metabolic markers: a longitudinal study in children (EarlyBird 38). *Diabetes Care* 2009;32:468–73.

[114]   Shultz SP, Dahiya R, Leong GM, Rowlands DS, Hills AP, Byrne NM. Muscular strength, aerobic capacity, and adipocytokines in obese youth after resistance training: A pilot study. *Australas Med J* 2015;8:113–20.

[115] Lopes WA, Leite N, da Silva LR, Brunelli DT, Gaspari AF, Radominski RB, Chacon-Mikahil MP, Cavaglieri CR. Effects of 12 weeks of combined training without caloric restriction on inflammatory markers in overweight girls. *J Sports Sci* 2016;34:1902–12.

[116] Reinehr T, Roth CL, Alexy U, Kersting M, Kiess W, Andler W. Ghrelin levels before and after reduction of overweight due to a low-fat high-carbohydrate diet in obese children and adolescents. *Int J Obes (Lond)* 2005;29:362–8.

[117] Corgosinho FC, Ackel-D'Elia C, Tufik S, Damaso AR, de Piano A, Sanches Pde L, Campos RM, Silva PL, Carnier J, Tock L, Andersen ML, Moreira GA, Pradella-Hallinan M, Oyama LM, de Mello MT. Beneficial effects of a multifaceted 1-year lifestyle intervention on metabolic abnormalities in obese adolescents with and without sleep-disordered breathing. *Metab Syndr Relat Disord* 2015;13:110–8.

[118] Racil G, Ben Ounis O, Hammouda O, Kallel A, Zouhal H, Chamari K, Amri M. Effects of high vs. moderate exercise intensity during interval training on lipids and adiponectin levels in obese young females. *Eur J Appl Physiol* 2013;113:2531–40.

[119] Inoue DS, De Mello MT, Foschini D, Lira FS, De Piano Ganen A, Da Silveira Campos RM, De Lima Sanches P, Silva PL, Corgosinho FC, Rossi FE, Tufik S, Damaso AR. Linear and undulating periodized strength plus aerobic training promote similar benefits and lead to improvement of insulin resistance on obese adolescents. *J Diabetes Complications* 2015;29:258–64.

[120] Campos RM, de Mello MT, Tock L, Silva PL, Masquio DC, de Piano A, Sanches PL, Carnier J, Corgosinho FC, Foschini D, Tufik S, Damaso AR. Aerobic plus resistance training improves bone metabolism and inflammation in adolescents who are obese. *J Strength Cond Res* 2014;28:758–66.

[121] Damaso AR, da Silveira Campos RM, Caranti DA, de Piano A, Fisberg M, Foschini D, de Lima Sanches P, Tock L, Lederman HM, Tufik S, de Mello MT. Aerobic plus resistance training was more effective in improving the visceral adiposity, metabolic profile and inflammatory markers than aerobic training in obese adolescents. *J Sports Sci* 2014;32:1435-–45.

[122] Jensen DE, Nguo K, Baxter KA, Cardinal JW, King NA, Ware RS, Truby H, Batch JA. Fasting gut hormone levels change with modest weight loss in obese adolescents. *Pediatr Obes* 2015;10:380–7.

[123] Rouhani MH, Kelishadi R, Hashemipour M, Esmaillzadeh A, Surkan PJ, Keshavarz A, Azadbakht L. The impact of a low glycemic index diet on inflammatory markers and serum adiponectin concentration in adolescent overweight and obese girls: a randomized clinical trial. *Horm Metab Res* 2016;48:251–6.

[124] Janczyk W, Lebensztejn D, Wierzbicka-Rucinska A, Mazur A, Neuhoff-Murawska J, Matusik P, Socha P. Omega-3 Fatty acids therapy in children with nonalcoholic Fatty liver disease: a randomized controlled trial. *J Pediatr* 2015;166:1358-63 e1–3.

[125] Machado AM, de Paula H, Cardoso LD, Costa NM. Effects of brown and golden flax-seed on the lipid profile, glycemia, inflammatory biomarkers, blood pressure and body composition in overweight adolescents. *Nutrition* 2015;31:90–6.

[126] Clarson CL, Mahmud FH, Baker JE, Clark HE, McKay WM, Schauteet VD, Hill DJ. Metformin in combination with structured lifestyle intervention improved body mass index in obese adolescents, but did not improve insulin resistance. *Endocrine* 2009;36:141–6.

[127] Kendall D, Vail A, Amin R, Barrett T, Dimitri P, Ivison F, Kibirige M, Mathew V, Matyka K, McGovern A, Stirling H, Tetlow L, Wales J, Wright N, Clayton P, Hall C. Metformin in obese children and adolescents: the MOCA trial. *J Clin Endocrinol Metab* 2013;98:322–9.

[128] Kaas A, Pfleger C, Hansen L, Buschard K, Schloot NC, Roep BO, Mortensen HB, Hvidore Study Group on Childhood D. Association of adiponectin, interleukin (IL)-1ra, inducible protein 10, IL-6 and number of islet autoantibodies with progression patterns of type 1 diabetes the first year after diagnosis. *Clin Exp Immunol* 2010;161:444–52.

[129] Galler A, Gelbrich G, Kratzsch J, Noack N, Kapellen T, Kiess W. Elevated serum levels of adiponectin in children, adolescents and young adults with type 1 diabetes and the impact of age, gender, body mass index and metabolic control: a longitudinal study. *Eur J Endocrinol* 2007;157:481–9.

[130] Hong HR, Ha CD, Kong JY, Lee SH, Song MG, Kang HS. Roles of physical activity and cardiorespiratory fitness on sex difference in insulin resistance in late elementary years. *J Exerc Nutrition Biochem* 2014;18:361–9.

[131] Boodai SA, Cherry LM, Sattar NA, Reilly JJ. Prevalence of cardiometabolic risk factors and metabolic syndrome in obese Kuwaiti adolescents. *Diabetes Metab Syndr Obes* 2014;7:505–11.

5

Human Gut Microbiota and Obesity During Development

Tomás Cerdó, Alicia Ruiz and Cristina Campoy

Abstract

Obesity, particularly in children and adolescents, has become a significant public health problem that has reached "epidemic" status worldwide. The etiology of obesity is complex and involves lifestyle factors that are challenging to modify. The intestinal microbiota contribute to protection against pathogens, maturation of the immune system, and metabolic welfare of the host but, under some circumstances, can contribute to the pathogenesis of certain diseases. Over the last decade, novel evidence from animal and human studies has identified associations between human intestinal bacteria and host metabolism and obesity. Infancy is a critical period in the development of the gut microbiota: initial colonization is influenced not only by a number of early-life exposures, including birth mode, infant nutrition, or antibiotic use, but also by maternal factors during pregnancy, including maternal BMI, nutrition, gut microbial composition, and drug exposure, among others. Thus, an adequate nutritional and microbial environment during the perinatal period and early life may provide windows of opportunity to reduce the risk of obesity and overweight in our children by using targeted strategies aimed to modulate the gut microbiota during early life.

Keywords: obesity, gut microbiota, early life, pregnancy, prebiotics, probiotics, antibiotics

1. Introduction

Obesity has become a major global health challenge because of the established health risks and substantial increases in prevalence. Urgent global action and leadership is needed to help countries to more effectively intervene [1]. This increase runs in parallel to an increase in the obesity during pregnancy; moreover, due to the adverse effects that this condition has on both the mother's and offspring's health, infant obesity has become a highlight topic of study [2].

It is well known that the physiology during pregnancy differs between obese and normal-weight women. Obesity is associated with increased insulin resistance, adverse effects in implantation and placentation processes, growth, development and metabolism alterations of the fetus, and even impact on the offspring gut microbiota [3].

Until now, studies focused on the origins of obesity were oriented towards dietary excesses (processed sugars, fat, and proteins) [4] or host genes [5]. But recent studies have shown changes in gut microbiota associated to different diseases, like obesity, metabolic syndrome, or type I [6] and type II diabetes [7]. The community of microorganisms living in a specific environment is known as microbiota. These microorganisms include bacteria, Archaea, viruses, and some unicellular eukaryotes [8]. The collective genomes of the microorganism that constitute the microbiota are known as microbiome [9]. The normal gut microbiota imparts specific function in host nutrient metabolism, xenobiotics, and drug metabolism, maintenance of structural integrity of the gut mucosal barrier, immunomodulation, and protection against pathogens [10]. In fact, some of these microorganisms residing in the gut encode proteins involved in functions important for the host's health, such as enzymes required for the hydrolysis of otherwise indigestible dietary compounds, and the synthesis of vitamins [9]. Since the 1990s, our knowledge of the complexity of this ecosystem has increased due to the advances in culture-independent techniques. These new techniques are fast, facilitate high throughput, and identify organisms that are uncultured to date and present in the gut microbiota; recently, by using these techniques, it has been shown that alterations in the gut microbiota composition and function are associated with certain disease states, such as obesity [11]. With the increase in knowledge about gut microbiome functions, it is becoming increasingly more possible to develop novel diagnostic, prognostic, and most important therapeutic strategies based on gut microbiota manipulation.

Focused on obesity, it has been shown that certain bacteria metabolize different nutrients more efficiently than others, increasing the absorption of calories from the diet and the amount of energy usable for the host, which contributes to fat deposition [12]. Many studies have been performed in order to link this disease with changes in the composition of the intestinal microbiota [13]. Several studies have shown increased ratio in the proportion of *Firmicutes/Bacteroidetes* in genetically obese mice (ob/ob) and obese humans [14, 15]. However, other studies have failed to confirm these findings and showed variable patterns in the composition of the microbiota in obese humans [13]. Within the studies cited above, it is clear that the gut microbiota plays a role in obesity and metabolic disease, but it is difficult to draw definitive conclusions about the importance of certain bacterial groups. It is therefore very important to identify the active bacteria that cause dysbiosis in the gut microbiota in order to design therapeutic strategies for long-term protection against obesity. Quantitative and qualitative alterations in the composition of the gut microbiome could lead to pathological dysbiosis.

The microbiota colonization of the maternal intestine influences offspring's metabolic and immune system development [16]. Besides, although the microbiota-gut-brain axis is not a new concept [17], in the last years there are growing interest in studying the influence of the microbiota in children neurodevelopment by analyzing the microbiome impact on eating behavior, infant cognitive function, and brain structure and function [18]. However, the mechanisms by which maternal microbiota may contribute to health programming in the offspring are still unknown. The type of delivery (vaginal or caesarean section), diet [breast milk or formula], and antibiotics exposure have an influence on the offspring's immune system that may promote the development of chronic inflammation, leading to allergies, autoimmune diseases, like diabetes mellitus or rheumatoid arthritis, or noncommunicable diseases such obesity and their comorbidities in children [19–21].

In the present chapter, we aimed to update the knowledge about the factors involved in gut microbiota establishment during perinatal life, infancy and early childhood, and the relationship to obesity development.

2. Maternal environment

There is evidence for the importance of the prenatal period in the health and development of offspring throughout childhood and adult life [22].

In the periconceptional period, and during pregnancy and lactation is necessary to acquire the total nutrient requirements, which are associated with mother's lifestyles and health [23]. These requirements include specific amounts of iron, vitamins (D, C, and B), calcium, folic acid, essential fatty-acids, and others, which will increase along pregnancy [24]. Furthermore, it has been demonstrated that bad habits like smoking, use of illegal drugs, consumption of caffeine and alcohol, or overweight/underweight are related to conceiving problems [25].

During the first trimester of pregnancy, the mother is under anabolism, increasing maternal fat and nutrients storage to meet the fetus-placental and maternal requirements during gestation and lactation [26]. When a deficit or overabundance of nutrients arrives to the fetus, it has to adapt itself to the new metabolic status, changing its physiology and metabolism constantly [27].

It is noteworthy that due to fetal programing, obesity may become a self-perpetuating problem, because children of obese mothers may themselves be vulnerable to becoming obese and more likely to have offspring who share this vulnerability, but the mechanisms behind this association are not fully elucidated [28].

One hypothesis to explain the influence of the mothers' weight on their children is the transmission of obesogenic microbes from mother to her offspring; in this situation is also very important the etiology of such maternal obesity and others factors like socioeconomic status or environmental factors [29].

On the other hand, a meta-analysis including nine studies has shown an increased risk of stillbirth in obese pregnant women compared to normal-weight pregnant women [30].

It has been demonstrated that a high body mass index (BMI) and an excessive weight gain during pregnancy are associated with disturbances in the maternal gut microbiota, which will influence the development of gut microbiota in the infant [31].

Infant gut microbiota will not be only influenced by mother's BMI, but also by the mode of delivery [32]. A study indicated that excess maternal prepregnancy weight is associated with differences in neonatal acquisition of microbiota during vaginal delivery, enriched in genus *Bacteroides* and depleted in genus *Enterococcus, Acinetobacter, Pseudomonas*, and *Hydrogenophilus* [33].

Subsequent to delivery, it has been shown that the type of feeding is one of the major factors modulating infants gut microbiota and it will be discussed in Section 4.

The establishment of the microbial community allows the maturation of the immune system as it has been demonstrated in germ-free (GF) animal models, where commensal microorganisms are required for the development of a fully functional immune system, which affects many physiological processes within the host [34].

In conclusion, the mother environment influences the offspring phenotype of her offspring, independently of his genotype. So, not only genetics will influence offspring gut microbiota development, but also mother's lifestyle before, during, and after pregnancy.

3. Gut colonization and microbiota establishment in infancy

The first few weeks of life are very important for the gut colonization in the infant. This process will be influenced by maternal factors (weight gain during pregnancy, BMI, nutrition, microbiome composition), intrauterine state (microbiota of amniotic fluid), type of delivery (caesarean or vaginal), type of feeding later (breast milk or infant formula), and antibiotic exposure, among others (**Figure 1**).

Traditionally, the placenta had been considered a sterile organ but current studies have reported the existence of a placental microbiome [35–37]. Although the origin of the bacteria colonizing the placenta is unclear, it has been shown that the microbial community is represented by members of nonpathogenic bacteria from the phylum *Proteobacteria, Firmicutes, Bacteriodetes, Fusobacteria*, and *Tenericutes* [38].

Recently, placenta microbiota has been associated with preeclampsia development during pregnancy and with preterm birth, which highlights the importance of the close relationship between the microbiota and pregnancy [39]. A placental dysbiosis during pregnancy as a consequence of excess weight gain could have a major influence on the colonization and establishment of gut microbiota community on the infant [40].

Because these findings are very recent, the effects of the bacterial profile modification by probiotic supplementation during pregnancy and the effects on placental microbiome modulation are still unknown and further studies are needed.

After birth, it is known that meconium is not sterile and harbors a particular microbial community, characterized by a higher abundance of *Firmicutes* compared to *Proteobacteria* in early fecal samples [41].

A study showed that the mode of delivery (caesarean or vaginal) did not affect the diversity of the microbiota from meconium, in contrast, these samples presented a lower species diversity

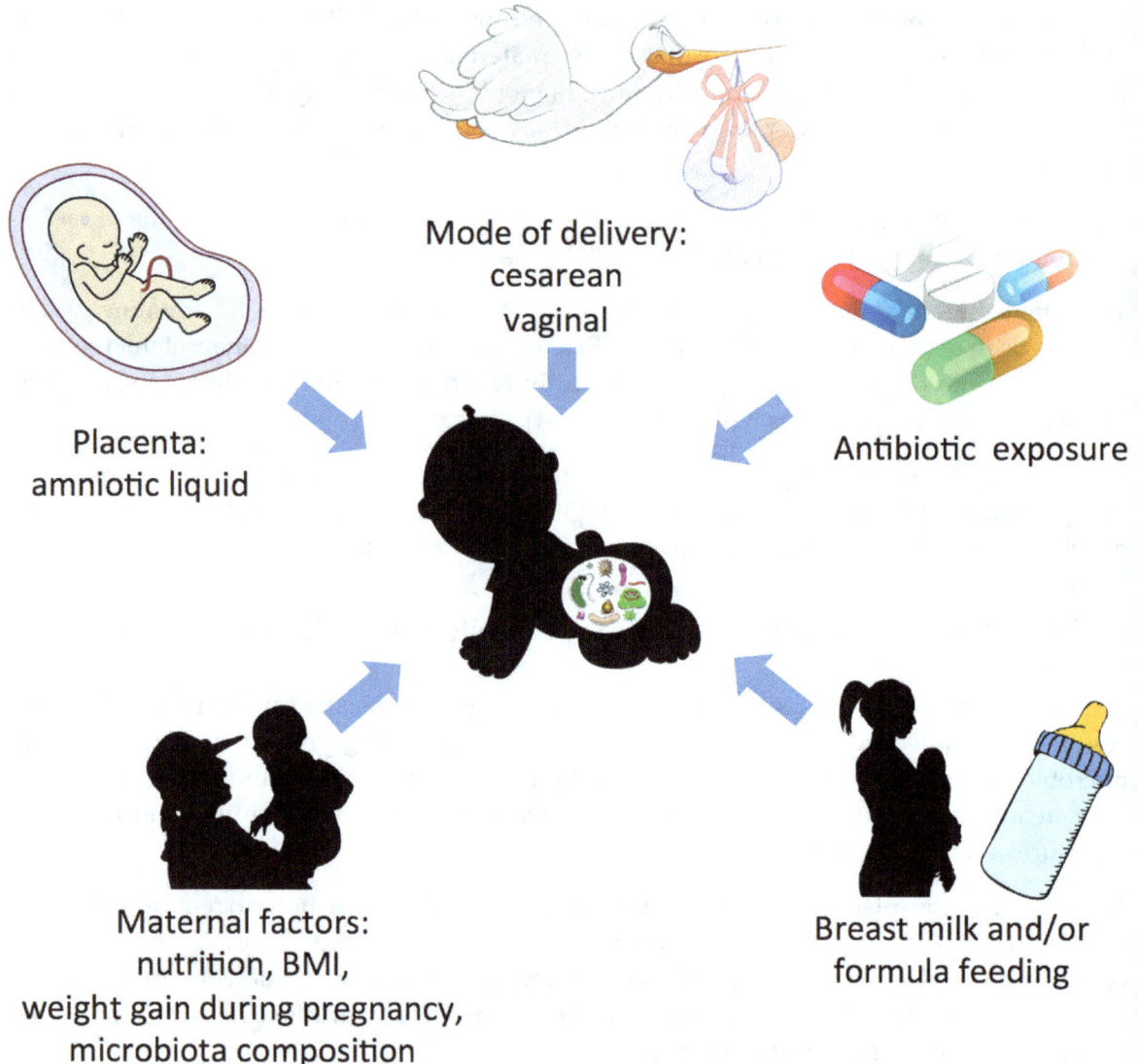

Figure 1. Maternal and environmental elements affecting the onset and modulation of the gut microbiota in the newborn infant. A plethora of factors during pregnancy can negatively influence the neonate's gut microbiota composition and function. Furthermore, environmental factors, such as mode of delivery and feeding modality can significantly drive the neonate's gut microbiota.

and a higher variation among samples in comparison with adult feces [42]. These results indicate that the microbial contact during perinatal life may imprint the offspring microbiota and immune system in preparation for the much larger inoculum transferred during vaginal delivery and breast-feeding.

As mentioned in the previous section, the mode of delivery is going to favor the establishment of a specific microbiota. Previous studies have demonstrated that gut microbiota of infant born through vaginal delivery is similar to maternal gut and vaginal microbiota; conversely, the infants born by caesarean section have a gut community more similar to bacteria from maternal skin or the hospital environment [43].

Regarding the mode of delivery, epidemiological studies suggest that caesarean delivery is associated with increased risk of overweight and obesity later in life [44]. A study has found that caesarean section delivery was associated with adiposity at 6 weeks of age, being this association stronger in children born from obese mothers and having higher risk of obesity and overweight at 11 years old [45]. Although the mode of delivery may affect the colonization of the intestinal microbiota in the baby and will increase the risk for later obesity development, it has been found that perinatal exposition of the infant born by caesarean section respect to the vaginal discharge, can partially restore its gut microbiota and resembles to babies born by vaginal delivery avoiding the problems that this entails [46].

The microbiota of the babies by the end of the first year of life presents a different microbial profile in comparison to adults. The initial gut composition of the infant is simple, dynamic, and very unstable and undergoes marked fluctuations influenced by external factors [47]. At the beginning, the gut environment is aerobic, but through colonization, the oxygen level is reduced generating a suitable environment for the growth of anaerobes [48]. The intestinal microbiota of neonates is characterized by low diversity and a relative dominance of facultative anaerobes of the phyla *Proteobacteria* and *Actinobacteria* [49]. After birth, the phyla *Firmicutes* and *Bacteroidetes* increase their diversity and dominance, reaching over 3 years old a total resemblance to the adult in terms of composition and diversity [50]. These results indicate that dietary intake during the first 1500 days of life is a critical factor in the establishment of gut microbiota community and its role in the development of obesity is a matter of research and discussion.

4. Type of infant feeding

Another important factor modulating microbial colonization in infants is the type of feeding. The diet during early life will influence on the establishment and composition of the gut microbiota during childhood and even adult life [51]. Breast milk meets the infant's needs by providing nutrients appropriate to the infant's developmental stage, as well as growth factors, antimicrobial peptides, and proteins to support their developing immune system. Even though breast milk provides all the necessary nutrients for a suitable development of the baby, many babies cannot take it for several reasons and they are fed with infant formulas. Infant formulas provide a greater weight gain and increase the risk of obesity, hypertension, and diabetes [52]. Therefore, it is necessary to continue studying the composition and the positive effects of breast milk versus milk infant formula in order to better understand the beneficial role of breast milk on offspring's health to improve the outcomes in the formula-fed infants.

Breast-feeding brings clear short-term benefits for child health by reducing mortality and morbidity from infectious diseases. There is evidence on the effects on child health and growth of exclusive breast-feeding for 6 months. Kramer et al. showed that infants who were exclusively breast-fed for 6 months experienced lower morbidity from gastrointestinal and allergic diseases, while showing nondeficits in growth rates to non–breast-fed children [53]. Based on such evidence, WHO and UNICEF recommend that every infant should be exclusively breast-fed for the first 6 months of their life; continued breast-feeding for up to 2 years or longer is also recommended [54]. Also, there is evidence of long-term benefits of breast-feeding such as increased school achievement and performance in intelligence tests, reduced mean blood pressure, lower total cholesterol, and a lower prevalence of overweight and obesity leading to lower incidence of inflammatory bowel diseases, type 2 diabetes, and obesity later in life [54, 55].

Human milk is a dynamic fluid that contains many hundreds to thousands of distinct bioactive molecules that confers beneficial properties for infants. Human milk changes in composition from colostrum to late lactation, and varies within feeds, diurnally, and between mothers [56].

The composition of this complex mixture differs also during the lactation period, from colostrum through transitional to mature milk. Colostrum is produced during the first days of postpartum, it contains high amounts of secretory IgA, lactoferrin, leukocytes, and epidermal growth factor. Transitional milk typically occurs from 5 days to 2 weeks postpartum, it shares some of the characteristics of colostrum but there is an increase in milk production to support the nutritional and developmental needs of the rapidly growing infant. By 4–6 weeks postpartum, human milk is considered fully mature and it remains stable in composition over the course of lactation [57–59]. Thus, infant formula should adapt to different physiological and nutritional needs of the growing baby.

Regarding the gut microbiota acquisition, the first colonizers of the infant gut are facultative anaerobes including *Staphylococcus*, *Streptococcus*, *Escherichia coli*, and *Enterobacteria* that will be later replaced by strict anaerobes that dominate the gastrointestinal tract, primarily *Clostridium*, *Bifidobacterium spp.*, and *Bacteroides* [60]. This change in dominant taxa representation can be attributed to the introduction of breast milk or formula-feeding, signifying the first diet-related colonization event in the infant gut microbiome [61, 62]. Breast milk has been shown to be an excellent and continuous source of potentially beneficial and commensal bacteria, including *Staphylococci*, *Streptococci*, *lactic acid bacteria*, and *Bifidobacteria*, with bacterial cell numbers reaching 103–105 ml^{-1} of breast milk. Although the commensals' origin is unknown, it is inevitable that bacterial from mother's skin are transferred to the baby during breast-feeding, but there is also other hypothesis wherein bacteria from the maternal gut may reach the mammary glands via maternal dendritic cells and macrophages [63]. More than 700 species of bacteria have now been identified in human colostrum and breast milk, including multiple species of lactic acid bacteria as well as species typically colonizing the oral cavity of infants [64].

The presence of *Bifidobacteria* in breast milk is important for the colonization of the infant gut, since it mediates the activation of IgA-producing plasma cells in the human neonatal intestine. It is well established that a gut microbiota dominated by *Bifidobacteria* typifies that of the healthy breast-fed infant [65]. There are conflicting results regarding differences in the relative abundance of these bacteria between breast- and formula-fed infants. Many studies have reported that formula-fed infants display dominance of *Bifidobacterium spp.* similar to what has been observed in breast-fed infants [61, 66]. However, another study reported approximately double the count of *Bifidobacterium* in breast-fed infants compared to those formula-fed [67].

Comparisons between breast-fed and formula-fed infants show that breast-fed infants tend to contain a more uniform population of gut microbes dominated by *Bifidobacteria* and *Lactobacillus* [67], whereas formula-fed infants exhibit higher proportions of *Bacteroides, Clostridium, Streptococcus, Enterobacteria*, and *Veillonella spp.* [66–69].

Although infant formulas have evolved greatly during last years, a formula providing exactly the same benefits than human milk has not yet been developed. Among others, human milk contains substantial quantities of complex nondigestible oligosaccharides (known as human milk oligosaccharides, HMOs). HMOs are considered a type of prebiotics as they promote the growth and proliferation of beneficial commensals and, consequently, prevent pathogen colonization of the infant gut and exert positive health effects [70]. Thus, the chemical composition of breast milk does influence the gut microbiome through supplying oligosaccharides that are selectively utilized by specific bacteria in the gut [60].

Another way to modify the gut microbiome is by the administration of probiotics. Probiotics are defined as "live microorganisms which when administered in adequate amounts, confer a health benefit to the host" [71]. *Lactobacillus* and *Bifidobacterium* species isolated from human milk are the most commonly used probiotic strains. They exert beneficial properties in the gut by suppressing the proliferation of pathogenic microbes, has been extensively studied [72]. For this reason, another area of research regarding formula enrichment is in HMOs and probiotics and their effects on the infant gut microbiota.

Certain gut-associated bacterial populations such as *Bifidobacterium spp.* possess gene clusters dedicated to the metabolism of HMOs [73, 74]. Degradation of these compounds produces lactate and short-chain fatty acids (SCFA), which in turn generates an acidic environment that prevents pathogen invasion [75]. Besides *Bifidobacteria*, HMOs may be consumed by other species such as *Bacteroides spp.* (e.g., *Bacteroides* fragilis and *Bacteroides vulgatus*) that consumes a broad range of HMO glycans [76]. Thus, HMOs play an important role in the gut colonization of the infants.

Among the most common prebiotics are fructo-oligosaccharides (FOS), galacto-oligosaccharides (GOS), inulin, and lactulose. The prebiotic mixture of 90% GOS plus 10% FOS has been assessed to be safe when added to infant formula [77]. Several randomized controlled trials have been made to evaluate the efficacy and safety of prebiotic supplementation in infant formulas [78, 79]. After compiling data of these trials into a meta-analysis, weight gain [weighted mean difference 1.07 g/day] was significantly higher among formula-fed infants supplemented with prebiotics compared to the placebo group [80]. In addition, a large number of clinical trials in term of infants have shown controversial results related to the increase in *Bifidobacteria* in feces due to supplementation of infant formula with GOS and FOS. A systematic review published by Rao et al. [78] reported that some of the randomized controlled trials (RCTs) showed a trend of increasing *Bifidobacteria* counts in formula supplemented fed infants, and another systematic review published by Mugambi et al. [81] failed to show the increase in *Bifidobacteria* or *Lactobacillus* or the decrease of pathogens in infants fed with prebiotic supplemented formula.

Nonetheless, there are promising results from studies which have assessed the effect of prebiotic supplemented formulas on the gut microbiota of infants. Prebiotics are able to change gut metabolic activity, bring stool consistency, and defecation frequency closer to that of breast-fed infants. Other outcomes included better weight gain and softer stools, and a significant reduction in stool pH for infants who received prebiotic supplementation [78, 81]. Moreover, prebiotics have been used to prevent or treat obesity. Compared to probiotics, human studies with prebiotics have shown more promising results in obesity management, with reductions in body weight and fat mass in adults [82–84] in contrast with results from meta-analysis mentioned above, where the supplementation with prebiotics was significantly associated to a higher weight gain [80].

In the last years there is a growing interest in the simultaneous administration of prebiotics and probiotics, what is termed "symbiotic." There are a few recent studies which have assessed the effect of symbiotic supplementation on the infant health. The ESPGHAN Committee on Nutrition showed an increase in stool frequency for three types of symbiotic (*B. longum* BL999 plus GOS/FOS, *B. longum* BL999 plus *L. rhamnosus* LPR plus GOS/FOS, and *L. paracasei* subsp. paracasei plus *B. animalis subsp. lactis* plus GOS) [79]. Also, Ringel-Kulka et al. showed that a yogurt with the probiotic bacteria *Bifidobacterium* animalis subspecies lactis (BB-12) and the prebiotic inulin significantly reduced days of fever, improved social and school functioning, and increased frequency of bowel movements in healthy children attending child care centers [85]. Regarding to obesity interventions with symbiotic, Safavi et al. [86] found that treatment of overweight children with a symbiotic mixture of the prebiotic, FOS, in combination with seven probiotic strains was associated with a decreased BMI z-score compared to placebo.

Studies suggest that pre-, probiotic, and symbiotic supplementation may be beneficial in the prevention and management of disease where the gut microbiota has a key role (e.g., necrotizing enterocolitis, gastroenteritis, or obesity). Although these studies show promising beneficial effects, the long-term risks or health benefits of pre- and probiotic supplementation are not clear as results from single studies need to be replicated in well-defined RCTs. Nonetheless, there is active research on functional food that contains pre-, probiotics, and symbiotics supplementation because they can influence not only the microbiota favoring the growth of beneficial microorganisms, but also the mucosal immune system associated to the gut [87].

5. Childhood exposure to antibiotics

Exposure to antibiotics during infancy and childhood use to begin very early. Two different studies showed that >30% of women with a delivery had done systemic antibiotic treatments during pregnancy [88, 89]. Although the effects of antibiotic exposure during pregnancy on acquisition of infants' microbiota have not been established, maternal antibiotic exposure is relevant since infants' microbiota is taken at least in part from their mothers. In addition, prenatal antibiotic exposure has been shown to have effects on the birth weight of neonates and is associated with increased risk of obesity and related metabolic sequelae later in life [90, 91].

After birth, a number of neonates, particularly premature infants, receive antibiotics to prevent or treat bacterial infections. Fjalstad et al. showed that 2.3% of all live-born term infants received intravenous antibiotics in the population, they analyzed from 2009 to 2011 [92].

Higher prescription rates were shown in preterm or term infants with relevant clinical problems. In a study involving neonates admitted to the neonatal intensive care unit in U.S. from 2005 to 2010, more than 88% of extremely low birth weight infants were administrated antibiotics [93].

Over the last decade, several national and international health institutions have made an enormous effort to decrease antibiotic use in the pediatric population by educating parents about the futility of treating viral infections with antibiotics and about concerns of antibiotic resistance [94, 95]. But, despite a recent reduction, widespread antibiotic use in infants and children remains a relevant health problem in the entire industrialized world, mainly because most prescriptions were frequently inappropriate [96].

However, even in countries in which the prescribing pattern usually adheres to national guidelines with respect to the choice of antibiotics, antibiotics are still largely prescribed to children, particularly to very young children [97–100].

In addition to antibiotic exposure for infection prevention and therapy, children could potentially be substantially exposed to antibiotics through the food supply chain or, more rarely, drinking water [101].

5.1. Evidence from animals

In last 50 years, farmers have been using low doses of antibiotics to promote growth and feed efficiency of pigs, cows, sheep, and poultry [102]. Different antibiotics have been demonstrated to have these effects independently of its class, chemical structure, and mode of action and spectrum of activity. Moreover, the effects on growth are greater when animals receive antibiotics early in life than if the exposure occurs later in life [103–105].

Also, studies in mice using multiple types of antibiotics have further confirmed this association, as well as identifying early life as the key period for microbe-mediated programing of host metabolism [106, 107].

Experiments with germ-free animal models have provided direct evidence of the key role of the microbiota in the association between low doses of antibiotics exposure and growth promotion. In 1963, Coates et al. showed that in germ-free chicken antibiotics alone have no growth promoting effects [108]. Recently, Cox et al. showed that germ-free mice who received the microbiota from mice treated with low dose penicillin gained more weight and fat mass than mice colonized with microbiota from control animals [107].

Then, there are two main findings from these experiments. First, early life is a critical time for metabolic development of the host, and second, the microbiome has a key role in this process and its disturbance duty to antibiotic exposure at this time affects the course of growth and development [109].

5.2. Epidemiologic evidence

There is epidemiologic evidence that exposure to antibiotics in early life is associated with increased risk of excess adiposity. Recently, epidemiological studies have shown that this phenomenon can also occur in humans starting in the fetal stage of life. In that sense, Mueller et al. observed in a U.S. cohort that the administration of antibiotics to women in the last two trimesters of pregnancy increased 84% the risk of obesity in children at 7 years old compared to children born to mothers without antibiotics administration at the same period [110]. Also, Mor et al. observed similar results in a study performed in Denmark where they showed that prenatal exposure to systemic antibacterials was associated with an increased risk of overweight and obesity at school age, and this association varies by birth weight [111].

After birth, the exposure to antibiotics has been associated to obesity due to the analysis of different human cohorts in various countries. In a Danish mother-child pairs cohort, Ajslev et al. showed antibiotic exposure in children during the first 6 months was associated with an increased risk of being overweight at 7 years of age; the effect was stronger in boys than in girls. In a U.K. cohort, Trasande et al. showed that antibiotic use in the first 6 months of life was associated with increased BMI at 10, 20, and 38 months of age [19]. Both studies also determined that maternal BMI was a contributing factor for the development of obesity following exposure to antibiotics in early life, with increased effects seen in children with mothers of normal weight compared with children from mothers who were overweight. Also, Azad et al. in a study of Canadian infants showed that antibiotics administered in the first year of life increased the likelihood of a child being overweight at 9 years and 12 years of age being almost seen in boys [112], which was consistent with the previous results from Ajslev et al. In a U.S. cohort, Bailey at al. observed that repeated exposure to broad-spectrum anti-biotics at ages 0–23 months was associated with early childhood obesity. Importantly, this observation was associated with the use of broad-spectrum antibiotics, but not with the use of narrow-spectrum antibiotics.

Finally, in a multicenter, multicountry, cross-sectional study (The International Study of Asthma and Allergies in Childhood Phase III) Murphy et al. observed a significant interaction between sex and early-life antibiotic exposure. Exposure to antibiotics during the first 12 months of life was associated with a small increase in BMI in boys aged 5–8 years but not in girls in this large international cross-sectional survey.

Colonization of neonate's gut microbiota relies on vertical transmission from the mother at the time of delivery; thus, during pregnancy or early-life exposure to antibiotics could have effects on weight later in life by disturbing the proper establishment of the gut microbiota.

5.3. Antibiotic exposure and dysbiosis in children

Prospective studies have showed that changes in gut microbiota in early life may precede the development of overweight and obesity [113, 114].

In particular, some bacterial taxa has been associated with the risk of obesity development, regarding to this, a high abundance of intestinal *Bifidobacteria* in early life appears to be asso-ciated with lower risk of overweight [114, 115], whereas high amounts of *Bacteroides fragilis* increase the risk of obesity development [113]. Thus, likely factors that exert an impact on gut microbiota composition and functionality in early life may also modulate the risk of obesity development.

Therefore, antibiotic exposure during childhood can reduce the phylogenetic diversity and microbial load of the gut microbiota [116].

Regarding preterm infants it has been shown that treatment with amoxicillin and gentamicin during the first week of life reduced the bacterial diversity and raised the relative abundance of *Enterobacter* in the second and third weeks of life compared to preterm infants not exposed to antibiotics [117].

Moreover, administration of penicillin, ampicillin, cephalexin, gentamicin, amikacin, erythromycin, vancomycin, clindamycin, and teichomycin to preterm infants has been associated with a decrease in the relative abundance of *Bifidobacteriaceae, bacilli*, and *Lactobacillales spp.*, commonly linked with a healthy status and an increase in the presence of potentially pathogenic *Enterobacteriaceae* [117–119]. Besides short-term-effects, the dysbiosis produced by antibiotics administration in infants may produce long-term effects like the persistence of the risk of obesity development. It has been observed that 3 months after of antibiotics persists the microbiota disruption [120]. However, antibiotic administration to neonates has been linked to several critical clinical conditions in which modification of the microbiota composition is thought to play a relevant role, in diseases such as necrotizing enterocolitis and sepsis [121, 122].

Antibiotic treatments in early life can lead to long-term alterations in microbiota composition that result in changes to host metabolic functions, particularly during development, increasing the risk of obesity [109].

Author details

Tomás Cerdó[1, 2, 3], Alicia Ruiz[1, 3] and Cristina Campoy[1, 2, 3, 4*]

*Address all correspondence to: ccampoy@ugr.es

1 EURISTIKOS Excellence Centre for Paediatric Research, University of Granada, Granada, Spain

2 Department of Paediatrics, School of Medicine, University of Granada, Granada, Spain

3 Centre for Biomedical Research, University of Granada, Granada, Spain

4 CIBERESP: National Network of Research in Epidemiology and Public Health, Institute Carlos III, Valencia, Spain

References

[1] Ng M, Fleming T, Robinson M, Thomson B, Graetz N, Margono C, et al. Global, regional, and national prevalence of overweight and obesity in children and adults during 1980–2013: a systematic analysis for the global burden of disease study 2013. Lancet (London, England). 2014;384(9945):766–781.

[2]   Ogburn PL. Obesity and gestational diabetes in pregnancy: an evolving epidemic. Journal of Perinatal Medicine. 2016;44(4):361–362.

[3]   Malhotra N, Sharma E, Malhotra J, Bora NM. Obesity in obstetric intensive care patient. Principles of Critical Care in Obstetrics Part IV: Springer; 2016. pp. 317–321.

[4]   Spreadbury I. Comparison with ancestral diets suggests dense acellular carbohydrates promote an inflammatory microbiota, and may be the primary dietary cause of leptin resistance and obesity. Diabetes, Metabolic Syndrome and Obesity: Targets and Therapy. 2012;5:175–189.

[5]   Hollopeter G, Erickson J, Palmiter R. Role of neuropeptide Y in diet-, chemical-and genetic-induced obesity of mice. International Journal of Obesity. 1998;22(6):506–512.

[6]   Murri M, Leiva I, Gomez-Zumaquero JM, Tinahones FJ, Cardona F, Soriguer F, et al. Gut microbiota in children with type 1 diabetes differs from that in healthy children: a case-control study. BMC Medicine. 2013;11(1):1.

[7]   Marchesi JR, Adams DH, Fava F, Hermes GDA, Hirschfield GM, Hold G, et al. The gut microbiota and host health: a new clinical frontier. Gut. 2015:gutjnl-2015-309990.

[8]   Sekirov I, Russell SL, Antunes LCM, Finlay BB. Gut microbiota in health and disease. Physiological Reviews. 2010;90(3):859–904.

[9]   D'Argenio V, Salvatore F. The role of the gut microbiome in the healthy adult status. Clinica Chimica Acta. 2015;451:97–102.

[10] Jandhyala SM, Talukdar R, Subramanyam C, Vuyyuru H, Sasikala M, Reddy DN. Role of the normal gut microbiota. World Journal of Gastroenterology: WJG. 2015;21(29):8787.

[11] Fraher MH, O'Toole PW, Quigley EMM. Techniques used to characterize the gut microbiota: a guide for the clinician. Nature Reviews Gastroenterology and Hepatology. 2012;9(6):312–322.

[12] Turnbaugh PJ, Bäckhed F, Fulton L, Gordon JI. Diet-induced obesity is linked to marked but reversible alterations in the mouse distal gut microbiome. Cell Host & Microbe. 2008;3(4):213–223.

[13] Tagliabue A, Elli M. The role of gut microbiota in human obesity: recent findings and future perspectives. Nutrition, Metabolism, and Cardiovascular Diseases: NMCD. 2013;23(3):160–168.

[14] Ley RE, Turnbaugh PJ, Klein S, Gordon JI. Microbial ecology: human gut microbes associated with obesity. Nature. 2006;444(7122):1022–1023.

[15] Ley RE, Backhed F, Turnbaugh P, Lozupone CA, Knight RD, Gordon JI. Obesity alters gut microbial ecology. Proceedings of the National Academy of Sciences of the United States of America. 2005;102(31):11070–11075.

[16] Collado MC, Cernada M, Neu J, Pérez-Martínez G, Gormaz M, Vento M. Factors influencing gastrointestinal tract and microbiota immune interaction in preterm infants. Pediatric Research. 2015;77(6):726–731.

[17] Track NS. The gastrointestinal endocrine system. Canadian Medical Association Journal. 1980;122(3):287.

[18] Cerdó T, García-Valdés L, Altmäe S, Ruíz-Rodríguez A, Suárez A, Campoy C. Role of microbiota function during early life and children neurodevelopment Aricule in press. Trends in Food Science & Technology xxx (2016); 1–16.

[19] Trasande L, Blustein J, Liu M, Corwin E, Cox L, Blaser M. Infant antibiotic exposures and early-life body mass. International Journal of Obesity. 2013;37(1):16–23.

[20] Dominguez-Bello MG, Costello EK, Contreras M, Magris M, Hidalgo G, Fierer N, et al. Delivery mode shapes the acquisition and structure of the initial microbiota across multiple body habitats in newborns. Proceedings of the National Academy of Sciences. 2010;107(26):11971–11975.

[21] Murphy EF, Cotter PD, Hogan A, O'Sullivan O, Joyce A, Fouhy F, et al. Divergent metabolic outcomes arising from targeted manipulation of the gut microbiota in diet-induced obesity. Gut. 2013;62(2):220–226.

[22] DiPietro JA. Maternal stress in pregnancy: considerations for fetal development. Journal of Adolescent Health. 2012;51(2):S3–S8.

[23] Kaiser L, Allen LH. Position of the American Dietetic Association: nutrition and life-style for a healthy pregnancy outcome. Journal of the American Dietetic Association. 2008;108(3):553–561.

[24] Gardiner PM, Nelson L, Shellhaas CS, Dunlop AL, Long R, Andrist S, et al. The clinical content of preconception care: nutrition and dietary supplements. American Journal of Obstetrics and Gynecology. 2008;199(6):S345–S56.

[25] Temel S, van Voorst SF, Jack BW, Denktaş S, Steegers EA. Evidence-based preconceptional lifestyle interventions. Epidemiologic Reviews. 2014;36(1):19–30.

[26] Lain KY, Catalano PM. Metabolic changes in pregnancy. Clinical Obstetrics and Gynecology. 2007;50(4):938–948.

[27] De Boo HA, Harding JE. The developmental origins of adult disease (Barker) hypothesis. Australian and New Zealand Journal of Obstetrics and Gynaecology. 2006;46(1):4–14.

[28] Leddy MA, Power ML, Schulkin J. The impact of maternal obesity on maternal and fetal health. Reviews in Obstetrics and Gynecology. 2008;1(4):170–178.

[29] Galley JD, Bailey M, Dush CK, Schoppe-Sullivan S, Christian LM. Maternal obesity is associated with alterations in the gut microbiome in toddlers. PLoS One. 2014;9(11): e113026.

[30] Chu SY, Kim SY, Lau J, Schmid CH, Dietz PM, Callaghan WM, et al. Maternal obesity and risk of stillbirth: a metaanalysis. American Journal of Obstetrics and Gynecology. 2007;197(3):223–238.

[31] Collado MC, Isolauri E, Laitinen K, Salminen S. Distinct composition of gut microbiota during pregnancy in overweight and normal-weight women. The American Journal of Clinical Nutrition. 2008;88(4):894–899.

[32] Gritz EC, Bhandari V. The human neonatal gut microbiome: a brief review. Frontiers in Pediatrics. 2015;3:17.

[33] Mueller NT, Shin H, Pizoni A, Werlang IC, Matte U, Goldani MZ, et al. Birth mode-dependent association between pre-pregnancy maternal weight status and the neonatal intestinal microbiome. Scientific Reports. 2016;6.

[34] Smith K, McCoy KD, Macpherson AJ, editors. Use of axenic animals in studying the adaptation of mammals to their commensal intestinal microbiota. Seminars in Immunology: Elsevier; April 2007;19(2):59–69.

[35] DiGiulio DB, Gervasi M, Romero R, Mazaki-Tovi S, Vaisbuch E, Kusanovic JP, et al. Microbial invasion of the amniotic cavity in preeclampsia as assessed by cultivation and sequence-based methods. Journal of Perinatal Medicine. 2010;38(5):503–513.

[36] Lee SE, Romero R, Lee SM, Yoon BH. Amniotic fluid volume in intra-amniotic inflammation with and without culture-proven amniotic fluid infection in preterm premature rupture of membranes. Journal of Perinatal Medicine. 2010;38(1):39–44.

[37] Romero R, Hassan SS, Gajer P, Tarca AL, Fadrosh DW, Bieda J, et al. The vaginal microbiota of pregnant women who subsequently have spontaneous preterm labor and delivery and those with a normal delivery at term. Microbiome. 2014;2(1):1.

[38] Aagaard K, Ma J, Antony KM, Ganu R, Petrosino J, Versalovic J. The placenta harbors a unique microbiome. Science Translational Medicine. 2014;6(237):237ra65-ra65.

[39] Amarasekara R, Jayasekara RW, Senanayake H, Dissanayake VH. Microbiome of the placenta in pre-eclampsia supports the role of bacteria in the multifactorial cause of pre-eclampsia. Journal of Obstetrics and Gynaecology Research. 2015;41(5):662–669.

[40] Antony KM, Ma J, Mitchell KB, Racusin DA, Versalovic J, Aagaard K. The preterm placental microbiome varies in association with excess maternal gestational weight gain. American Journal of Obstetrics and Gynecology. 2015;212(5):653. e1-e16.

[41] Moles L, Gomez M, Heilig H, Bustos G, Fuentes S, de Vos W, et al. Bacterial diversity in meconium of preterm neonates and evolution of their fecal microbiota during the first month of life. PLoS One. 2013;8(6):e66986.

[42] Hu J, Nomura Y, Bashir A, Fernandez-Hernandez H, Itzkowitz S, Pei Z, et al. Diversified microbiota of meconium is affected by maternal diabetes status. PLoS One. 2013;8(11):e78257.

[43] Martin R, Makino H, Yavuz AC, Ben-Amor K, Roelofs M, Ishikawa E, et al. Early-life events, including mode of delivery and type of feeding, siblings and gender, shape the developing gut microbiota. PLoS One. 2016;11(6):e0158498.

[44] Kuhle S, Tong O, Woolcott C. Association between caesarean section and childhood obesity: a systematic review and meta-analysis. Obesity Reviews. 2015;16(4):295–303.

[45] Blustein J, Attina T, Liu M, Ryan A, Cox L, Blaser M, et al. Association of caesarean delivery with child adiposity from age 6 weeks to 15 years. International Journal of Obesity. 2013;37(7):900–906.

[46] Dominguez-Bello MG, De Jesus-Laboy KM, Shen N, Cox LM, Amir A, Gonzalez A, et al. Partial restoration of the microbiota of cesarean-born infants via vaginal microbial transfer. Nature Medicine. 2016;22: 250–253.

[47] Dogra S, Sakwinska O, Soh S-E, Ngom-Bru C, Brück WM, Berger B, et al. Rate of establishing the gut microbiota in infancy has consequences for future health. Gut Microbes. 2015;6(5):321–325.

[48] Fouhy F, Ross RP, Fitzgerald GF, Stanton C, Cotter PD. Composition of the early intestinal microbiota: knowledge, knowledge gaps and the use of high-throughput sequencing to address these gaps. Gut Microbes. 2012;3(3):203–220.

[49] Bäckhed F. Programming of host metabolism by the gut microbiota. Annals of Nutrition and Metabolism. 2011;58(Suppl. 2):44–52.

[50] Eckburg PB, Bik EM, Bernstein CN, Purdom E, Dethlefsen L, Sargent M, et al. Diversity of the human intestinal microbial flora. Science (New York, NY). 2005;308(5728):1635–1638.

[51] Nylund L, Satokari R, Salminen S, de Vos WM. Intestinal microbiota during early life - impact on health and disease. The Proceedings of the Nutrition Society. 2014;73(4): 457–469.

[52] Timby N, Domellöf E, Hernell O, Lönnerdal B, Domellöf M. Neurodevelopment, nutrition, and growth until 12 mo of age in infants fed a low-energy, low-protein formula supplemented with bovine milk fat globule membranes: a randomized controlled trial. The American Journal of Clinical Nutrition. 2014;99(4):860–868.

[53] Kramer MS, Kakuma R. The optimal duration of exclusive breastfeeding. Protecting Infants through Human Milk: Springer; 2004. Section II, pp. 63–77.

[54] World Health O, Unicef. Global strategy for infant and young child feeding: World Health Organization; 2003.

[55] Le Huërou-Luron I, Blat S, Boudry G. Breast- v. formula-feeding: impacts on the digestive tract and immediate and long-term health effects. Nutrition Research Reviews. 2010;23(01):23–36.

[56] Ballard O, Morrow AL. Human milk composition: nutrients and bioactive factors. Pediatric Clinics of North America. 2013;60(1):49–74.

[57] Kulski JK, Hartmann PE. Changes in human milk composition during the initiation of lactation. The Australian Journal of Experimental Biology and Medical Science. 1981;59(1):101–114.

[58] Field CJ. The immunological components of human milk and their effect on immune development in infants. The Journal of Nutrition. 2005;135(1):1–4.

[59] Castellote C, Casillas R, Ramírez-Santana C, Pérez-Cano FJ, Castell M, Moretones MG, et al. Premature delivery influences the immunological composition of colostrum and transitional and mature human milk. The Journal of Nutrition. 2011;141(6):1181–1187.

[60] Turroni F, Peano C, Pass DA, Foroni E, Severgnini M, Claesson MJ, et al. Diversity of bifidobacteria within the infant gut microbiota. PLoS One. 2012;7(5):e36957.

[61] Harmsen HJ, Wildeboer-Veloo AC, Raangs GC, Wagendorp AA, Klijn N, Bindels JG, et al. Analysis of intestinal flora development in breast-fed and formula-fed infants by using molecular identification and detection methods. Journal of Pediatric Gastroenterology and Nutrition. 2000;30(1):61–67.

[62] Jost T, Lacroix C, Braegger CP, Chassard C. New insights in gut microbiota establishment in healthy breast fed neonates. PLoS One. 2012;7(8):e44595.

[63] Jost T, Lacroix C, Braegger CP, Rochat F, Chassard C. Vertical mother-neonate transfer of maternal gut bacteria via breastfeeding. Environmental Microbiology. 2014;16(9): 2891–2904.

[64] Cabrera-Rubio R, Collado MC, Laitinen K, Salminen S, Isolauri E, Mira A. The human milk microbiome changes over lactation and is shaped by maternal weight and mode of delivery. The American Journal of Clinical Nutrition. 2012;96(3):544–551.

[65] Gueimonde M, Laitinen K, Salminen S, Isolauri E. Breast milk: a source of bifidobacteria for infant gut development and maturation? Neonatology. 2007;92(1):64–66.

[66] Fallani M, Young D, Scott J, Norin E, Amarri S, Adam R, et al. Intestinal microbiota of 6-week-old infants across Europe: geographic influence beyond delivery mode, breast-feeding, and antibiotics. Journal of Pediatric Gastroenterology and Nutrition. 2010;51(1):77–84.

[67] Bezirtzoglou E, Tsiotsias A, Welling GW. Microbiota profile in feces of breast- and formula-fed newborns by using fluorescence in situ hybridization (FISH). Anaerobe. 2011;17(6):478–482.

[68] Adlerberth I, Wold AE. Establishment of the gut microbiota in Western infants. Acta Paediatrica (Oslo, Norway: 1992). 2009;98(2):229–938.

[69] Favier CF, Vaughan EE, De Vos WM, Akkermans AD. Molecular monitoring of succession of bacterial communities in human neonates. Applied and Environmental Microbiology. 2002;68(1):219–226.

[70] German JB, Freeman SL, Lebrilla CB, Mills DA. Human milk oligosaccharides: evolution, structures and bioselectivity as substrates for intestinal bacteria. Nestle Nutrition Workshop Series Paediatric Programme. 2008;62:205–218.

[71] Sanders ME. Probiotics: definition, sources, selection, and uses. Clinical Infectious Diseases. 2008;46(Suppl. 2):S58–S61.

[72] Hill C, Guarner F, Reid G, Gibson GR, Merenstein DJ, Pot B, et al. Expert consensus document. The International Scientific Association for Probiotics and Prebiotics consensus statement on the scope and appropriate use of the term probiotic. Nature Reviews Gastroenterology & Hepatology. 2014;11(8):506–514.

[73] Ward RE, Ninonuevo M, Mills DA, Lebrilla CB, German JB. In vitro fermentability of human milk oligosaccharides by several strains of bifidobacteria. Molecular Nutrition & Food Research. 2007;51(11):1398–1405.

[74] Sela DA, Mills DA. Nursing our microbiota: molecular linkages between bifidobacteria and milk oligosaccharides. Trends in Microbiology. 2010;18(7):298–307.

[75] Yu ZT, Chen C, Kling DE, Liu B, McCoy JM, Merighi M, et al. The principal fucosylated oligosaccharides of human milk exhibit prebiotic properties on cultured infant microbiota. Glycobiology. 2013;23(2):169–177.

[76] Marcobal A, Sonnenburg JL. Human milk oligosaccharide consumption by intestinal microbiota. Clinical Microbiology and Infection: The Official Publication of the European Society of Clinical Microbiology and Infectious Diseases. 2012;18 (Suppl. 4):12–15.

[77] Food ESCo. Additional statement on the use of resistant short chain carbohydrates (oligofurctosyl-saccharose and oligogalactosyl-lactose) in infant formula and in follow-on formula. EC Scientific Committee on Food; Brussels, Belgium. 2001.

[78] Rao S, Srinivasjois R, Patole S. Prebiotic supplementation in full-term neonates: a systematic review of randomized controlled trials. Archives of Pediatrics & Adolescent Medicine. 2009;163(8):755–764.

[79] Braegger C, Chmielewska A, Decsi T, Kolacek S, Mihatsch W, Moreno L, et al. Supplementation of infant formula with probiotics and/or prebiotics: a systematic review and comment by the ESPGHAN committee on nutrition. Journal of Pediatric Gastroenterology and Nutrition. 2011;52(2):238–250.

[80] Koleva PT, Bridgman SL, Kozyrskyj AL. The infant gut microbiome: evidence for obesity risk and dietary intervention. Nutrients. 2015;7(4):2237–2260.

[81] Mugambi MN, Musekiwa A, Lombard M, Young T, Blaauw R. Synbiotics, probiotics or prebiotics in infant formula for full term infants: a systematic review. Nutrition Journal. 2012;11(1):1.

[82] Lyon M, Wood S, Pelletier X, Donazzolo Y, Gahler R, Bellisle F. Effects of a 3-month supplementation with a novel soluble highly viscous polysaccharide on anthropometry and blood lipids in nondieting overweight or obese adults. Journal of Human Nutrition and Dietetics: The Official Journal of the British Dietetic Association. 2011;24(4):351–359.

[83] Parnell JA, Reimer RA. Weight loss during oligofructose supplementation is associated with decreased ghrelin and increased peptide YY in overweight and obese adults. The American Journal of Clinical Nutrition. 2009;89(6):1751–1759.

[84] Yang HY, Yang SC, Chao JC, Chen JR. Beneficial effects of catechin-rich green tea and inulin on the body composition of overweight adults. The British Journal of Nutrition. 2012;107(5):749–754.

[85] Ringel-Kulka T, Kotch JB, Jensen ET, Savage E, Weber DJ. Randomized, double-blind, placebo-controlled study of synbiotic yogurt effect on the health of children. The Journal of Pediatrics. 2015;166(6):1475–81. e3.

[86] Safavi M, Farajian S, Kelishadi R, Mirlohi M, Hashemipour M. The effects of synbiotic supplementation on some cardio-metabolic risk factors in overweight and obese children: a randomized triple-masked controlled trial. International Journal of Food Sciences and Nutrition. 2013;64(6):687–693.

[87] Latulippe ME, Meheust A, Augustin L, Benton D, Berčík P, Birkett A, et al. ILSI Brazil International Workshop on Functional Foods: a narrative review of the scientific evidence in the area of carbohydrates, microbiome, and health. Food & Nutrition Research. 2013;57.

[88] Verani JR, McGee L, Schrag SJ. Prevention of perinatal group B streptococcal disease: Revised guidelines from CDC, 2010: Department of Health and Human Services, Centers for Disease Control and Prevention; 2010.

[89] Broe A, Pottegard A, Lamont RF, Jorgensen JS, Damkier P. Increasing use of antibiotics in pregnancy during the period 2000–2010: prevalence, timing, category, and demographics. BJOG: An International Journal of Obstetrics and Gynaecology. 2014;121(8):988–996.

[90] Vidal AC, Murphy SK, Murtha AP, Schildkraut JM, Soubry A, Huang Z, et al. Associations between antibiotic exposure during pregnancy, birth weight and aberrant methylation at imprinted genes among offspring. International Journal of Obesity. 2013;37(7):907–913.

[91] Jepsen P, Skriver MV, Floyd A, Lipworth L, Schønheyder HC, Sørensen HT. A population-based study of maternal use of amoxicillin and pregnancy outcome in Denmark. British Journal of Clinical Pharmacology. 2003;55(2):216–621.

[92] Fjalstad JW, Stensvold HJ, Bergseng H, Simonsen GS, Salvesen B, Rønnestad AE, et al. Early-onset sepsis and antibiotic exposure in term infants: a nationwide population-based study in Norway. The Pediatric Infectious Disease Journal. 2016;35(1):1–6.

[93] Hsieh EM, Hornik CP, Clark RH, Laughon MM, Benjamin DK, Smith PB. Medication use in the neonatal intensive care unit. American Journal of Perinatology. 2014;31(09):811–822.

[94] Lieberman JM. Appropriate antibiotic use and why it is important: the challenges of bacterial resistance. The Pediatric Infectious Disease Journal. 2003;22(12):1143–1151.

[95] Besser RE. Antimicrobial prescribing in the United States: good news, bad news. Annals of Internal Medicine. 2003;138(7):605–606.

[96] Hersh AL, Jackson MA, Hicks LA, Brady MT, Byington CL, Davies HD, et al. Principles of judicious antibiotic prescribing for upper respiratory tract infections in pediatrics. Pediatrics. 2013;132(6):1146–1154.

[97] Pottegård A, Broe A, Aabenhus R, Bjerrum L, Hallas J, Damkier P. Use of antibiotics in children: a Danish nationwide drug utilization study. The Pediatric Infectious Disease Journal. 2015;34(2):e16-e22.

[98] Holstiege J, Garbe E. Systemic antibiotic use among children and adolescents in Germany: a population-based study. European Journal of Pediatrics. 2013;172(6):787–795.

[99] Blix HS, Engeland A, Litleskare I, Rønning M. Age-and gender-specific antibacterial prescribing in Norway. Journal of Antimicrobial Chemotherapy. 2007;59(5):971–976.

[100] Schneider-Lindner V, Quach C, Hanley JA, Suissa S. Secular trends of antibacterial prescribing in UK paediatric primary care. Journal of Antimicrobial Chemotherapy. 2011;66(2):424–433.

[101] Martin MJ, Thottathil SE, Newman TB. Antibiotics overuse in animal agriculture: a call to action for health care providers. American Journal of Public Health. 2015;105(12):2409–2410.

[102] Jukes TH, Williams WL. Nutritional effects of antibiotics. Pharmacological Reviews. 1953;5(4):381–420.

[103] Gaskins HR, Collier CT, Anderson DB. Antibiotics as growth promotants: mode of action. Animal Biotechnology. 2002;13(1):29–42.

[104] Butaye P, Devriese LA, Haesebrouck F. Antimicrobial growth promoters used in animal feed: effects of less well known antibiotics on gram-positive bacteria. Clinical Microbiology Reviews. 2003;16(2):175–188.

[105] Muir LA. Mode of action of exogenous substances on animal growth—an overview. Journal of Animal Science. 1985;61(Suppl. 2):154–180.

[106] Cho I, Yamanishi S, Cox L, Methé BA, Zavadil J, Li K, et al. Antibiotics in early life alter the murine colonic microbiome and adiposity. Nature. 2012;488(7413):621–626.

[107] Cox LM, Yamanishi S, Sohn J, Alekseyenko AV, Leung JM, Cho I, et al. Altering the intestinal microbiota during a critical developmental window has lasting metabolic consequences. Cell. 2014;158(4):705–721.

[108] Coates ME, Fuller R, Harrison GF, Lev M, Suffolk SF. A comparision of the growth of chicks in the Gustafsson germ-free apparatus and in a conventional environment, with and without dietary supplements of penicillin. British Journal of Nutrition. 1963;17(01):141–150.

[109] Cox LM, Blaser MJ. Antibiotics in early life and obesity. Nature Reviews Endocrinology. 2015;11(3):182–190.

[110] Mueller NT, Whyatt R, Hoepner L, Oberfield S, Dominguez-Bello MG, Widen EM, et al. Prenatal exposure to antibiotics, cesarean section and risk of childhood obesity. International Journal of Obesity. 2015;39:665–670.

[111] Mor A, Antonsen S, Kahlert J, Holsteen V, Jørgensen S, Holm-Pedersen J, et al. Prenatal exposure to systemic antibacterials and overweight and obesity in Danish schoolchildren: a prevalence study. International Journal of Obesity. 2015;39(10):1450–1455.

[112] Azad MB, Bridgman SL, Becker AB, Kozyrskyj AL. Infant antibiotic exposure and the development of childhood overweight and central adiposity. International Journal of Obesity. 2014;38(10):1290–1298.

[113] Vael C, Verhulst SL, Nelen V, Goossens H, Desager KN. Intestinal microflora and body mass index during the first three years of life: an observational study. Gut Pathogens. 2011;3(1):8.

[114] Kalliomaki M, Collado MC, Salminen S, Isolauri E. Early differences in fecal microbiota composition in children may predict overweight. The American Journal of Clinical Nutrition. 2008;87(3):534–538.

[115] Dogra S, Sakwinska O, Soh SE, Ngom-Bru C, Bruck WM, Berger B, et al. Dynamics of infant gut microbiota are influenced by delivery mode and gestational duration and are associated with subsequent adiposity. mBio. 2015;6(1).

[116] Principi N, Esposito S. Antibiotic administration and the development of obesity in children. International Journal of Antimicrobial Agents. 2016;47(3):171–177.

[117] Greenwood C, Morrow AL, Lagomarcino AJ, Altaye M, Taft DH, Yu Z, et al. Early empiric antibiotic use in preterm infants is associated with lower bacterial diversity and higher relative abundance of Enterobacter. The Journal of Pediatrics. 2014;165(1):23–29.

[118] Tanaka S, Kobayashi T, Songjinda P, Tateyama A, Tsubouchi M, Kiyohara C, et al. Influence of antibiotic exposure in the early postnatal period on the development of intestinal microbiota. FEMS Immunology & Medical Microbiology. 2009;56(1):80–87.

[119] Arboleya S, Sánchez B, Milani C, Duranti S, Solís G, Fernández N, et al. Intestinal microbiota development in preterm neonates and effect of perinatal antibiotics. The Journal of Pediatrics. 2015;166(3):538–544.

[120] Vangay P, Ward T, Gerber JS, Knights D. Antibiotics, pediatric dysbiosis, and disease. Cell Host & Microbe. 2015;17(5):553–564.

[121] Leach ST, Lui K, Naing Z, Dowd SE, Mitchell HM, Day AS. Multiple opportunistic pathogens, but not pre-existing inflammation, may be associated with necrotizing enterocolitis. Digestive Diseases and Sciences. 2015;60(12):3728–3734.

[122] Berrington JE, Stewart CJ, Cummings SP, Embleton ND. The neonatal bowel microbiome in health and infection. Current Opinion in Infectious Diseases. 2014;27(3):236–243.

6

Obesity and its Influence on Mediators of Inflammation: Clinical Relevance of C-Reactive Protein in Obese Subjects

Emilio González-Jiménez

Abstract

The rising prevalence of overweight and obesity in the world has been described as a global pandemic, with marked variations across countries in the levels and trends in overweight and obesity with distinct regional patterns. Concern about the health risks associated with rising obesity has become nearly universal. In this chapter, a systematic review that was conducted in four databases (Web of Science, MEDLINE, Scopus, CINAHL), using the MeSH terms [obesity, inflammation, disease management, C-reactive protein (CRP)] is presented. Based on the above, the aims of this work are to provide information on the relationship between obesity and circulating levels of CRP, to describe the basic chemical structure and functions, and to analyze its clinical usefulness in obese patients. The available scientific evidence justifies the need to include determining the values of high-sensitivity C-reactive protein (hs-CRP) among clinical screening tests on obese subjects to evaluate the cardiovascular risk, among other risks.

Keywords: obesity, inflammation, C-reactive protein, clinical relevance, cardiovascular risk

1. Introduction

The rising prevalence of overweight and obesity in the world has been described as a global pandemic at all stages of life worldwide [1]. Overweight and obesity are defined as abnormal or excessive fat accumulation that may impair health with serious health complications and increases the risks of morbidity and the prevalence of several health complications, such as type-2 diabetes, hypertension, atherosclerosis, dyslipidemia, prothrombotic state, insulin resistance, cardiovascular disease, metabolic syndrome, and various types of cancers [2]. A complex interaction between the environmental factors, genetic predisposition, and human behavior is the cause of the current obesity pandemic [3]. Obesity has been linked strongly with metabolic abnormalities including increased blood pressure [4], increased blood sugar [5], and lipid profile abnormalities [6]. Furthermore, obesity has been predisposed to metabolic abnormalities via inflammatory process [7]. In the state of obesity, the pro-inflammatory adipokines, derived from adipose tissue, are overexpressed, increased production, and secretion of inflammatory mediators: interleukin 6 (IL-6) and tumor necrosis factor alpha (TNF-α) [8, 9]. The increased circulatory levels of inflammatory mediators particularly IL-6 have been associated with hepatocyte stimulation to synthesize and produce a low-grade systemic inflammation marker C-reactive protein (CRP) [8]. This protein was discovered in 1930 by Tillet and Francis, being insulated in the serum of patients with acute inflammatory processes. Upon its discovery, it was thought that C-reactive protein levels could be a pathogenic secretion for its high levels in patients with multiple pathologies. Finally, the discovery of its synthesis and secretion in the liver closed this discussion [10]. Currently, PCR serum represents an effective clinical indicator of infectious and inflammatory processes in the body, and therefore, it can be used to determine the risk of heart disease and to predict metabolic syndrome and diabetes mellitus [11]. In this sense, the systemic inflammation represented by increased level of high-sensitivity CRP (hs-CRP) has been classified as a characteristic feature and an essential cause of many illness conditions including metabolic syndrome [12], atherosclerosis [13], coronary heart disease [14], and cancers [15]. Based on the above, the aims of this work were to provide information on the relationship between obesity and circulating levels of CRP, to describe the basic chemical structure and functions, and to analyze its clinical usefulness in obese patients.

2. Overall structure

CRP is a protein of the pentraxins group, which is distinguished by its conformation in the space, presenting pentameric form of annular disc (see **Figure 1**). Structurally, it is composed of five identical subunits unglycosylated and linked by noncovalent bonds that depend of calcium binding to exert their action [16]. From a functional perspective, the active forms of PCR are the pentameric or native structure (p-n-PCR or PCR) and the monomeric isoform (m-PCR). This latter is formed by a dissociation process of the p-PCR. The monomeric isoform may appear linked to membranes or free in plasma, changing their functions in each case [17]. The pentameric isoform has two faces, one with ability to adhere to the phosphatidylcholine in the presence of calcium ions [18], while the other presents adhesion sites for complement component C1q and Fc receptors. The existence of five subunits with capacity to bind together phosphatidylcholine determines its high avidity for phosphatidylcholine [18]. This interaction occurs during the identification of microorganisms such as bacteria, fungi, and parasites showing phosphatidylcholine in their membrane [19]. Once identified pathogens, adherence to C1q occurs on the other side of the pentamer, activating partially the complement pathway and adhering to factor H [17]. This mechanism is a first defensive barrier in our organism against certain pathogens.

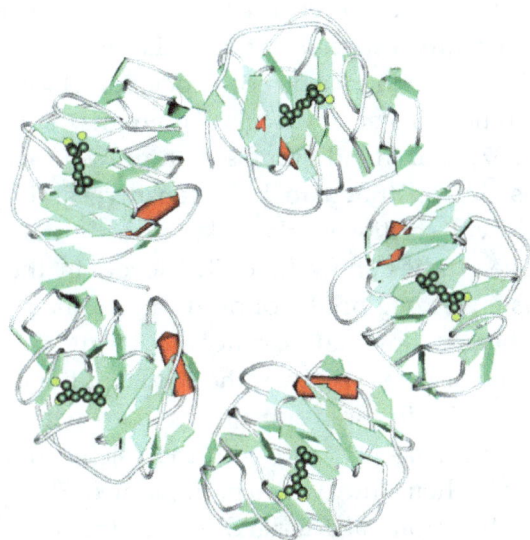

Figure 1. Crystal structure of C-reactive protein complexed with phosphocholine from Thompson et al. [50].

3. Functions and clinical significance in obese subjects

CRP is synthesized in hepatocytes in response to stimulation of interleukin 6 (IL-6) [20], being their serum concentrations higher among obese subjects [21]. It is an acute phase reactant protein whose plasma levels are elevated rapidly during a tissue damage or aggression and according to the intensity, reaching its peak in 24–48 h. This increase is due to an increase in the plasma concentration of IL-6, which is produced by macrophages [22], endothelial cells, T cells, and adipocytes [23]. When the inflammatory process ceases, within a period of 3–7 days, the CRP returns to normal values.

PCR is deposited in anatomical locations in which inflammatory processes occur, as in the intima of arteries [24]. In this location, PCR could participate in LDL capture by macrophages in atherosclerotic plaque and thus be related to the development of atherosclerosis [25, 26]. Also, it is known that CRP directly induces the production of other inflammatory cells and decreases the expression of nitric oxide synthase [27], participating actively in the atherogenic process. The first evidence of the relationship between circulating CRP levels and the development of coronary artery disease were published in 1954, showing an elevated CRP levels in patients with acute myocardial infarction [28]. However, it will be during the decade of the nineties when studies show the independent prognostic value of CRP in primary and secondary prevention of coronary artery disease [29, 30]. Currently, by the ultrasensitive method [31], it can be detected levels of hs-CRP required to the prediction of cardiovascular risk [32]. Based on this method, the American Heart Association (AHA) [33] recommends the following ranges for predicting cardiovascular risk: <1.0 mg/L low risk, 1.1–3.0 mg/L moderate risk, and 3.1–10.0 mg/L high risk. hs-CRP values in the above ranges have shown sensitivity and specificity for early detection of vascular events, not just in coronary arteries, also in the peripheral circulation and brain in obese subjects [34]. Thus, in the study by Jager et al. [35] on a population of 2484 individuals, researchers concluded that CRP was an important predictive value for cardiovascular mortality, especially in association with other risk factors such as obesity. Other recent studies have shown a direct association between elevated plasma levels of hs-CRP and the occurrence of cardiovascular accidents, both in individuals without cardiovascular disease [36, 37], and in individuals with previous cardiovascular disease [38]. In this sense, hs-CRP has demonstrated to be a sensitive and specific marker for early identification of individuals with cardiovascular risk, especially among obese subjects [39]. On the other hand, prospective studies show that CRP levels in the general population and especially in obese subjects is a strong predictor of future coronary events, stroke, peripheral artery disease, congestive heart failure, and cardiovascular mortality in general [40], with a continuous gradient of cardiovascular risk over the whole of their serum levels. In addition, serum levels of CRP may be an indicator of subclinical atherosclerosis, correlating its concentration with intima-media thickness [41] and with the calcification degree of the coronary arteries [42]. Pande et al. [43], in their study with a population of 3000 patients, described higher levels of CRP in patients with peripheral arterial disease. Ridker et al. [44], from a population greater than 13,000 subjects and assessing different inflammatory markers, including CRP, also found a statistically significant correlation between CRP levels and the risk of peripheral arterial disease. In addition, in a five-year follow-up in a small cohort of 150 patients, the authors conclude that those subjects who developed peripheral artery disease had higher average CRP values during the monitoring period. In this sense, Vainas et al. [45], in a sample greater than 300 patients with peripheral arterial disease, they conclude that the severity of peripheral arterial disease was correlated with serum CRP levels.

In the recent study, Gaillard et al. [46] were studied 1116 pregnant women with obesity. The study was developed during the second trimester of pregnancy and evaluated the serum levels of CRP in the mothers and fetus's fat mass. The authors concluded that higher second-trimester maternal CRP level was associated with higher mid-childhood overall and central adiposity.

Other studies have shown that the obesity is a negative prognostic factor after diagnosis of breast cancer [47]. There are evidences that propose a greater amount of adipose tissue will increase the susceptibility of the patients to metastasis development [48]. Several mechanisms have been proposed to explain the adverse effect of obesity on survival among women with breast cancer, including alteration in cytokines profiles such as CRP [49]. In this sense, alteration in acute phase proteins such us CRP in obese patients may exaggerate the inflammation status [47]. Owing to the fact that the inflammation has the potential to prone the patients toward later distant metastasis, it is necessary to regulate and control the levels of CRP among other cytokines. Nevertheless, the exact mechanisms in which obesity and CRP levels may influence breast cancer are not well known and need more research for its clarifying [47].

4. Conclusions

In conclusion, the available scientific evidence justifies the need to include determining the values of hs-CRP among clinical screening tests on obese subjects to evaluate the cardiovascular risk, among other risks. CRP is an important clinical parameter in the early detection of atherosclerotic disease and thus for the prevention of cardiovascular disease in people with obesity. Its possible influence as an inflammation marker in the prognosis of cancer patients is another important aspect that needs further study. However, even considering the scientific evidence, new prospective studies are necessary with larger populations to acquire solid and extrapolable results to citizenship.

Author details

Emilio González-Jiménez[*]

Address all correspondence to: emigoji@ugr.es

Department of Nursing, Faculty of Health Science, University of Granada, Spain

References

[1] Poskitt EM. Childhood obesity in low- and middle-income countries. Paediatr Int Child Health. 2014;34(4):239–249.

[2] Boura-Halfon S, Zick Y. Phosphorylation of IRS proteins, insulin action, and insulin resistance, Am J Physiol Endocrinol Metab. 2009;296(4):E581–E591.

[3] Enes CC, Slater B. Obesity in adolescence and its main determinants. Rev Bras Epidemiol. 2010;13(1):163–171.

[4] Kalantari S. Childhood cardiovascular risk factors, a predictor of late adolescent overweight. Adv Biomed Res. 2016;5:56.

[5] Yamamoto K, Okazaki A, Ohmori S. The relationship between psychosocial stress, age, BMI, CRP, lifestyle, and the metabolic syndrome in apparently healthy subjects. J Physiol Anthropol. 2011;30(1):15–22.

[6] Talavera-Garcia E, Delgado-Lista J, Garcia-Rios A, Delgado-Casado N, Gomez-Luna P, Gomez-Garduño A, Gomez-Delgado F, Alcala-Diaz JF, Yubero-Serrano E, Marin C, Perez-Caballero AI, Fuentes-Jimenez FJ, Camargo A, Rodriguez-Cantalejo F, Tinahones FJ, Ordovas JM, Perez-Jimenez F, Perez-Martinez P, Lopez-Miranda J. Influence of obesity and metabolic disease on carotid atherosclerosis in patients with coronary artery disease (CordioPrev Study). PLoS One. 2016;11(4):e0153096.

[7] González-Jiménez E, Schmidt-Riovalle J, Sinausía L, Carmen Valenza M, Perona JS. Predictive value of ceruloplasmin for metabolic syndrome in adolescents. Biofactors. 2016;42(2):163–170.

[8] Ellulu MS, Khaza'ai H, Rahmat A, Patimah I, Abed Y. Obesity can predict and promote systemic inflammation in healthy adults. Int J Cardiol. 2016;215:318–324.

[9] Karastergiou K, Mohamed-Ali V. The autocrine and paracrine roles of adipokines. Mol Cell Endocrinol. 2010;318(1):69–78.

[10] Gómez Gerique JA. Protein C reactive as a marker of any type of inflammation. Clin Invest Arterioscl. 2006;18(3):96–98.

[11] Ridker PM. A test in context: high-sensitivity C-reactive protein. J Am Coll Cardiol. 2016;67(6):712–723.

[12] Hosseinzadeh-Attar MJ, Golpaie A, Foroughi M, Hosseinpanah F, Zahediasl S, Azizi F. The relationship between visfatin and serum concentrations of C-reactive protein, interleukin 6 in patients with metabolic syndrome. J Endocrinol Invest. 2016; 39(8):917–22.

[13] Shimoda M, Kaneto H, Yoshioka H, Okauchi S, Hirukawa H, Kimura T, Kanda-Kimura Y, Kohara K, Kamei S, Kawasaki F, Mune T, Kaku K. Influence of atherosclerosis-related risk factors on serum high-sensitivity C-reactive protein levels in patients with type 2 diabetes: comparison of their influence in obese and non-obese patients. J Diabetes Investig. 2016;7(2):197–205.

[14] Chen YC, Shen CT, Wang NK, Huang YL, Chiu HH, Chen CA, Chiu SN, Lin MT, Wang JK, Wu MH. High sensitivity C reactive protein (hs-CRP) in adolescent and young adult patients with history of Kawasaki disease. Zhonghua Minguo Xin Zang Xue Hui Za Zhi. 2015;31(6):473–477.

[15] Kinoshita A, Onoda H, Imai N, Nishino H, Tajiri H. C-Reactive protein as a prognostic marker in patients with hepatocellular carcinoma. Hepatogastroenterology. 2015;62(140):966–970.

[16] Manfredi AA, Rovere-Querini P, Barbara Botazzi B, Garlanda C, Alberto Mantovani A. Pentraxins, humoral innate immunity and tissue injury. Curr Opin Inmunol. 2008;20:538–544.

[17] Mihlan M, Stippa S, Józsi M, Zipfel PF. Monomeric CRP contributes to complement control in fluid phase and on cellular surfaces and increases phagocytosis by recruiting factor H. Cell Death Differ. 2009;16(12):1630–1640.

[18] Szalai AJ. The biological functions of C-reactive protein. Vascul Pharmacol. 2002;39(3): 105–107.

[19] Moalli F, Jaillon S, Inforzato A, Sironi M, Bottazzi B, Mantovani A, Garlanda C. Pathogen recognition by the long pentraxin PTX3. J Biomed Biotechnol. 2011;2011:830421.

[20] Volanakis JE. Human C-reactive protein: expression, structure and function. Mol Immunol. 2001;38(2–3):189–197.

[21] Ebrahimi M, Heidari-Bakavoli AR, Shoeibi S, Mirhafez SR, Moohebati M, Esmaily H, Ghazavi H, Saberi Karimian M, Parizadeh SM, Mohammadi M, Mohaddes Ardabili H,

Ferns GA, Ghayour-Mobarhan M. Association of serum hs-CRP levels with the presence of obesity, diabetes mellitus, and other cardiovascular risk factors. J Clin Lab Anal. 2016;8. doi:10.1002/jcla.21920 In press.

[22] Pepys MB, Hirschfield GM. C-reactive protein: a critical update. J Clin Invest. 2003;111(12):1805–1812.

[23] Lau DC, Dhillon B, Yan H, Szmitko PE, Verma S. Adipokines: molecular links between obesity and atheroslcerosis. Am J Physiol Heart Circ Physiol. 2005;288 (5):2031–2041.

[24] Rader D. Inflammatory markers of coronary risk. N Engl J Med. 2000;343:1178–1182.

[25] Zwaka TP, Hombach V, Torzewski J. C-reactive protein-mediated low density lipopro-tein uptake by macrophages. Circulation. 2001;103:1194–1197.

[26] Chiu FH, Chuang CH, Li WC, Weng YM, Fann WC, Lo HY, Sun C, Wang SH. The association of leptin and C-reactive protein with the cardiovascular risk factors and metabolic syndrome score in Taiwanese adults. Cardiovasc Diabetol. 2012;11:40. doi: 10.1186/1475-2840-11-40)

[27] Lagrand WK, Visser CA, Hermens WT, Niessen HW, Verheugt FW, Wolbink GJ, Hack CE. C-reactive protein as a cardiovascular risk factor: more than an epiphenomenon? Circulation. 1999;100:96–102.

[28] Kroop IG, Shackman NH. Levels of C-reactive protein as a measure of acute myocardial infarction. Proc Soc Exp Biol Med. 1954;86:95–97.

[29] The Emerging Risk Factors Collaboration. C-reactive protein concentration and risk of coronary heart disease, stroke, and mortality: an individual participant metaanalysis. Lancet. 2010;375:132–140.

[30] Schiele F, Meneveau N, Seronde MF, Chopard R, Descotes-Genon V, Dutheil J, Bassand JP, Reseau de Cardiologie de Franche Comte. C-reactive protein improves risk predic-tion in patients with acute coronary syndromes. Eur Heart J. 2010;31:290–297.

[31] Ridker PM. High-sensitivity C-reactive protein potential adjunct for global risk assessment in the primary prevention of cardiovascular disease. Circulation. 2001;103:1813–1818.

[32] Koening W, Löwel H, Baumert J, Meisinger C. C-reactive protein modulates risk prediction based on the Framingham score. Circulation. 2004;109:1349–1353.

[33] Pearson TA, et al. New AHA/CDC guidelines support the use of usCRP testing in intermediate risk CVD patients. Circulation. 2003;107:499–511.

[34] Rifai N, Ridker PM. Proposed cardiovascular risk assessment algorithm using high sensitivity C-reactive protein and Lipid screen. Clin Chem. 2001;47(1):28–30.

[35] Jager A, Van Hinsberg VWM, Kostense PJ, Emeis JJ, Yudkin JS, Nijpels G, Dekker JM, Heine RJ, Bouter LM, Stehouwer CDA. Von Willebrand Factor, C-reactive protein, and

5-years mortality in diabetic and nondiabetic subjects. Arterioscler Thromb Vasc Biol. 1999;19:3071.

[36] Berezin AE, Kremzer AA, Martovitskaya YV, Samura TA, Berezina TA, Zulli A, Klimas J, Kruzliak P. The utility of biomarker risk prediction score in patients with chronic heart failure. Int J Clin Exp Med. 2015;8(10):18255–18264.

[37] Tsai SS, Lin YS, Lin CP, Hwang JS, Wu LS, Chu PH. Metabolic syndrome-associated risk factors and high-sensitivity C-reactive protein independently predict arterial stiffness in 9903 subjects with and without chronic kidney disease. Medicine (Baltimore). 2015;94(36):e1419.

[38] Coto GD, Ibañez A. Diagnostic and therapeutic protocol of neonatal sepsis. Bol Pediatr. 2006;46(Suppl 1):125–134.

[39] Nissen SE, Tuzcu EM, Schoenhagen P, Crowe T, Sasiela WJ, Tsai J, Orazem J, Magorien RD, O'Shaughnessy C, Ganz P; Reversal of atherosclerosis with aggressive lipid lowering (REVERSAL) investigators. Statin therapy, LDL cholesterol, C-reactive protein and coronary artery disease. N Engl J Med. 2005;352:29–38.

[40] Ridker PM. Clinical application of C-reactive protein for cardiovascular disease detection and prevention. Circulation. 2003;107:363–369.

[41] Wang TJ, Nam BH, Wilson PW, Wolf PA, Levy D, Polak JF, D'Agostino RB, O'Donnell CJ. Association of C-reactive protein with carotid atherosclerosis in men and women: the Framingham Heart Study. Arterioscler Thromb Vasc Biol. 2002;22:1662–1667.

[42] Wang TJ, Larson MG, Levy D, Benjamin EJ, Kupka MJ, Manning WJ, Clouse ME, D'Agostino RB, Wilson PW, O'Donnell CJ. C-reactive protein is associated with subclinical epicardial coronary calcification in men and women: the Framingham Heart Study. Circulation. 2002;106:1189–1191.

[43] Pande RL, Perlstein TS, Beckman JA, Creager MA. The association of insulin resistance and inflammation with peripheral arterial disease: the National Health and Nutrition Examination Survey 1999–2004. Circulation. 2008;118:33–41.

[44] Ridker PM, CushmanM, Stampfer MJ, Tracy RP, Hennekens CH. Plasma concentration of C reactive protein and risk of developing peripheral vascular disease. Circulation. 1998;97:425–428.

[45] Vainas T, Stassen FR, de Graaf R, Twiss EL, Herngreen SB, Welten RJ, van den Akker LH, van Dieijen-Visser MP, Bruggeman CA, Kitslaar PJ. C-reactive protein in peripheral arterial disease: relation to severity of the disease and to future cardiovascular events. J Vasc Surg. 2005;42:243–251.

[46] Gaillard R, Rifas-Shiman SL, Perng W, Oken E, Gillman MW. Maternal inflammation during pregnancy and childhood adiposity. Obesity (Silver Spring). 2016; 24(6):1320–7.

[47] Babaei Z, Moslemi D, Parsian H, Khafri S, Pouramir M, Mosapour A. Relationship of obesity with serum concentrations of leptin, CRP and IL-6 in breast cancer survivors. J Egypt Natl Canc Inst. 2015;27(4):223–229.

[48] Iyengar NM, Hudis CA, Dannenberg AJ. Obesity and inflammation: new insights into breast cancer development and progression. Am Soc Clin Oncol Educ Book. 2013; 33: 46–51.

[49] Ravishankaran P, Karunanithi R. Clinical significance of preoperative serum interleukin-6 and C-reactive protein level in breast cancer patients. World J Surg Oncol. 2011;9:18.

[50] Thompson D, Pepys MB, Wood SP. The physiological structure of human C-reactive protein and its complex with phosphocholine. Structure. 1999;7(2):169–177.

7

Immunometabolism in Obesity

Efrain Chavarria-Avila,

Rosa-Elena Navarro-Hernández,

Milton-Omar Guzmán-Ornelas,

Fernanda-Isadora Corona-Meraz,

Sandra-Luz Ruíz-Quezada and

Mónica Vázquez-Del Mercado

Abstract

Immunometabolism is a current issue that has shown relevance in recent years, because the way we understand the adipose tissue has shifted from simply being a site of energy storage to a very active endocrine organ, which dysregulation has a major impact on other systems, especially on the immune one. Understanding the molecular basis of the regulation of adipose tissue is essential to look for alternatives in the treatment and prognosis of obesity in future generations. In this regard, it is described that the immune system has great importance in physiological processes of adipose tissue and vice versa. The main objective of this chapter is to describe the relationship between the immune system and metabolism, emphasizing dysregulation when obesity is present. Upon completion of this chapter, the reader will be able to understand the relationship between the immune system and metabolism, in normal and obesity states; also, will identify the chronic state of low-grade inflammation as the main etiological factor of obesity co-morbidities, such as insulin resistance, diabetes mellitus, osteoarthritis and susceptibility to some kinds of cancer, among others.

Keywords: immunometabolism, cytokines, adipokines, chemokines, low-grade inflammation, miRNAs

1. Introduction

Inmmunometabolism has been defined as the interphase between metabolism and immune response [1, 2], in which, adipose tissue plays a key role. Leptin was the first molecule described linking the immune system with metabolism. The first leptin function described was appetite control; however, nowadays it has been described with multiple permissive functions, like immune homeostasis, among others (**Figure 1**) [3]. On innate and adaptive immune response cells, leptin can mainly increase cytokine expression, cell surface adhesion molecules and chemokine receptors [3, 4]. Additional to leptin, free fatty acid receptors family (FFARs) has been reported to be expressed on key cell types regulating both: energy homoeostasis and inflammatory responses [2]. Obesity induces changes in gut microbiota, it has been reported that *Bacteroidetes* and *Firmicutes* phyla produce high levels of the short chain free fatty acids (SCFAs) C2–C4 which are the main agonists for FFAR2 [5]; at the same time, microbiota can influence innate and adaptive immune responses [6, 7]. These examples make clear the inter-relation between metabolism and the immune system. We will focus along this chapter in alterations of this interphase due to the presence of obesity.

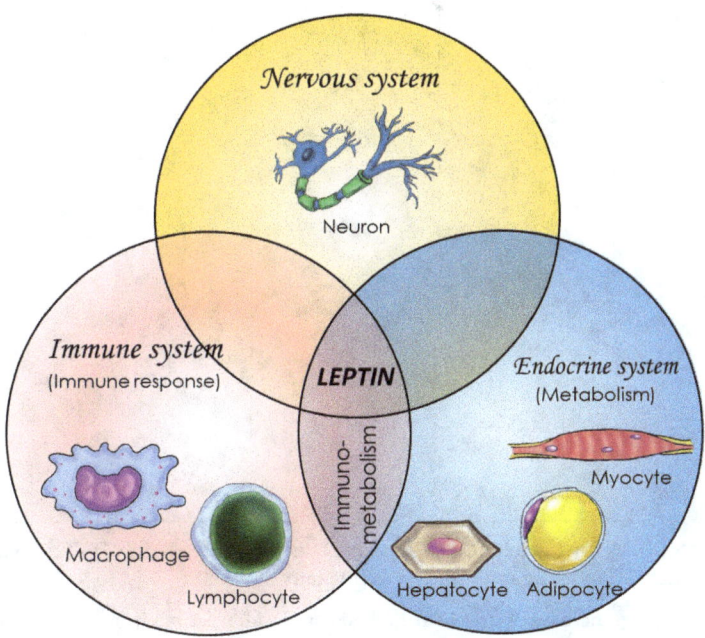

Figure 1. Neuroendocrine immune system.

2. Immunometabolism characteristics on normal weight range and obese individuals

Immune cell status in normal weight range (lean) individuals is mostly anti-inflammatory; this environment needs a continual production of type 2 cytokines (i.e. interleukin (IL)-5 and IL-13).

On the other hand, the presence of obesity is associated with a low-grade inflammation state characterized by increased pro-inflammatory cytokine production (i.e. tumour necrosis factor (TNF)-α, IL-1β and IL-6) (**Table 1**) [10, 24].

Component	Changes respect to normal weight range
Cells	
White adipocytes [8]	↑↑↑
Brown adipocytes [8]	↓
M1 [9]	↑↑
M2 [9]	↓↓
Mast cells [10]	↑
Eosinophils [10]	↓
Non-cytotoxic ILCs (NK) [11]	↑↑
ILC1s [11]	↑
ILC2s [12]	↓
Molecules	
Th-1 cytokines [13]	↑
Th-2 cytokines [13]	↑
Leptin [14, 15]	↑↑
Adiponectin [16]	↓↓
Resistin [17]	↑
Chemerin [18]	↑
CCL2 [19]	↑
FFA [20]	↑
Glucose [21]	↑↑
Insulin [20]	↑/↓↓↓
Cholesterol [21]	↑
Microbiote	
Bacteroidetes sp. [22]	↓
Actinobacteria sp. [22]	↑
Faecalibacterium prausnitzii [23]	↓

M1: macrophages associated with Th-1 cytokines; M2: macrophages associated with Th-2 cytokines; ILC1s: innate lymphoid cells type 1; CCL2: C-C motif ligand 2 and FFA: free fatty acids.

*During obesity onset, an insulin increase occurs (insulin resistance), after a time it frequently progress to exhaustion of β-cells.

Table 1. Changes on immunometabolic components due to obesity.

2.1. Adipose tissue-resident cells

Adipose tissue is a specialized connective one, white adipose tissue (WAT) is the most abundant in adult human (~85%) by its distribution, it can be classified in subcutaneous or visceral (omental, mesenteric and retroperitoneal accumulation). Besides WAT, there exist two more types: brown adipose tissue (BAT) and bone marrow adipose tissue (BMAT), each one have singular cellular composition, anatomical location and pathophysiological properties [25].

In lean individuals, macrophages count for around 5% of WAT's cells depots, in obesity conditions, macrophages increase as much as 50% [1]; nevertheless, besides quantitative changes, there also occurs qualitative ones. The main function of macrophages (or initially described) have been phagocytosis, however, nowadays, they are recognized as a heterogeneous population with multiple functions [1, 2].

2.1.1. Adipocytes

Three types of adipocytes have been described: white, beige (brite, brownish) and brown adipocytes; these are different in structure and metabolism [26]. The terms white and brown came from the appearance of tissues when stained with immunohistochemistry against UCP-1 [27, 28].

White adipocytes are specialized cells, arising from a Myf5$^-$ preadipocyte lineage, which have a unilocular large lipid droplet and comprise predominantly the WAT [8, 26]. Many functions are attributed for these cells such as insulation and physical protection of the viscera, thermal insulation, reservoir of stored energy in form of triglycerides and regulation of fat release and storage. Beyond these functions, white adipocytes produce and secrete several molecules (adipokines), including leptin, resistin, retinol binding protein 4 (RBP4), fibroblast grown factor 21 (FGF21) and adiponectin mainly. Endocrine communication of adipose tissue is bidirectional, white adipocytes also respond to hormonal signals to induce lipolysis and release free fatty acids (FFAs) into the circulation, for oxidation or storage by other tissues [8, 26].

Brown adipocytes are multilocular with small lipid droplets and express uncoupling protein-1 (UCP-1) [26], emerge from Myf5$^+$ precursor lineage and are developmentally more related to skeletal muscle cells than to white adipocytes. The amount and location of brown adipocytes changes throughout life, in the early years, the number of reservoirs is higher and is mainly located in breastbone, interscapular space and retroperitoneal level; whereas in adults, it decreases and can only find deposits in carotid bodies, aortic bodies and adrenal gland. The main function of these adipocytes is thermogenesis, keeping temperature homeostasis in cold. This is because brown adipocytes possess a large number of mitochondria, and these in turn, express UCP-1 in the inner membrane. This protein decouples the electron transport chain, making it more inefficient, thus the number of ATPs produced decreases and energy is dissipated as heat [29, 30].

The name brite is the result of combining brown (br) and white (ite), since this kind of adipocytes was described to be morphologically similar to white adipocytes but at the same time, they expressed minimum levels of UCP-1 [26]. The discovery of this kind of cells challenged the initial idea of WAT and BAT as two different tissues [31, 32], and opened the possibility of considering them as a single adipose organ [33]. Beige adipocytes arise in subcutaneous white adipose tissue from precursors expressing CD137 and transmembrane protein 26, under the condition of low temperatures or β-adrenergic-receptor stimulation. When the stimulus stops, the cells appear to return to white cells, however, upon re-stimulation respond as beige adipocytes [10]. This phenomenon has encouraged the ability to control the differentiation of adipose tissue by increasing energy expenditure to reduce the accumulation of energy in the form of triglycerides, including WAT change to BAT (browning of WAT) under pathological conditions in humans was reported [34, 35]. We should learn more about browning control (on and off) to avoid presentation of undesired effects (i.e. cachexia, atherosclerosis and hepatic steatosis) [27, 36].

2.1.2. Macrophages

Macrophages were reported by Elie Metchnikoff in 1884. For many decades, they were considered to be a homogeneous lineage with a main function, phagocytosis. Now they are recognized as very plastic immune cells with multiple functions, because of this, their population is highly heterogeneous and difficult to classify, but two main phenotypes (subtypes) are generally accepted: classically (M1) or alternatively (M2) activated [37, 38].

The M1 phenotype is promoted by T-helper 1 (Th1) cytokines (i.e. interferon (IFN)-γ) or by pathogen-associated molecular patterns (PAMPs) (i.e. LPS) and is characterized by the production of pro-inflammatory cytokines (IL-6, TNF-α, IFN-γ, IL-1β, IL-12 and IL-23), chemokines promoting inflammatory infiltrate (CXCL9,10,11,13, CCL8, 15, 19, 20), and expressed on surface high levels of MHCII, CD80, CD86 and CD11c, among other markers (i.e. Ly6C, CD11b, CD62L, CCR2, CX3CR1 and CCR5). In nucleus, STAT1 and IRF5 are the consensus transcription factors [37, 38].

In contrast, T-helper 2 (Th2) cytokines (i.e. IL-4, IL-10 and IL-13) drive the M2 phenotype, with high phagocytic capacity, and secrete extracellular matrix components, angiogenic and chemotactic factors (CCL17, 18, 22, 24), anti-inflammatory cytokines (IL-10) and the transforming growth factor β (TGF-β), then M2 activates expression of immunosuppressive factors and the peroxisome proliferator-activated receptor gamma (PPARγ) that promotes tissue remodelling and helps to resolve inflammation [37, 38].

Generally, in lean individuals, M2 exists in the WAT; however, the accumulation of adipose tissue leads to increased number of macrophages, besides, the macrophages display M1 phenotype. There are two possible explanations for this phenomenon: (1) environmental factors present in adipose tissue of obese individuals causes a switch in phenotype from M2 to M1; (2) on the other hand, the increase in chemokines (such as CCL2) promotes the recruitment of circulating monocytes and due to the low-grade inflammation state they differentiate to M1 [10, 37].

2.1.3. Eosinophils and mast cells

To maintain the M2 polarization of WAT- residents macrophages, a constant production of IL-4 is necessary. It is speculated that the eosinophils present in the WAT are the main source [8, 10, 12]. Studies in normal weight mice showed that there are a lot of infiltrated eosinophils, which are a major source of IL-4. Moreover, their amount decreased in obese mice no matter what the origin is (genetic as ob/ob or high fat diet) [8, 10, 12], however, there are no reports in humans. Mast cells unlike eosinophils, increases their number in WAT of humans with diabetes mellitus type 2 or obesity, there are reports in fed mice with high fat diet, linking these cells with an increasing adiposity and insulin resistance [8, 10].

2.1.4. Innate lymphoid cells

In recent years, studies have been published to identify innate lymphoid cells (ILCs), all members of this new family are characterized by a similar lymphocyte morphology, however, lack markers on its surface that identifies them as another immune cell type, because this is defined as lacking cells lineage markers (Lin⁻) [39]. The ILCs come from two development pathways: (1) the first called cytotoxic ILCs, integrated by classic NK; (2) on the other hand, we have non-cytotoxical ILCs. The last group is subdivided into three types: ILC1s, ILC2s and ILC3s; they express T-bet, GATA-3 and ROR-γT, respectively, which is the main difference between them. ILCs can directly communicate with several varieties of cells and regulate immunity, inflammation and homeostasis in different tissues [8, 39].

ILC2s plays an important role in the regulation of glucose metabolism, lipid storage and redox balance in lean individuals. It accomplishes these by communicating with other immune cells associated with the type 2 immune axis (i.e. M2, eosinophils and invariant natural killer T) and participates in cross-talk with adipocytes [8, 39]. These cells produce cytokines associated with lymphocyte T-helper 2, cytokines that are required for immunity against helminths, allergic inflammation and tissue repair [8].

In contrast, it was found that cytotoxic ILCs (individuals and mice) and non-cytotoxic ILC1s (mice) are increased in visceral adipose tissue when obesity is present, accompanied by an increase in the production of interferon gamma, the latter contributes to change of the phenotype of macrophages to M1, thus, favours an inflammatory environment and increased recruitment of immune cells type 1 axis [8, 10, 12].

2.2. Adipokines

Adipose tissue was considered just an energy (triglycerides) storage site until obesity arises as a health problem worldwide. Adipose tissue came to the fore as an active secretory organ involved in various physiological and pathophysiological processes. Adipokines is a term used to identify molecules released from adipose tissue; some of them are secreted by others tissues (i.e. TNF-α, IL-1A, -1β, -5, -6, -8, 10, -15, -18) and certain are mainly or exclusively synthetized by adipocytes (i.e. leptin, adiponectin, resistin), these adipokines deserve that proposed term adipokinome [40, 41].

2.2.1. Leptin

Leptin is an adipokine secreted principally by white adipose tissue that regulates food intake and energy expenditure; furthermore, it also plays an important role in glucose homeostasis, immunity and fertility among others [42, 43]. Leptin exerts its action through leptin receptors, which are transmembrane proteins, members of the class I cytokine receptor superfamily, their pathway involves JAK/STAT, PI3K, MAPK/ERK systems, and PKC [42, 43]. There are six (a–f) isoforms of the leptin receptor generated by alternative splicing, b-isoform is the longest one, and have all the signalling motifs; moreover, it is the most expressed in diverse cell lineages (i.e. adipocytes, myocytes, immune cells, neurons) permitting to leptin act in autocrine, paracrine and endocrine ways [44, 45].

Leptin production is proportional to the amount of adipose tissue; so, in subjects within a normal range weight, increasing leptin levels suppresses the need to eat by inhibiting the release of orexigenic neuropeptides (e.g. neuropeptide Y and Agouti-related protein) in the arcuate nucleus of hypothalamus, while obese individuals do not have this physiological response, a state called 'leptin resistance' [46].

It has been proposed that the establishment of this condition is a consequence of the combination of three main mechanisms: diminished intracellular leptin-receptor signalling, abnormal transport of leptin across the blood-brain barrier and development programming disorders; however, the molecular mechanisms by which lesser sensitivity to leptin is present in obesity have not yet been defined [46, 47].

2.2.2. Adiponectin

Adiponectin is a multifunctional and multi-named adipokine (adipocyte complement-related protein of 30 kDa, Acrp30; gelatin binding protein of 28 kDa, GBP-28; adipose most abundant gene transcript 1, apM1), coded by *ADIPOQ* gene, is a major adipocyte-secreted protein and is down-regulated in obesity and its co-morbidities. Adiponectin regulates metabolic homeostasis by acting on organs such as the brain, kidney, liver, pancreas and skeletal muscle by exerting potent insulin-sensitizing, anti-atherogenic and anti-inflammatory activities [8, 48].

Adiponectin is synthesized as a monomer, however, suffers extensive post-translational modifications to form trimers, hexamers and high molecular weight species (HMW, 12–18 monomers) before being secreted by adipocytes. Recent evidence suggests that depending on the degree of multimerization, different biological effects have been obtained [49, 50].

Biological activity of adiponectin is mainly mediated by binding to one of its two adiponectin receptors: AdipoR1 and AdipoR2. These receptors are differentially expressed, and adiponectin shows distinct affinity to them according to its multimerization degree [51]. AdipoR1 is most commonly found in skeletal muscle and binds preferably to low molecular weight species (trimers and hexamers), whereas AdipoR2 is abundant in liver and binds easily to HMW adiponectin [49, 51]. Liver and skeletal muscle have a crucial role in the IR process, therapeutic effect of thiazolidinediones is in part due to the enhanced expression of adiponectin and its receptors through PPAR-γ activation [52].

2.2.3. Resistin

Resistin was described in mice as the responsible molecule of IR; however in humans, results were not conclusive, in part because its specific receptor has not been identified yet. It is an adipokine that stimulates the synthesis of pro-inflammatory cytokines among which are: TNF-α, IL-1, IL-6 and IL-12; in various types of cells through pathway-dependent signalling nuclear factor (NF)-κB [17, 53]. It also induces increased expression of adhesion molecules (i.e. VCAM-1, ICAM-1) and chemokines (i.e. CX3CL1, CX3CR1) in human endothelial cells [17, 53].

Various studies report positive correlations of serum resistin levels with the amount of body fat, however, other studies have found no correlation [53–55]. The most important association of circulating resistin levels reported is with C-reactive protein, which could be a marker of systemic inflammation [53].

2.2.4. Chemerin

It is secreted by adipocytes; it is closely associated with amount and distribution of adipose tissue. As a chemoattractant protein, chemerin acts as a ligand for the coupled G-receptor protein (ChemR23) and participates in both adaptive and innate immunity [56]. In humans, chemerin gene (*RRARES2*) is highly expressed in WAT and to a lesser extent in liver and lungs. On immune cells, chemerin is known to stimulate chemotaxis of dendritic cells, macrophages and natural killer (NK) cells. Meanwhile, its receptor, ChemR23 gene (*CMKLR1*), is expressed in dendritic cells, monocyte/macrophages and endothelial cells [18, 56, 57]. ChemR23 is involved in the differentiation of adipocytes and increased intracellular glucose or lipids promote its expression [18].

The interaction of chemerin/ChemR23 has been shown to reduce cytokines, chemokines and phagocytosis, proving to be important in the inflammatory process associated with obesity [18, 57]. In this context, chemerin/ChemR23 axis has been shown to impact IR development, which influences the clinical course and severity of obesity-related diseases.

As has been exposed, dysregulation of adipokinome due to accumulation of adipose tissue in obesity establishes and perpetuates a vicious circle from which emerges the chronic low-grade inflammation state.

2.3. Low-grade inflammation state in obesity

Inflammation is a physiological response to a stimulus (i.e. injury or infection) described by Celsus and Galen and is characterized by five classical signs: pain, heat, redness, swelling and loss of function [58, 59]. The inflammation resolution is an active process influenced, in part, by the time and especially regulated by the formation of a group of lipid mediators, which are identified as LXs, protectins and resolvins [60].

The low-grade inflammation state is a term used to define the activation of the vascular endothelium and presence of inflammatory cells in the absence of the five classical signs (subclinical) [61]. This state is due, at least initially, to adipose tissue hypertrophy present in obese individuals because different pathological processes occurs (i.e. fatty acids in excess, hypoxia, cell infiltration and activation of the inflammasome), this pro-inflammatory state is chronic in obesity and now is considered the etiologic agent of its co-morbidities [58, 62]. Effects of this 'unresolved' inflammation state can be appreciated in other context not explored here, but in which we cannot ignore the nervous system [63, 64]; these three: metabolism, immunity and nervous system are so interdependent that now they are considered as branches of a higher hierarchical level, the neuroendocrine-immune system.

2.3.1. Recruitment of immune cells to adipose tissue

The corresponding number of immune cells in adipose tissue is increased in obesity, mainly due to circulating cells' recruitment, when compared to lean individuals. [10, 65]. The main infiltrating cells are monocytes, however, other cell types such as NK, LB and LT may also migrate principally [10, 65, 66]. The infiltrated cells promote a positive feedback loop for a chronic low-grade inflammation state.

A key molecule for this recruitment of macrophages is CCL2 chemokine (formerly MCP-1), its expression displays positive correlation with the amount of adipose tissue [10, 19, 67], which is produced by macrophages and other cell types after stimulation. *In vitro* studies have shown that free fatty acids and TNF-α can stimulate production in chemotactic molecules of adipocytes [68].

CCL2 is the most important chemoattractant in the recruitment of monocytes, but possibly not the only one, mice fed with high-fat diets also showed an increase in expression of leukotriene B4 (LTB4) in muscle, liver and adipose tissue [10].

3. Insulin resistance: a direct consequence of immunometabolic imbalance

Insulin resistance (IR) is a condition characterized by the inability of cells to appropriately respond to insulin, which results in prolonged systemic hyperglycemia. It was considered a pathology since the 1930s, however, it was the development of insulin quantification assays and methodologies to estimate its biological action, as well as large epidemiology studies, which allowed to define the magnitude of the problem and the clinical implications.

3.1. Insulin resistance classification

The gold standard for IR assessment is the 'Hyperinsulinaemic-euglycaemic clamp' described by DeFronzo et al. [69]. However, this technique is hard to perform, time consuming, invasive and expensive; therefore, it is prohibitive for large studies. Because of this, numerous indexes have been developed and validated as surrogates, one of the most used is the 'Homeostasis Model Assessment of Insulin Resistance' (HOMA-IR) described by Matthews et al. that kept a correlation of 69 and 88% with euglycaemic and hyperglycaemic clamp, respectively [70].

Cut-offs and conditions has been tested to improve IR individuals classification; Stern et al. compiled demographics, clinical, laboratory and anthropometrics data of 2321 subjects studied with the euglycaemic insulin clamp technique and determined that with a combination of two simple rules: (1) HOMA-IR > 3.60 and (2) BMI > 27.5 kg/m^2; individuals can be classified as insulin-resistant with a sensitivity and specificity of 84.9 and 78.7%, respectively [71].

3.2. Insulin resistance aetiology

Establishment of IR arises from the interaction between environmental factors (principally obesity), and predisposition genes that confer susceptibility.

At the cellular level, there are two main mechanisms responsible of IR development: (1) cellular stress in the endoplasmic reticulum, and in the mitochondria of adipocytes, hepatocytes and myocytes; and (2) release of pro-inflammatory cytokines, principally, TNF-α and IL-6 by activation of the Toll-like receptor 4 (TLR-4) on the surface of infiltrated macrophages of white adipose tissue and liver [72, 73]. Obtained data point towards multiple triggering paths for this processes to be started, however, it is the obesity-associated chronic low-grade inflammation the most linked one [72, 73].

Moreover, in obesity, the amount and the size of adipocytes increase (hyperplasia and hypertrophy); furthermore, macrophage infiltration in white adipose tissue is higher and these processes together deregulate the secretion of adipokines. One of them, adiponectin, is negatively correlated with WAT accumulation (as mentioned before), this diminishes insulin signalling, already affected by the pro-inflammatory milieu. To add complexity to the IR phenomenon, they have been recently described novel mechanisms of immunometabolic regulation, the miRNAs.

4. Novel mechanisms involved on immunometabolic regulation: miRNAs

The microRNAs (miRNAs) were discovered in 1993 by Lee, Feinbaum and Ambros, when it was shown that their expression involves negative regulation at the post-transcriptional level and their biogenesis was a result of two unrelated molecular routes.

About miRNAs biogenesis, the non-coding region into the genes is transcribed, hence a small non-coding RNA is obtained, these molecules synchronized the downregulation of protein expression both at the transcriptional and translational levels. However, upregulation of translation has also been reported. In the negative regulation processes, the miRNAs bind to their complementary sites within the 3'-untranslated regions (UTRs) of target mRNA throughout sequence recognition, resulting in mRNA translational repression or degradation of the mRNA transcripts [74, 75].

The miRNAs are a kind of non-coding RNA of specific genes, whose products are single-stranded RNA molecules between 19 and 25 nucleotides, their sequences were identified by Northern blot analysis, microarrays or the real-time PCR method. Nucleotide sequences of miRNAs are reported in miRBase registry (http://mirbase.org/), and the correct nomenclature is discussed by several authors [76, 77].

4.1. microRNAs biogenesis

The molecular biosynthesis process of microRNAs involving multiple pathways however is possible to characterize a general mechanism, in which sequential routes of a particular method are identified (**Figure 2**):

1. miRNAs are transcribed in the cell nucleus by the RNA polymerase II, based on three main gene sequences: intronic regions, polycistronic clusters or from intergenic areas; the molecules obtained are called pri-miRNAs.

2. pri-miRNAs are improved by RNasa type III (Drosha) to become pre-miRNA, which is recognized by the XPO5 and RanGTP complex and transported to the cytoplasm through a nuclear pores [78].

3. The pre-miRNA, once it reaches in the cell cytoplasm, Dicer cleaves the double-stranded fragment and releases the loop, the miRNA duplex is unrolled and loaded into the complex miRISC [78].

4. Once it is loaded into the RISC complex, the mature miRNA is capable of associating with the mRNA target.

Subsequently when the mature miRNA is formed, their function will be to recognize by 3'UTR complementary sequences in the target mRNA. The level of coincidence in these sequences determines the degree of regulation of transcription, with one of two options, when the sequence of the complex is 100% complementary to the sequence in the region of the target (perfect complementarity), leading to denaturation and degradation of mRNA, while incomplete complementarity triggers silencing of mRNA through different molecular mechanisms, as repression of translation, degradation and/or sequestration of target [78, 79].

Since its deregulation has been related to different illnesses and it is estimated that more than 60% of the human genes expression are regulated by microRNAs [80].

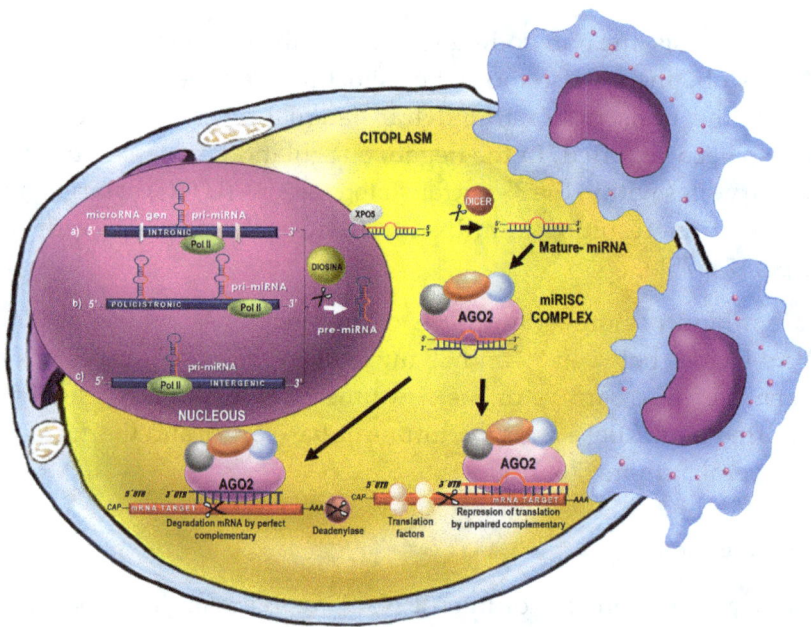

Figure 2. miRNA biogenesis. MicroRNA is transcribed by the polymerase II from (a) genes, (b) polycistronic clusters and (c) intronic regions. These pri-miRNAs are processed by the RNase Drosha which shortens them. The pre-miRNA formed is transported to cytoplasm by the XPO5 and then Dicer cleaves the loop leaving a double chain fragment that is recognized for the miRISC complex and targets the mRNA. POL II: polymerase II; XPO5: exportin 5; AGO2: argonaute protein 2; UTR: untranslated region; CAP: caperuse and AAAA: poly A chain.

4.2. microRNAs structural forms

For the reason that miRNAs are produced from the differential gene expression, heterogeneous structures are obtained with different length and nucleotide sequences. Sequences of two biochemically stable forms with asymmetrical structural motifs, the immature form (pre-miRNA) and the mature form (miRNA) have been reported.

The pre-miRNAs have a length of more 60 nucleotides, obtained from pri-miRNAs by the division in the union on the opposite side of the double chain loop. The recurrent structure is a double-helix that ends in a loop that joins both chains, the chain that goes from 5' to 3' and the chain of the direction from 3' to 5', which are 100% non-complementary and the length varies according to the mature stage due to the cuts made by the enzymes [81]. This double chain contains a monophosphate group in the end 5', and a free OH group in end 3'.

The mature microRNAs are approximately of 18–25 nucleotides in length, and differ from one another in their nucleotide sequence and length. Finally, two chains are generated in sense (5') and antisense (3') directions, emerging from the 5' arm of the hairpin microRNA or 3' arm of the microRNA hairpin, these sequences are called -5p or -3p, respectively. Generally, only one of them is dominant while the other is considered as a minor product, due to the intracellular concentration. However, both sequences are functional, as this depends on the tissue and species in which they are located [76, 82].

4.3. The functional diversity of miRNAs

The study of miRNAs is relevant because it has been involved in diverse functions and their expression levels have been associated with different diseases, such as insulin resistance, diabetes, atherosclerosis or cancer. While the new miRNAs sequence is identified, their participation in biological processes at the molecular level is to be defined. The mechanisms described include adipocyte differentiation, metabolic integration and appetite regulation [80, 83].

Among the metabolic diseases associated with the expression of miRNAs, their role in diabetes mellitus type 2 has been described, where it was shown that the miR-375 is directly involved in the regulation of insulin secretion. These data suggest their participation in the metabolic pathways and the possible association with inflammatory markers and their expression in individuals with phenotypic characteristics associated with obesity inflammation [84].

On the other hand, the miRNAs can also be found in the soluble form and it is important to remark that they are stable in serum for long periods of time due to two mechanisms, formation of a complex of ribonucleoprotein with argonaut proteins and the addition of exosomes and micro-particles. Besides, it has been discovered that HDLc can transport miRNAs in the plasma and take them to the target cells where they will be captured [85].

Related to their location in the serum of the miRNAs mature form, Slack has proposed two hypotheses: first, the miRNAs of tissues can be present in the circulation as a result of cell death and lysis, and second, the tissue cells actively secrete miRNAs in their microenvironment, where they get into the blood vessels so that they get their way up the circulation, so that it has been also suggested their potential usage as markers for different diseases [86].

Due to the strong correlation between the expression patterns of miRNAs and the state of the diseases, that has been showed not only in animal models but also in human patients, the miRNAs have been considered as promising candidates for the next generation of biomarkers.

4.4. miRNAs and immunometabolism

It is important to recognize that metabolic diseases have a strong immune component derived from inflammation and oxidative stress in which microRNAs regulate different ways (**Figure 3**).

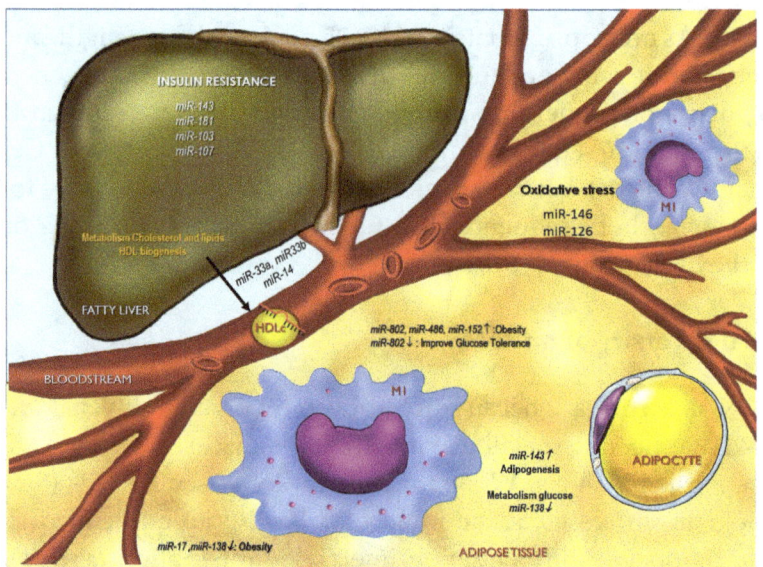

Figure 3. miRNA and immunometabolism. In immunometabolism, the microRNAs have an important role in regulation of different levels of metabolism. Further, the oxidative stress is the link between inflammation and obesity, since the accumulation of adipose tissue stimulates the expression of inflammation markers allowing the establishment of pathologies like DM2 and insulin resistance. Otherwise, there are microRNAs that improve glucose tolerance and lipid metabolism. M1: macrophages phenotype 1; HDLc: high-density lipoprotein cholesterol and miR: microRNA.

In diabetes mellitus type 2 patients, associations of miR-146 and miR-126 with markers of endoplasmic reticulum stress and inflammation as well as decreased miR-20b, miR-21, miR-24, miR-15a, miR-126, miR-191, miR-197, miR-223, miR-320 and miR-486 have been reported. Evenly, in obesity, the miR-152 increases, whereas miR-17 and miR-138 decreases [75, 87, 88].

With regard to metabolic functions in the skeletal muscle and the deregulation of the miRNA species, it is known that it can lead to deep alterations of glucose and the lipid metabolism in the adipose tissue, which is an important metabolic regulator. Regarding this, it has been shown that the expression of miR-14 decreases the levels of triacylglycerol and diacylclycerol, so that miR-14 could be an important lipid regulator in this level, besides other involved miRNAs such as miR-143 [89], miR-181a [90], miR-103 and miR-107 [91] have all been shown to affect hepatic insulin sensitivity, and more recently, miR-802 has been shown to be increased with obesity and that its reduction improves glucose tolerance and insulin action [92].

According to the association between obesity and the fatty acids different microRNAs have been associated, among them miR33a and miR33b, which are found in the intronic regions of the genes *SREBF2* and *SREBF1* that code for the transcription factors SREBP2 and SREBP1 and control the expression of the genes involved on the synthesis of cholesterol and fatty acids [93].

miR33a/b act as suppressing genes that oppose the functions of SREBP, for instance, the cholesterol efflux and the oxidation of fatty acids; so that under low-cholesterol conditions the transcription of SREBP2 and the regulation of the genes involved in the synthesis of cholesterol and absorption is activated, therefore, co-transcription of miR-33a acts in exporting cell cholesterol inhibiting the transcription of ABCA1 [93].

On the other hand, it is known that high levels of free fatty acids (FFA) and different adipokines, such as leptin and resistin, have a strong regulator role in other microRNAs; while expression of miR-143 can modulate the differentiation of the preadipocytes by increasing the storing of lipids, likewise, inhibition of miR-143 blocks differentiation of adipocytes through the kinase 5 regulator of extracellular signals (ERK5) [94].

5. Perspectives

At present, it seeks to make the value of clinical information available further effective, favouring a comprehensive approach to identify novel early biomarkers in the development of obesity and its co-morbidities.

In obesity, the biologic representative hallmark is the establishment of a subclinical chronic low-grade inflammatory process, promoted by the dysregulation of the immune system cells resident of white adipose tissue. Antagonistically, an underlying molecular mechanism induced by BAT control (hypermetabolism) can be developed. The understanding of both processes may allow the identification of early biomarkers with therapeutic aim of mitigate or eliminate the associated immunometabolic effects.

Researchers have focused their efforts on finding new biomarkers in obesity, based on the concept that a biomarker is identified as a qualitatively and/or quantitatively measurable biological parameter, which can be characterized as an indicator of health status versus disease, and also it serves as a marker for susceptibility or to stratify the relative risk in the general population.

The importance of a novel early biomarker is that it can have a high diagnostic or prognostic value in the context of development, establishment and progression of obesity and its co-morbidities. Because cut-off values are established in the biomarker validation process, it can be identified as a 'distorted indicator and differentiated predecessor' of clinical manifestations, with the possibility of aid at establishment, a classification in the progression of co-morbidities and severity of obesity.

As a consequence, from discovery to clinical application, an ideal early biomarker need run into the following characteristic: be easily accessible by using a sampling procedure minimally invasive, therefore, samples of blood, urine and saliva are excellent sources of choice.

In this contextual group of ideas, miRNAs that are transported to target cells through the bloodstream, are relatively stable and easily removed from blood serum have been identified. They are associated with metabolic risk and dysregulation of the immune system when white adipose tissue increases, and they are postulated as candidates of 'novel early biomarkers', due to their ability to become acquainted with the progression of the pathogenic process of obesity.

Author details

Efrain Chavarria-Avila[1,2,4,5], Rosa-Elena Navarro-Hernández[1,2,3,5], Milton-Omar Guzmán-Ornelas[1,2], Fernanda-Isadora Corona-Meraz[1,2], Sandra-Luz Ruíz-Quezada[2,3] and Mónica Vázquez-Del Mercado[1,5,6,7*]

*Address all correspondence to: dravme@hotmail.com

1 Institute for Rheumatology Research and MuscleSkeletal System, CUCS, University of Guadalajara, Guadalajara, Jalisco, Mexico

2 UDG-CA-701, Research Group on Immunometabolism and Emerging Diseases, Health Sciences School, Guadalajara, Jalisco, Mexico

3 UDG-CA-817, Research Group on Genomics and Biomedicine, Department of Farmacy and Biology, University of Guadalajara, Exact Sciences and Engineering School, Marcelino García Barragán Boulevard, Guadalajara, Jalisco, Mexico

4 Deparment of Philosophical, Methodological, and Instrumental Disciplines, University of Guadalajara, Health Sciences School, Guadalajara, Jalisco, Mexico

5 Department of Molecular Biology and Genomics, University of Guadalajara, Health Sciences School, Guadalajara, Jalisco, Mexico

6 Rheumatology Service PNPC 004086, CONACyT, Internal Medicine Division, Civil Hospital Dr. Juan I. Menchaca, Guadalajara, Jalisco, Mexico

7 UDG-CA-703, Research Group on Immunology and Rheumatology, University of Guadalajara, Health Sciences School, Guadalajara, Jalisco, Mexico

References

[1] Ferrante, A.W., Jr., *The immune cells in adipose tissue.* Diabetes Obes Metab, 2013. 15 Suppl 3: pp. 34–38.

[2] Alvarez-Curto, E. and G. Milligan, *Metabolism meets immunity: The role of free fatty acid receptors in the immune system.* Biochem Pharmacol, 2016. 114: pp. 3–13.

[3] Procaccini, C., C. La Rocca, F. Carbone, V. De Rosa, M. Galgani, and G. Matarese, *Leptin as immune mediator: Interaction between neuroendocrine and immune system.* Dev Comp Immunol, 2016. (16) pp. 30183-3, in press.

[4] Mejia, P., J.H. Trevino-Villarreal, C. Hine, E. Harputlugil, S. Lang, E. Calay, et al., *Dietary restriction protects against experimental cerebral malaria via leptin modulation and T-cell mTORC1 suppression.* Nat Commun, 2015. 6: p. 6050.

[5] Maslowski, K.M., A.T. Vieira, A. Ng, J. Kranich, F. Sierro, D. Yu, et al., *Regulation of inflammatory responses by gut microbiota and chemoattractant receptor GPR43.* Nature, 2009. 461(7268): pp. 1282–1286.

[6] Thaiss, C.A., N. Zmora, M. Levy, and E. Elinav, *The microbiome and innate immunity.* Nature, 2016. 535(7610): pp. 65–74.

[7] Honda, K. and D.R. Littman, *The microbiota in adaptive immune homeostasis and disease.* Nature, 2016. 535(7610): pp. 75–84.

[8] Brestoff, J.R. and D. Artis, *Immune regulation of metabolic homeostasis in health and disease.* Cell, 2015. 161(1): pp. 146–160.

[9] Liu, P.S., Y.W. Lin, F.H. Burton, and L.N. Wei, *M1-M2 balancing act in white adipose tissue browning—a new role for RIP140.* Adipocyte, 2015. 4(2): pp. 146–148.

[10] Lackey, D.E. and J.M. Olefsky, *Regulation of metabolism by the innate immune system.* Nat Rev Endocrinol, 2016. 12(1): pp. 15–28.

[11] Klose, C.S. and D. Artis, *Innate lymphoid cells as regulators of immunity, inflammation and tissue homeostasis.* Nat Immunol, 2016. 17(7): pp. 765–774.

[12] O'Sullivan, T.E., M. Rapp, X. Fan, O.E. Weizman, P. Bhardwaj, N.M. Adams, et al., *Adipose-resident group 1 innate lymphoid cells promote obesity-associated insulin resistance.* Immunity, 2016. 45(2): pp. 428–441.

[13] McLaughlin, T., L.F. Liu, C. Lamendola, L. Shen, J. Morton, H. Rivas, et al., *T-cell profile in adipose tissue is associated with insulin resistance and systemic inflammation in humans.* Arterioscler Thromb Vasc Biol, 2014. 34(12): pp. 2637–2643.

[14] Ronnemaa, T., S.L. Karonen, A. Rissanen, M. Koskenvuo, and V.A. Koivisto, *Relation between plasma leptin levels and measures of body fat in identical twins discordant for obesity.* Ann Intern Med, 1997. 126(1): pp. 26–31.

[15] Chavarria-Avila, E., M. Vazquez-Del Mercado, E. Gomez-Banuelos, S.L. Ruiz-Quezada, J. Castro-Albarran, L. Sanchez-Lopez, et al., *The impact of LEP G-2548A and LEPR Gln223Arg polymorphisms on adiposity, leptin, and leptin-receptor serum levels in a Mexican mestizo population*. Biomed Res Int, 2015. 2015: p. 539408.

[16] Mangge, H., G. Almer, M. Truschnig-Wilders, A. Schmidt, R. Gasser, and D. Fuchs, *Inflammation, adiponectin, obesity and cardiovascular risk*. Curr Med Chem, 2010. 17(36): pp. 4511–4520.

[17] Park, H.K. and R.S. Ahima, *Resistin in rodents and humans*. Diabetes Metab J, 2013. 37(6): pp. 404–414.

[18] Mariani, F. and L. Roncucci, *Chemerin/chemR23 axis in inflammation onset and resolution*. Inflamm Res, 2015. 64(2): pp. 85–95.

[19] Guzman-Ornelas, M.O., M.H. Petri, M. Vazquez-Del Mercado, E. Chavarria-Avila, F.I. Corona-Meraz, S.L. Ruiz-Quezada, et al., *CCL2 serum levels and adiposity are associated with the polymorphic phenotypes -2518A on CCL2 and 64ILE on CCR2 in a Mexican population with insulin resistance*. J Diabetes Res, 2016. 2016: p. 5675739.

[20] Arner, P. and M. Ryden, *Fatty acids, obesity and insulin resistance*. Obes Facts, 2015. 8(2): pp. 147–155.

[21] Giannini, S., G. Bardini, I. Dicembrini, M. Monami, C.M. Rotella, and E. Mannucci, *Lipid levels in obese and nonobese subjects as predictors of fasting and postload glucose metabolism*. J Clin Lipidol, 2012. 6(2): pp. 132–138.

[22] Turnbaugh, P.J., M. Hamady, T. Yatsunenko, B.L. Cantarel, A. Duncan, R.E. Ley, et al., *A core gut microbiome in obese and lean twins*. Nature, 2009. 457(7228): pp. 480–484.

[23] Remely, M., E. Aumueller, C. Merold, S. Dworzak, B. Hippe, J. Zanner, et al., *Effects of short chain fatty acid producing bacteria on epigenetic regulation of FFAR3 in type 2 diabetes and obesity*. Gene, 2014. 537(1): pp. 85–92.

[24] Winer, S. and D.A. Winer, *The adaptive immune system as a fundamental regulator of adipose tissue inflammation and insulin resistance*. Immunol Cell Biol, 2012. 90(8): pp. 755–762.

[25] Hardouin, P., T. Rharass, and S. Lucas, *Bone marrow adipose tissue: To be or not to be a typical adipose tissue?* Front Endocrinol (Lausanne), 2016. 7: p. 85.

[26] Bartness, T.J. and V. Ryu, *Neural control of white, beige and brown adipocytes*. Int J Obes Suppl, 2015. 5(Suppl 1): pp. S35–S39.

[27] Abdullahi, A. and M.G. Jeschke, *White adipose tissue browning: A double-edged sword*. Trends Endocrinol Metab, 2016. 27(8): pp. 542–552.

[28] Mulya, A. and J.P. Kirwan, *Brown and beige adipose tissue: Therapy for obesity and its comorbidities?* Endocrinol Metab Clin North Am, 2016. 45(3): pp. 605–621.

[29] Marzetti, E., E. D'Angelo, G. Savera, C. Leeuwenburgh, and R. Calvani, *Integrated control of brown adipose tissue.* Heart Metab, 2016. 69: pp. 9–14.

[30] Porter, C., D.N. Herndon, M. Chondronikola, T. Chao, P. Annamalai, N. Bhattarai, et al., *Human and mouse brown adipose tissue mitochondria have comparable UCP1 function.* Cell Metab, 2016. 24(2): pp. 246–255.

[31] Loncar, D., L. Bedrica, J. Mayer, B. Cannon, J. Nedergaard, B.A. Afzelius, et al., *The effect of intermittent cold treatment on the adipose tissue of the cat. Apparent transformation from white to brown adipose tissue.* J Ultrastruct Mol Struct Res, 1986. 97(1–3): pp. 119–129.

[32] Marquie, G., J. Duhault, P. Hadjiisky, P. Petkov, and H. Bouissou, *Diabetes mellitus in sand rats (Psammomys obesus): Microangiopathy during development of the diabetic syndrome.* Cell Mol Biol, 1991. 37(6): pp. 651–667.

[33] Cinti, S., *The adipose organ.* Prostaglandins Leukot Essent Fatty Acids, 2005. 73(1): pp. 9–15.

[34] Petruzzelli, M., M. Schweiger, R. Schreiber, R. Campos-Olivas, M. Tsoli, J. Allen, et al., *A switch from white to brown fat increases energy expenditure in cancer-associated cachexia.* Cell Metab, 2014. 20(3): pp. 433–447.

[35] Sidossis, L.S., C. Porter, M.K. Saraf, E. Borsheim, R.S. Radhakrishnan, T. Chao, et al., *Browning of subcutaneous white adipose tissue in humans after severe adrenergic stress.* Cell Metab, 2015. 22(2): pp. 219–227.

[36] Lizcano, F. and D. Vargas, *Biology of beige adipocyte and possible therapy for type 2 diabetes and obesity.* Int J Endocrinol, 2016. 2016: p. 9542061.

[37] Castoldi, A., C. Naffah de Souza, N.O. Camara, and P.M. Moraes-Vieira, *The macrophage switch in obesity development.* Front Immunol, 2015. 6: p. 637.

[38] Kratz, M., B.R. Coats, K.B. Hisert, D. Hagman, V. Mutskov, E. Peris, et al., *Metabolic dysfunction drives a mechanistically distinct proinflammatory phenotype in adipose tissue macrophages.* Cell Metab, 2014. 20(4): pp. 614–625.

[39] Artis, D. and H. Spits, *The biology of innate lymphoid cells.* Nature, 2015. 517(7534): pp. 293–301.

[40] Poulos, S.P., D.B. Hausman, and G.J. Hausman, *The development and endocrine functions of adipose tissue.* Mol Cell Endocrinol, 2010. 323(1): pp. 20–34.

[41] Trayhurn, P. and I.S. Wood, *Adipokines: Inflammation and the pleiotropic role of white adipose tissue.* Br J Nutr, 2004. 92(3): pp. 347–355.

[42] Pan, H., J. Guo, and Z. Su, *Advances in understanding the interrelations between leptin resistance and obesity.* Physiol Behav, 2014. 130: pp. 157–169.

[43] Procaccini, C., E. Jirillo, and G. Matarese, *Leptin as an immunomodulator.* Mol Aspects Med, 2012. 33(1): pp. 35–45.

[44] Mullen, M. and R.R. Gonzalez-Perez, *Leptin-induced JAK/STAT signaling and cancer growth.* Vaccines (Basel), 2016. 4(3): pp. E26, epub.

[45] Reis, B.S., K. Lee, M.H. Fanok, C. Mascaraque, M. Amoury, L.B. Cohn, et al., *Leptin receptor signaling in T cells is required for Th17 differentiation.* J Immunol, 2015. 194(11): pp. 5253–5260.

[46] Rehman Khan, A. and F.R. Awan, *Leptin resistance: A possible interface between obesity and pulmonary-related disorders.* Int J Endocrinol Metab, 2016. 14(1): p. e32586.

[47] Yang, X.N., C.Y. Zhang, B.-W. Wang, S.G. Zhu, and R.M. Zheng, *Leptin signalings and leptin resistance.* Sheng Li Ke Xue Jin Zhan, 2015. 46(5): pp. 327–333.

[48] Caselli, C., *Role of adiponectin system in insulin resistance.* Mol Genet Metab, 2014. 113(3): pp. 155–160.

[49] Simpson, F. and J.P. Whitehead, *Adiponectin — it's all about the modifications.* Int J Biochem Cell Biol, 2010. 42(6): pp. 785–788.

[50] Liu, M. and F. Liu, *Regulation of adiponectin multimerization, signaling and function.* Best Pract Res Clin Endocrinol Metab, 2014. 28(1): pp. 25–31.

[51] Yamauchi, T., M. Iwabu, M. Okada-Iwabu, and T. Kadowaki, *Adiponectin receptors: A review of their structure, function and how they work.* Best Pract Res Clin Endocrinol Metab, 2014. 28(1): pp. 15–23.

[52] DeFronzo, R.A., *Insulin resistance, lipotoxicity, type 2 diabetes and atherosclerosis: The missing links. The Claude Bernard Lecture 2009.* Diabetologia, 2010. 53(7): pp. 1270–1287.

[53] Huang, X. and Z. Yang, *Resistin, obesity and insulin resistance: The continuing disconnect between rodents and humans.* J Endocrinol Invest, 2016. 39(6): pp. 607–615.

[54] Chavarria-Avila, E., S.L. Ruiz Quezada, M.O. Guzman-Ornelas, J. Castro-Albarran, M.E. Aguilar Aldrete, M. Vasquez-Del Mercado, et al., *Association of resistin gene 3'UTR +62G>A polymorphism with insulin resistance, adiposity and the adiponectin-resistin index in Mexican population.* Nutr Hosp, 2013. 28(6): pp. 1867–1876.

[55] Bilir, B.E., S. Guldiken, N. Tuncbilek, A.M. Demir, A. Polat, and B. Bilir, *The effects of fat distribution and some adipokines on insulin resistance.* Endokrynol Pol, 2016. 67(3): pp. 277–282.

[56] Zabel, B.A., M. Kwitniewski, M. Banas, K. Zabieglo, K. Murzyn, and J. Cichy, *Chemerin regulation and role in host defense.* Am J Clin Exp Immunol, 2014. 3(1): pp. 1–19.

[57] Ernst, M.C. and C.J. Sinal, *Chemerin: At the crossroads of inflammation and obesity.* Trends Endocrinol Metab, 2010. 21(11): pp. 660–667.

[58] Minihane, A.M., S. Vinoy, W.R. Russell, A. Baka, H.M. Roche, K.M. Tuohy, et al., *Low-grade inflammation, diet composition and health: Current research evidence and its translation.* Br J Nutr, 2015. 114(7): pp. 999–1012.

[59] Rather, L.J., Disturbance of function (functiolaesa): The legendary fifth cardinal sign of inflammation, added by Galen to the four cardinal signs of Celsus. Bull N Y Acad Med, 1971. 47(3): pp. 303–22.

[60] Neuhofer, A., M. Zeyda, D. Mascher, B.K. Itariu, I. Murano, L. Leitner, et al., *Impaired local production of proresolving lipid mediators in obesity and 17-HDHA as a potential treatment for obesity-associated inflammation.* Diabetes, 2013. 62(6): pp. 1945–1956.

[61] Devaux, B., D. Scholz, A. Hirche, W.P. Klovekorn, and J. Schaper, *Upregulation of cell adhesion molecules and the presence of low grade inflammation in human chronic heart failure.* Eur Heart J, 1997. 18(3): pp. 470–479.

[62] Pereira, S.S. and J.I. Alvarez-Leite, *Low-grade inflammation, obesity, and diabetes.* Curr Obes Rep, 2014. 3(4): pp. 422–431.

[63] Lasselin, J., E. Magne, C. Beau, A. Aubert, S. Dexpert, J. Carrez, et al., *Low-grade inflammation is a major contributor of impaired attentional set shifting in obese subjects.* Brain Behav Immun, 2016. 1591(16): pp. 30122–2, in press.

[64] Lasselin, J., M.K. Kemani, M. Kanstrup, G.L. Olsson, J. Axelsson, A. Andreasson, et al., *Low-grade inflammation may moderate the effect of behavioral treatment for chronic pain in adults.* J Behav Med, 2016. 39(5): pp. 916–24

[65] Bourlier, V. and A. Bouloumie, *Role of macrophage tissue infiltration in obesity and insulin resistance.* Diabetes Metab, 2009. 35(4): pp. 251–260.

[66] Harford, K.A., C.M. Reynolds, F.C. McGillicuddy, and H.M. Roche, *Fats, inflammation and insulin resistance: Insights to the role of macrophage and T-cell accumulation in adipose tissue.* Proc Nutr Soc, 2011. 70(4): pp. 408–417.

[67] Weisberg, S.P., D. McCann, M. Desai, M. Rosenbaum, R.L. Leibel, and A.W. Ferrante, Jr., *Obesity is associated with macrophage accumulation in adipose tissue.* J Clin Invest, 2003. 112(12): pp. 1796–1808.

[68] Patsouris, D., J.G. Neels, W. Fan, P.P. Li, M.T. Nguyen, and J.M. Olefsky, *Glucocorticoids and thiazolidinediones interfere with adipocyte-mediated macrophage chemotaxis and recruitment.* J Biol Chem, 2009. 284(45): pp. 31223–31235.

[69] DeFronzo, R.A., J.D. Tobin, and R. Andres, *Glucose clamp technique: A method for quantifying insulin secretion and resistance.* Am J Physiol, 1979. 237(3): pp. E214–E223.

[70] Matthews, D.R., J.P. Hosker, A.S. Rudenski, B.A. Naylor, D.F. Treacher, and R.C. Turner, *Homeostasis model assessment: Insulin resistance and beta-cell function from fasting plasma glucose and insulin concentrations in man.* Diabetologia, 1985. 28(7): pp. 412–419.

[71] Stern, S.E., K. Williams, E. Ferrannini, R.A. DeFronzo, C. Bogardus, and M.P. Stern, *Identification of individuals with insulin resistance using routine clinical measurements.* Diabetes, 2005. 54(2): pp. 333–339.

[72] Tinkov, A.A., A.I. Sinitskii, E.V. Popova, O.N. Nemereshina, E.R. Gatiatulina, M.G. Skalnaya, et al., *Alteration of local adipose tissue trace element homeostasis as a possible mechanism of obesity-related insulin resistance.* Med Hypotheses, 2015. 85(3): pp. 343–347.

[73] Chen, L., R. Chen, H. Wang, and F. Liang, *Mechanisms linking inflammation to insulin resistance.* Int J Endocrinol, 2015. 2015: p. 508409.

[74] Vienberg, S., J. Geiger, S. Madsen, and L.T. Dalgaard, *MicroRNAs in metabolism.* Acta Physiol (Oxf), 2016. DOI: 10.1111/apha.12681.

[75] Zampetaki, A., S. Kiechl, I. Drozdov, P. Willeit, U. Mayr, M. Prokopi, et al., *Plasma microRNA profiling reveals loss of endothelial miR-126 and other microRNAs in type 2 diabetes.* Circ Res, 2010. 107(6): pp. 810–817.

[76] Griffiths-Jones, S., H.K. Saini, S. van Dongen, and A.J. Enright, *miRBase: Tools for microRNA genomics.* Nucleic Acids Res, 2008. 36(Database issue): pp. D154–D158.

[77] Kozomara, A. and S. Griffiths-Jones, *miRBase: Integrating microRNA annotation and deep-sequencing data.* Nucleic Acids Res, 2011. 39(Database issue): pp. D152–D157.

[78] Aranda, J.F., J. Madrigal-Matute, N. Rotllan, and C. Fernandez-Hernando, *MicroRNA modulation of lipid metabolism and oxidative stress in cardiometabolic diseases.* Free Radic Biol Med, 2013. 64: pp. 31–39.

[79] Araldi, E. and E. Schipani, *MicroRNA-140 and the silencing of osteoarthritis.* Genes Dev, 2010. 24(11): pp. 1075–1080.

[80] Heneghan, H.M., N. Miller, and M.J. Kerin, *Role of microRNAs in obesity and the metabolic syndrome.* Obes Rev, 2010. 11(5): pp. 354–361.

[81] Starega-Roslan, J., J. Krol, E. Koscianska, P. Kozlowski, W.J. Szlachcic, K. Sobczak, et al., *Structural basis of microRNA length variety.* Nucleic Acids Res, 2011. 39(1): pp. 257–268.

[82] Yang, J.S., M.D. Phillips, D. Betel, P. Mu, A. Ventura, A.C. Siepel, et al., *Widespread regulatory activity of vertebrate microRNA* species.* RNA, 2011. 17(2): pp. 312–326.

[83] Gharipour, M. and M. Sadeghi, *Pivotal role of microRNA-33 in metabolic syndrome: A systematic review.* ARYA Atheroscler, 2013. 9(6): pp. 372–376.

[84] Poy, M.N., L. Eliasson, J. Krutzfeldt, S. Kuwajima, X. Ma, P.E. Macdonald, et al., *A pancreatic islet-specific microRNA regulates insulin secretion.* Nature, 2004. 432(7014): pp. 226–230.

[85] Li, Y. and K.V. Kowdley, *Method for microRNA isolation from clinical serum samples.* Anal Biochem, 2012. 431(1): pp. 69–75.

[86] Slack, F.J., *MicroRNAs regulate expression of oncogenes.* Clin Chem, 2013. 59(1): pp. 325–326.

[87] Lenin, R., A. Sankaramoorthy, V. Mohan, and M. Balasubramanyam, *Altered immuno-metabolism at the interface of increased endoplasmic reticulum (ER) stress in patients with type 2 diabetes.* J Leukoc Biol, 2015. 98(4): pp. 615–622.

[88] Wu, L., X. Dai, J. Zhan, Y. Zhang, H. Zhang, H. Zhang, et al., *Profiling peripheral microRNAs in obesity and type 2 diabetes mellitus.* APMIS, 2015. 123(7): pp. 580–585.

[89] Jordan, S.D., M. Kruger, D.M. Willmes, N. Redemann, F.T. Wunderlich, H.S. Bronneke, et al., *Obesity-induced overexpression of miRNA-143 inhibits insulin-stimulated AKT activation and impairs glucose metabolism.* Nat Cell Biol, 2011. 13(4): pp. 434–446.

[90] Zhou, Y.F., J.L. Fu, and Y.F. Guan, *MicroRNAs and diabetic nephropathy.* Sheng Li Ke Xue Jin Zhan, 2012. 43(5): pp. 351–355.

[91] Trajkovski, M., J. Hausser, J. Soutschek, B. Bhat, A. Akin, M. Zavolan, et al., *MicroRNAs 103 and 107 regulate insulin sensitivity.* Nature, 2011. 474(7353): pp. 649–653.

[92] Kornfeld, J.W., C. Baitzel, A.C. Konner, H.T. Nicholls, M.C. Vogt, K. Herrmanns, et al., *Obesity-induced overexpression of miR-802 impairs glucose metabolism through silencing of Hnf1b.* Nature, 2013. 494(7435): pp. 111–115.

[93] Rayner, K.J. and K.J. Moore, *MicroRNA control of high-density lipoprotein metabolism and function.* Circ Res, 2014. 114(1): pp. 183–192.

[94] Zhu, L., C. Shi, C. Ji, G. Xu, L. Chen, L. Yang, et al., *FFAs and adipokine-mediated regulation of hsa-miR-143 expression in human adipocytes.* Mol Biol Rep, 2013. 40(10): pp. 5669–5675.

8

The Omics of Obesity

Darren Henstridge and Kiymet Bozaoglu

Abstract

Obesity is a complex multi-faceted disease affecting billions of people worldwide. Traditionally, obesity was thought to be a consequence of having access to energy dense food and busy lifestyles that do not factor in sufficient physical activity. Although diet and exercise play a major role in obesity development, these are not the only contributors. It is widely accepted that genetic and epigenetic factors also play a major role in obesity development and these in turn affect the lipidome, metabolome and proteome. With new technological advances, it is now possible to delve into these specific areas to further understand the mechanisms involved in obesity development. These technologies are collectively termed "omics" technologies, and this chapter will summarise the recent advances in obesity and metabolism research and describe new technologies that have been used to identify mechanisms that play a major role in the development of obesity. In particular, we will examine the different omics platforms that are available and have been used to study obesity. Collectively, these studies will be fundamental in identifying new and effective treatment strategies.

Keywords: obesity, genomics, epigenomics, lipidomics, proteomics, metabolomics

1. Introduction

Obesity is a global epidemic and is on the rise at an alarming rate. It is estimated that 2.1 billion people worldwide are either obese or overweight, which is almost 30% of the world's population [1]. This increase in obesity also predisposes individuals to other comorbidities such as cardiovascular disease, type 2 diabetes and metabolic syndrome [2] and therefore is a major public health concern. Obesity has traditionally been thought of as a consequence of a "bad diet" (high energy intake) and/or a sedentary lifestyle (low energy expenditure) resulting in a positive energy balance that manifests itself in the form of energy storage within adipose tissue. While this is true, it is now apparent that this is a simplistic view, and there are many contributing factors that impact energy storage and utilisation. In recent years, significant advances in the understanding of obesity and metabolism have been made using "omic" technologies. "Omic" techniques involve the detection and identification of molecules within a given biological sample, whether it is derived from cells, a tissue sample or indeed an entire organ or organism. Primarily, omics studies have aimed to identify the genes (genomics), messenger RNA (mRNA) (transcriptomics), proteins (proteomics) and metabolites (metabolomics that encompasses lipids (lipidomics)) of a sample or a group of samples and how they differ from another sample or group. Other omics platforms are also important in the regulation of these pathways including the effect of epigenetics (the epigenome/epigenomics) on the function of genes and the role of the gut microbiota within a host (the microbiome/microbiomics) on metabolite production and energy harvest from food. "Omic" platforms are being utilised by researchers around the world to identify mechanisms that contribute to the development and maintenance of obesity, the evolution of obesity to metabolic diseases such as type 2 diabetes and to try and identify possible therapeutic avenues to treat obesity (**Figure 1**). This chapter focuses on discussing obesity from the level of the genes associated with obesity and their regulation by the epigenome right through to the proteomic, lipidomic and metabolomic level in studies from both human cohorts as well as studies conducted in pre-clinical models.

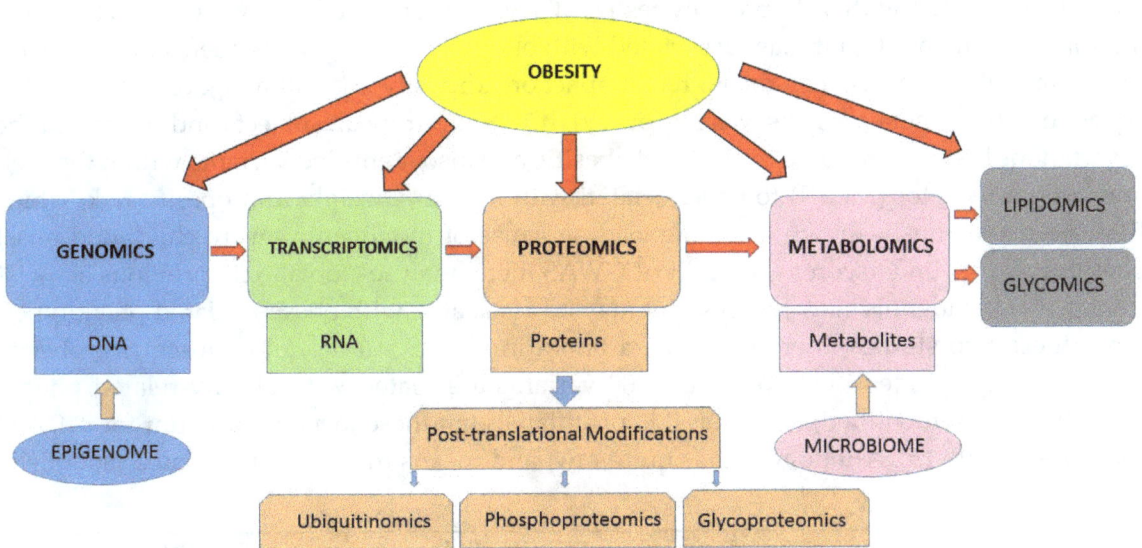

Figure 1. Flow chart representation of the various "omic" platforms used to study obesity. Further understanding of each of these stages will not only lead to a greater understanding of the pathogenesis of obesity and identification of therapeutic targets, but could potentially be used for prescription of personalized medicine (prevention and treatment). Data such as what is able to be obtained from lipidomic analysis may be utilized in the clinic to evaluate risk and monitor disease severity and provide prognostic information.

2. Genomics

While the global incidence of obesity is on the rise and is thought to be predominantly due to poor diet and sedentary lifestyles, it is also widely accepted that genetic and epigenetic factors also play an important role in obesity development. Twin studies have demonstrated that the heritability of obesity ranges from 40 to 70% [3], which clearly shows an important role of genetics in obesity and could depict which individuals are at higher risk of developing the disease. Therefore, it is empirical that we identify and understand the genetic regulation of obesity which will potentially lead to more targeted therapies to help stem this obesity epidemic.

2.1. Genome-wide association studies in obesity

With the completion of the Human Genome Project, it has been established that there are 20,000–25,000 genes within the human genome [4]. High-throughput genotyping technology coupled with The HapMap project [5] and 1000 Genomes Project [6] has made it possible to conduct genome-wide association studies (GWASs) to identify common variations in the genome that may be linked to diseases. The basis of GWAS is the detection of association of linkage disequilibrium (LD) between the causal variants and single-nucleotide polymorphisms (SNPs), which reduces the number of SNPs required to cover the whole genome. However, this is also a limitation as in the analyses a minor allele frequency of >5% is required, which means that only common SNPs will be identified. The very first large-scale SNP chip GWAS was performed by the Wellcome Trust Case Control Consortium in 1,924 type 2 diabetic (T2D) cases and 2,938 population controls from European samples and identified several variants associated with T2D phenotypes [7]. They also identified a novel gene, which was associated with obesity, fat mass associated with obesity (*FTO*). *FTO* has been shown to exert its primary effect on T2D risk through its impact on adiposity [8]. Following on from the discovery of *FTO*, a meta-analysis was performed in 16,876 European subjects and replicated the associations between variants in *FTO* and obesity, and also identified variants within the melanocortin-4 receptor (*MC4R*) to be associated with fat mass, weight and obesity risk, which have been previously shown to be the leading cause of monogenic severe childhood-onset obesity [9]. This underscores the merit of GWAS meta-analyses to validate previous associations as well as identify new regions that may be associated with obesity-related phenotypes. Since these two studies, there has been a boom in GWAS studies and subsequent obesity susceptibility loci identified. To date, ~200 variants associated with obesity-related phenotypes have been identified; however, it is postulated that these loci only account for <10% of the variance [10–15]. Although this is quite low, and means that 90% of variance remains to

Study population	Number of samples	Loci identified	Reference
European and African Americans	100,716	12 BMI loci identified; 4 were novel	[15]
European	52,140	6 loci associated with leptin, 5 independent of BMI	[14]
European	339,224	97 BMI loci identified	[11]
European, East Asian, South Asian, and African American	224,459	49 BMI loci identified; 33 were novel	[12]
European	47,541	3 new BMI loci	[13]
European	226,911	2 known and 6 novel BMI associated loci	[10]

Table 1. Summary of recent genome-wide meta-analyses of obesity.

be explained, they have provided us with an emerging wealth of knowledge of the genomic localisation, frequency and effect sizes, and potential functional implications that these loci may have. More recently, a number of meta-analyses of GWAS data have been performed and have identified new loci associated with body mass index (BMI) (**Table 1**). Surprisingly, these meta-analyses also replicated previously identified loci, which validate that these loci may be contributing to obesity and underscore the importance of performing GWASs in the first place.

3. Epigenomics

Epigenomics is the study of alterations to the transcriptional activity of genes in response to environmental stimuli *without* altering the DNA sequence. These alterations include methylation, histone modification as well as other changes in the chromatin structure that may affect the transcriptional regulation of a given gene. Importantly, these epigenetic modifications are thought to be an important link in the "missing heritability" hypothesis [16-18]. The concept of epigenetic regulation of obesity has become of great interest over the last decade and several studies have demonstrated that epigenetic modifications can occur very early in life which may predispose individuals to obesity later in life.

3.1. Early life epigenetic programming

In the late 1980s, Barker and Osmond were the first to describe that early life exposure to certain adverse conditions including over or under nutrition and stress may increase susceptibility to disease later in life [19]. Since then, there have been many studies, particular animal studies that have verified this hypothesis and have demonstrated that malnutrition (both excess and deprivation) during pregnancy is associated with increased fat deposition in the offspring and may also directly impact the oocytes in females and primordial germ cells of male foetuses [20, 21]. Furthermore, there is evidence that *in utero* over or under nutrition can affect DNA methylation, histone post-translational modification as well as gene expression of target genes involved in insulin signalling and fatty acid metabolism [22, 23]. Hence, this predisposes the offspring and the grand-offspring to obesity and related disorders. Therefore, epigenetic modifications are hypothesised to be trans-generational and have been shown to be reversible whereby specific epigenetic marks can be turned on or off depending on the stimuli (Bishop et al). Most of these studies have been performed in animal models including mice [24, 25], rats [26, 27], Macaque [28], drosophila [29] and sheep [23, 30, 31]. The effects of the *in utero* environment on foetal programming in humans have not been well explored. Two recent studies have investigated the effects of maternal nutrition before and during pregnancy on DNA methylation on the offspring. The first study, the Dutch Hunger Winter Study [22], examined the effects of prenatal exposure to famine on DNA methylation and was able to show an increased methylation in *LEP* and *IL10* and decreased methylation in *IGF2* and *INSIGF*; however, these subjects were obese, and therefore, it is not clear whether these changes occurred due to the maternal famine exposure or a response to increased BMI. The second study, the Gambian mother-child cohort, was a large randomised control trial which examined the effects of DNA methylation in response to maternal nutrition at conception and have demonstrated altered methylation in the offspring of these mothers and that these epigenetic changes were sex specific [32, 33]. A more recent randomised controlled study examined the effects of double blind peri-conceptional micronutrient supplementation in cord blood and observed sex-specific methylation changes which further supports the importance of *in utero* nutrition and the potential effects it may have on adiposity later in life (Dominguez-Salas, Moore et al. 2014). Another study, the AVON Longitudinal Study of parents and children, performed an epigenome-wide association analysis in 1,108 patients and found that the maternal underweight condition may be more influential on the DNA methylation of the offspring compared to the offspring from the maternal overweight mothers, while weight gain during pregnancy did not have much effect on DNA methylation in the offspring [34]. Although there is growing evidence of the effects of maternal nutrition on fatty acid metabolism and insulin signalling in humans later in life, there still remains some uncertainty and replication in large-scale population cohorts are warranted. The early detection of changes in the expression and epigenetic changes of candidate genes may provide biomarkers that will prevent or delay the onset of disease.

3.2. Human epigenome-wide association studies

Stemming from the animal epigenetic studies, there has been a recent incline in epigenome-wide association studies (EWAS) across different human populations. Most studies have focused more on site-specific differences in DNA methylation and its association with metabolic phenotypes, as it has been proposed to be a potential biomarker for clinical diagnosis and prognosis of disease [35]. A number of epigenetic marks related to obesity have been identified and replicated in other populations.

A study by Aslibeykan et al. (2015) performed an EWAS in CD4+ cells from frozen buffy coats from 991 healthy participants from the used Genetics of Lipid Lowering Drugs and Diet Network (GOLDN) study which identified eight differentially methylated sites associated with BMI, including cg00574958 (*CPT1A*), cg04332373 (*CD38*), cg17287155 (*AHRR*), cg26164488 (NA), cg07504977 (NA), cg14476101 (*PHGDH*), cg26680760 (NA) and cg26140475 (NA). They also identified four differentially methylated sites associated with waist circumference Cg00574958 (*CPT1A*), Cg04332373 (*CD38*), Cg14476101 (*PHGDH*) and cg25349939 (*GTDC1*) [36]. They replicated these methylation sites in whole blood from two independent cohorts—the Framingham Heart Study (FHS) (n = 1,935 case: control study, and n = 442 random samples) and the Atherosclerosis Risk in Communities (ARIC) study (n = 2,015 samples). A follow-up study in the ARIC study identified 76 BMI-related and 164 WC-related epigenetic marks mainly in *HIF3A*, *CPT1A* and *ABCG1* [37]. Thirty-seven of the BMI and one waist circumference mark were replicated in the GOLDN (n = 991 samples) and FHS (n = 2,377 samples) cohort. Another study identified 982 individual differentially methylated CpG sites between the insulin sensitive (IS) and insulin resistant (IR) groups. Of these sites, 538 were associated with unique genes with functions in cell adhesion, signal transduction and regulation of transcription and include *ADAM2*, *IGF2BP1*, *TBX5*, *HDACM*, *CD44* and *ZNF711*. These data are supportive of the close link between obesity and T2D and suggest the existence of a methylome map within Visceral adipose tissue (VAT) that may predispose individuals to IR and T2D [38].

Family studies are beneficial as they have the potential to identify causative candidate regions of differential DNA methylation. A study by Ali et al. (2016) used a discovery approach in 192 subjects from seven families from the Take off Pounds Sensibly Family Study of Epigenetics (TFSE), and then validated the initial differential methylation marks in an extended cohort of 1,052 subjects [39]. They identified and replicated three loci where methylation status was associated with BMI%, and these were located in the body of suppressor of cytokine signalling (*SOCS3*), 3' untranslated region of the zinc finger protein 771 (*ZNF771*) and at the transcription start site of LIM domain containing 2 (*LIMD2*) gene. Functional analyses were then performed in 330 subjects from the methylation analyses [39].

Examining promoter methylation patterns is thought to be a promising strategy for the use of early detection of disease (Laird 2003). Given that TNF*a* is pro-inflammatory cytokine elevated in obese subjects, Campion et al. (2009) investigated methylation patterns in the promoter region of TNF*a*. Methylation was measured in baseline peripheral blood mononuclear cells (PBMCs) from 24 patients who were put on an 8-week calorie restricted diet. Two differentially methylated promoter regions were assessed according to previous literature. The group of men who lost weight with the low calorie diet showed a significantly lower TNF*a* promoter methylation and that their baseline circulating TNF*a* levels were positively associated with total promoter methylation (Campion, Milagro et al. 2009). This demonstrates that examining promoter methylation may well be an important aspect in early detection and prognosis of disease.

3.3. Can PBMCs be used as a surrogate for epigenetic studies?

Despite progress in the epigenetic marks of obesity, there still remain some controversy in the use of peripheral blood mononuclear cells (PBMCs) as a surrogate for identification of epigenetic marks that may contribute to obesity development as there may be site-specific marks that may be missed. However, it is important to consider that with human studies, we are limited to tissues that we can readily access and the most commonly and easily accessible tissue to examine epigenetic modifications in humans is whole blood or PBMCs. This has been thought to have limitations in itself as it may not explain tissue-specific modifications that may be present. In light of this, many recent studies have examined epigenetic profiles in both PBMCs as well as subcutaneous adipose tissue (SAT). Once such study was from Arner et al. 2016, where they performed and EWAS using PBMCs, SAT and VAT in 80 obese women of which 40 insulin resistant and 40 insulin sensitive (Arner, Sahlqvist et al. 2016). They wanted to determine similarities of methylation status between the tissues and to determine whether PBMCs could be used as a marker of systemic IR. They were not able to show similar methylation sites between the PBMCs and adipose tissue and therefore concluded that CpG methylation in PBMCs does not reflect differential methylation sites in white adipose tissue (WAT). These data suggest that PBMCs may not be a suitable tissue for metabolic phenotyping of obese individuals. However, another study by Demarath et al. (2015) (described above) also measured methylation markers in SAT from their ARIC cohort and replicated 16 of these BMI markers (Demerath, Guan et al. 2015). Given that these associations remained in different ethnic cohorts as well as different tissue samples (whole blood vs. CD4 cells from buffy coat vs. adipose tissue) demonstrate that adiposity traits are associated with different methylation sites independent of tissue type or ethnicity. It is clear that more thorough investigations into tissue differences are required; however, this may not always be possible in some settings such as brain- or heart-related disorders.

3.4. Epigenetics and intervention studies

The variation in epigenetic patterns with obesity has raised some interest in the field. There have been several intervention studies that have investigated the role of obesity and weight-loss interventions on global and promoter specific DNA methylation patterns. A 6-month exercise intervention study using adipose tissue from 23 healthy men with a family history (or not) of T2D demonstrated a global increase of adipose tissue DNA methylation in response to the exercise intervention (Ronn, Volkov et al. 2013). Interestingly, the subjects with a family history of T2D had less CpG sites with a significant difference in methylation patterns in obesity-related genes in response to the 6-month exercise intervention (Ronn, Volkov et al. 2013). Another study examined methylation changes in subjects that underwent gastric band surgery and were able to demonstrate significant effects on promoter methylation. More interestingly, before the patients underwent surgery, they observed significant methylation changes in genes involved in metabolic pathways and mitochondrial function, however after surgery and subsequent weight loss, the expression of these same genes normalised to similar levels to non-obese subjects (Barres, Kirchner et al. 2013). An additional study examined epigenetic changes in a normal weight, obese and successful weight loss maintainers (maintained weight for 9 years) that consisted of 48 males and females and demonstrated that the successful weight-loss maintainer group had methylation patterns that resembled the normal weight group rather than the obese group, which shows that methylation changes can be reversed (Huang, Maccani et al. 2015).

In summary, these studies collectively validate an important role for epigenetic regulation in metabolic processes. Furthermore, epigenetic marks coupled with gene expression in candidate genes may offer new pharmacological targets to counteract these modifications and potentially help avert obesity and associated diseases.

4. Proteomics

While genetic regulation in a biological system is unequivocally vital to health and disease, mRNA transcript levels generally only partially correlate with protein expression [16]. Typically, transcript abundance explains approximately one- to two-thirds of the variance in protein levels, depending on the organism [16]. This is due to the fact that it is not only the transcription that determines protein abundance but also post-transcriptional factors such as RNA processing and stability, translation, protein stability/turnover and protein modification. So while transcription data can provide a starting point as to whether or not a protein will be found and its likely level of abundance in a given sample, changes in expression levels may not correlate to changes in protein levels. Consequently, proteomics is an important area of research to enable the characterisation of the proteome. Traditionally, the expression of individual proteins has been quantified using antibodies and techniques such as western blotting but today many proteins and the whole proteome of a sample can be assessed at once by using various mass spectrometry approaches. Proteins are regulated by a wide variety of chemical alterations after they have been translated. These post-translational modifications can include but is not limited to phosphorylation, ubiquitination, acetylation, glycosylation, nitrosylation, acetylation and methylation, and consequently, these are all sub-branches of proteomics.

4.1. Proteomic analysis in adipocyte cell culture models

Insulin plays a major role in the regulation of metabolic homeostasis. In adipose tissue, insulin-stimulated glucose uptake and the inhibition of lipolysis are two major functions of insulin. Quantitative phosphoproteomics using stable isotope labelling with amino acids in cell culture (SILAC) was used to interrogate the insulin signalling network in response to insulin stimulation in the 3T3-L1 adipocytes cell culture model [17]. The phosphoproteomics identified 37,248 phosphorylation sites that spanned 5705 proteins. Of these, around 15% were regulated by insulin demonstrating the complexity of the insulin signalling network in adipose cells [17]. A time course analysis also revealed a large variation in when phosphorylation events occur following insulin treatment, demonstrating the dynamic nature of the pathways. Novel mechanisms of the AKT-mTORC2 were also identified leading to the identification of SIN1 as an Akt substrate that contributes to the regulation of mTORC2 activity [17]. Proteomic analysis has also been useful in determining that large-scale changes to proteins that occur in 3T3-L1 cells during adipogenesis [18]. Wilson-Fritch et al. used mass spectrometry and database correlation analysis to describe a 20–30-fold increase in mitochondrial proteins during adipogenesis including proteins involved in fatty acid metabolism and those that are mitochondrial chaperones [18]. Further analysis revealed that the insulin-sensitising drug rosiglitazone (belonging to the thiazolidinedione (TZD) class of drug) also changes expression of mitochondria-related proteins which makes sense considering it is a known adipogenesis-inducing agent.

4.2. Proteomic changes in human obesity

The characterisation of protein expression in organs during obesity can help scientist unveil the biological impact of obesity and lead to a greater understanding of the condition. An interesting area of adipocyte biology is how the subcutaneous adipose tissue (fat found under the skin and largely around the hips, thighs and buttocks) is thought to be the more metabolically active and metabolically healthy type of fat and the visceral adipose tissue (central obesity) which is associated with metabolic dysfunction and disease differs. Via 2D-DIGE and mass spectrometry analysis, Perez-Perez and team investigated the protein differences in omental and subcutaneous adipose tissue of healthy obese individuals. These results identified 43 differentially expressed proteins including those that have been linked to lipid and glucose metabolism, lipid transport, protein synthesis and folding inflammation and the cellular stress response [19]. One way of getting proteomic information without the invasiveness of using adipose biopsies is to use peripheral blood mononuclear cells (PBMCs) as a surrogate tissue. Abu-Farha and colleagues utilised shotgun proteomics to examine the PBMC proteome in lean versus obese individuals [20]. About 1063 proteins were identified as common proteins between both groups (lean and obese participants), and of these, 47 were differentially expressed (by at least 1.5-fold). Of these 47, 18 were increased and 29 decreased in the obese group compared to lean. As adipose tissue is an endocrine organ that secretes substances (adipokines) that impact metabolism in other tissues, proteomic analysis of these factors is of interest. Human primary subcutaneous adipose tissue cells were cultured and tandem mass spectrometry used to analyse the secretome of the cells [21]. As well as the detection of a number of well-characterised adipokines-like adiponectin (validating the technique), this method leads to the identification of multiple serine protease inhibitors (called serpins) [21]. Using this proteomics approach and exposing the adipose cells to different metabolic states and treatments, may be a way to further elucidate the factors that are released by adipocytes, the quantities by which they are released and under which conditions they are released. This could pave the way for a greater understanding as to the endocrine effects of the adipocyte.

4.3. Animal models of obesity and alterations to the proteome

One way to look at the way obesity impacts biology and metabolism is to look at and study the white adipose tissue (WAT) itself. A global label-free phosphoproteomic screen of WAT in mice discordant for obesity due to high-fat feeding detected and quantified a total of 7696 peptides. Differential phosphorylation levels between groups were found at 282 phosphosites from 191 different proteins [22]. This data set identified phosphorylation changes in enzymes involved in metabolic pathways such as glucose and lipid homeostasis pathways, linking these proteins to disturbed metabolism [22]. Importantly, the authors were able to further dissect out the likely impact of adiposity by using the data set to provide predictions on upstream kinases that are likely affected. These predictions revealed well-known kinase families such as AMPK and AKT that have been heavily studied in metabolic dysregulation verifying their approach. It also identified others such as MRCKα and PAK 1 and 2 whose role is unknown in relation to obesity [22]. Thus, this sort of analysis has the potential to uncover novel pathways altered with obesity and how this alters adipocyte function.

We all know that some individuals seem to put on weight even though they consume a healthy, low-fat diet, whereas others eat all of the energy-dense junk food that they want and do not have any impact on their waistlines. As this would rule out calorie content as the driving force for this type of accumulation of adiposity, it is likely that there is an underlying susceptibility in these individuals. Xie and colleagues tried to replicate this in an animal study where they performed proteomic analysis on mice that were either obesity resistant or obesity prone [23]. Results indicated that ubiquinol-cytochrome c reductase core protein 1 (Uqcrc1) and Enolase 3 were decreased and monoglyceride lipase (MGLL) and glucose-6-phosphate dehydrogenase (G6PDH) were increased in the visceral adipose tissue of obesity-prone mice compared to obesity-resistant mice [23]. These proteins involved in energy metabolism, glycolysis and fat synthesis may provide a clue as to why visceral adipose tissue is more or less likely to store energy and expand.

Though adipose tissue is obviously important to study, other metabolic organs are also too important to study. Baiges et al. [24] investigated the effects of a high-fat diet (HFD) on the rat liver proteome. Analysis identified 1,131 liver proteins and demonstrated that a high-fat diet changed the expression of 90 of these proteins. As one would have hypothesised, many of these proteins are involved in glucose and lipid metabolism [24]. Proteomics can also be further enhanced by analysing sub-cellular compartments such as mitochondria. In a study comparing lean versus obese mice, Nesteruk et al. [25] purified isolated mitochondria from both liver and skeletal muscle and analysed mitochondrial-associated proteins via mass spectrometry. Analysis identified 1,675 liver and 704 muscle mitochondria-associated proteins and of these, 221 liver and 44 muscle proteins were differentially expressed between the lean and obese groups [25]. Analysis of"sub-proteomes" such as the ones at the mitochondrial proteome may be used more in the future to identify cellular compartment-specific changes associated with obesity. This type of analysis is also beneficial in the sense that it can increase the sensitivity of the process and allow the detection of lowly expressed proteins.

Looking into the future, the combination and integration of proteomics analysis with other"omic" platform analysis such as genomics, transcriptomics and metabolomics may provide a useful systems biology approach to further understand the regulation of whole-body fat mass.

5. Metabolomics

Metabolites are small molecules that can be measured in bodily fluids including blood and urine as well as in tissue samples. Of particular interest are low-molecular-weight metabolites that are involved in metabolic pathways where they act as substrates, intermediates or products. Such metabolites include hormones, fatty acids and amino acids [26]. Metabolomics therefore is the analysis of the metabolite profile in a given sample, cell or organ. There are a number of different subtypes of metabolomics including lipidomics, glycomics, fluxomics and peptidomics. While the genome and in turn the proteome set the scene as to what biological processes take place or are dominant in a cell, the actual activity and function encoded by the genes and proteins is carried out via metabolites [26]. Consequently, the metabolome is impacted by the accumulation of all the genetic variation, epigenetic status, gene and protein expression, enzymatic activity and environmental factors that are expressed in or exerted on an organism. Given that the large array of metabolites are formed in biological systems, this is a complex task. Most often, the techniques used to profile metabolomics are nuclear magnetic resonance spectroscopy (NMR) and gas chromatography mass spectrometry (GC-MS). In general, metabolomics is a high-throughput technology and while initial start-up costs of purchasing equipment and providing the infrastructure is expensive, once established, on a per-sample basis, it is relatively inexpensive. Short of this, there are many centres that specialise in metabolomic measures set up throughout the world. These centres often will provide metabolomics data on samples for a fee-for-service arrangement.

5.1. Metabolomic analysis in obese humans

For an in-depth description of the amino acid metabolism, lipid metabolism, carbohydrate metabolism and nucleotide metabolism-related metabolites that have been shown to be altered in the setting of obesity or diabetes or obesity with diabetes, we refer the readers to the review by Park et al. [27]. Herein, we will discuss some of these changes and provide a separate section on a popular sub-branch of metabolomics that concentrates on studying lipids (lipidomics). In the 1970s, it was demonstrated that obese individuals have higher circulating levels of numerous amino acids including branched-chain amino acids (BCAAs) [28]. Recently, utilising new analytical techniques, a number of studies have confirmed and expanded on these findings. In a study, utilising metabolomics and lipidomics of blood plasma and urine to investigate association of metabolites with adiposity, it was demonstrated that there were seven metabolites that were important in predicting visceral fat levels, which included the amino acids tyrosine and glutamine and the lipid species PC-O 44:6, PC-O 44:4, PC-O 42:4, PC-O 40:4 and PC-O 40:3 [29]. In an alternative study conducted in obese Japanese individuals, plasma levels of amino acids are found to be associated with visceral fat accumulation. These amino acids included levels of alanine, glycine, glutamate, tryptophan and tyrosine [30]. In a metabolomic profiling study of 74 obese and 67 lean individuals, a number of differences in fatty and amino acids were reported [31]. Levels of free fatty acids C14:0, C16:0, C16:1, C18:1, C20:4 remained elevated in obese as compared to lean subjects. Levels of eight amino acids increased in obese as compared to lean individuals including alanine, arginine, asparagine, glutamine, leucine, phenylalanine, tyrosine and valine while conversely one decreased (glycine). Four acylcarnitine species (C3, C5, C6 and C8:1) were higher in the samples from obese individuals [31]. The data suggested the existence of a (BCAA)-related metabolic signature in obesity and linking this to metabolic dysregulation, these changes were associated with insulin resistance [31].

Metabolomic profiling may assist in distinguishing different types of obesity. As metabolic abnormalities are associated with central obesity more so than they are with peripheral obesity, Gao et al. set out to identify via metabolomics whether serum metabolic markers differ in those with central versus peripheral obesity [32]. Five types of metabolites were verified to be higher in the central obesity group after multiple testing adjustments. These included the BCAAs leucine, isoleucine and valine as well as alpha-aminoadipic acid and propionylcarnitine (C3 acylcarnitine) [32]. These metabolites may provide a useful mechanistic insight into determining the difference between metabolically healthy peripheral obesity and metabolically unhealthy central obesity. Another way to discriminate against metabolically healthy obesity and metabolically abnormal obesity is to divide patients on the basis of whether they have any form of hyperglycemia, hypertension or dyslipidemia. Chen et al. conducted such study in obese individuals from a weight-loss clinic and could indeed identify differential metabolic profiles and metabolic pathways [33]. These groups differed in L-kynurenine, glycerophosphocholine (GPC), glycerol 1-phosphate, glycolic acid, tagatose, methyl palmitate and uric acid. The pathways that could distinguish between the obese metabolically healthy and unhealthy groups were pathways involved in fatty acid biosynthesis, phenylalanine metabolism, and valine, leucine and isoleucine degradation pathway [33].

Variants in the fat mass and obesity-associated gene FTO has been identified as a risk factor for the accumulation of fat mass and the development of obesity [8, 34]. By correlating metabolites after stratification for whether or not an individual is a carrier of the FTO risk allele, genetic FTO-induced changes in the metabolome can be assessed. Via utilising samples obtained as part of a Korean community-based cohort (KARE cohort), Kim et al. [35] used serum metabolite quantification by targeted metabolomics to correlate FTO-genotype with alterations to metabolites. This resulted in the analysis of 134 different metabolites (78 glycerophospholipids, 21 amino acids, 12 sphingolipids, 12 acylcarnitines, 10 biogenic amines and 1 hexose). Of these metabolites, the authors found that seven metabolites were associated with increased risk of obesity due to the presence of the rs9939609 FTO risk allele [35]. Most notably, of these seven metabolites, five were phosphatidylcholines (PCs) (C36:5, C36:6, C38:5, C38:5, C38:6 and C40:6) and these showed the strongest effect, while the monosaccharide (hexose) and amino acid (valine) were also associated. Similar future studies investigating the impact of genetic risk factors on the metabolome can provide insight into how genes impact metabolism and contribute to the development of obesity.

5.2. Metabolomic and obesity in animal models

Using mouse models that have had a genetic manipulation (knock-out, knock-down overexpression), metabolomics can be used to gain an idea as to the impact a genetic modification has on obesity or metabolic pathways. Neuroblast differentiation-associated protein AHNAK knock-out mice (AHNAK(-/-)) have been reported as having a phenotype whereby they have a strong resistance to high-fat diet-induced obesity. Consequently, Kim et al. [36] applied (1) H NMR-based metabolomics to compare the altered metabolites in the urine from high-fat diet (HFD) fed wild-type and AHNAK(-/-) mice. The profiling identified that the urinary metabolites of HFD-fed AHNAK(-/-) mice gave higher levels of methionine, putrescine, tartrate, urocanate, sucrose, glucose, threonine and 3-hydroxyisovalerate compared to wild-type mice suggesting that the resistance to the HFD-induced obesity may arise from alterations in amino acids [36]. Likewise, human ataxin-2 (ATXN2) knock-out mice display obesity, insulin resistance and dyslipidemia [37]. To understand the effects of the loss of ATXN2, Meierhofer and team used unbiased profiling approaches to quantify the global metabolome of ATXN2 knock-out mice with label-free mass spectrometry [38]. Significant down-regulated pathways for branched chain and other amino acid metabolism, fatty acids and citric acid cycle provided evidence for the biological function of ATXN2 and the potential mechanism via which the lean phenotype is maintained [38]. Thus, metabolomics used in combination with genetic models offers a viable way to determine biological significance of genes and improve understanding of cellular pathways.

6. Lipidomics

Lipidomic measurement is a sub-branch of metabolomics where the identification of lipid classes and species is made. Given obesity is a disease whereby lipids accumulate in adipose tissue to make large adipose tissue depots, lipidomics is an extremely relevant platform for the field. Typically, analysis can identify not only the different classes of lipid that are in a given sample, but also the molecular species that make up those different classes. Multiple approaches to performing lipidomics are available. Shotgun lipidomics refers to the process of identifying the lipidome of biological lipid extracts directly without the need for chromatographic purification. Targeted lipidomics involves the combination of liquid chromatography and stable isotope or non-physiological internal standards to provide quantification to hundreds of lipids. While untargeted lipidomics refers to the combination of liquid chromatography with high mass analysis to detect lipid species [39]. Numerous studies have investigated the lipidomic signature that is associated with increased fat mass in animal and human models.

6.1. Insights into human obesity from plasma lipidomics

Plasma lipidomic screening has been used to characterise the circulating lipids in obese compared to lean individuals to gain an insight into how obesity alters this parameter. In a study of monozygotic twins who differed in body weight by 10–25 kg, characterisation of lipid species in serum samples identified that obesity, independent of genetic influences, was associated with increases in lysophosphatidylcholine (LPC) lipids and decreases in ether phospholipids [40]. In an alternative study looking for plasma lipidomic associations with waist circumference used as a marker of central obesity, it was noted that dihydroceramides were associated with waist circumference, particularly the species 18:0, 20:0, 22:0 and 24:1, while two sphingomyelin species 31:1 and 41:1 were inversely associated with waist circumference [41]. In a study of 1,176 young individuals (20 years of age) in which 175 different plasma lipid metabolites were analysed, a positive association was found between waist circumference and seven sphingomyelins and five diacylphosphatidylcholines and negative association with two LPCs [42] while another study also demonstrated a reduction in numerous LPC species in the plasma of obese individuals [43]. Differences observed between studies could be due to the type of obesity in the different cohorts sampled. For example, obesity due to a high caloric intake could potentially result in a different lipidomic profile than what is observed in individuals who are obese due to a sedentary lifestyle. Other factors such as diet, sample preparation and age could also have an effect.

One potential use of plasma lipidomics is to use it as a diagnostic tool or monitoring tool in obese patients. By measuring the plasma lipidomic signature and correlating levels of various lipid species to risk factors of further disease such as region-specific adiposity or liver dysfunction, a panel of lipids may be identified to stratify at-risk patients [44]. A serum biomarker that predicts ectopic fat levels could be utilised in the clinic to track ectopic fat levels or conversely to track the effectiveness of interventions to decrease it. Currently, it is necessary to use expensive large-scale imaging technology to investigate ectopic lipid deposition. Even so, this only detects levels of triacylglycerols (TAGs) rather than other lipid metabolites that are found in lower abundance that have been implicated in causing metabolic dysfunction such as ceramides and diacylglycerols (DAGs). Alternatively, invasive biopsy procedures with analytical analysis can be used to identify the relative expression of these lipids. Given the relative ease of blood collection, plasma lipid profiling may provide an alternative avenue to provide a picture of tissue lipid levels if a predictor(s) can be identified.

In one study using shotgun lipidomics that captured 252 individual lipid species over 14 different classes, the authors aimed to link the circulating levels of blood plasma lipids to fat accumulated in various parts of the body including visceral adiposity and epicardial adipose tissue (EAT) (which are both cardiac disease risk factors) [44]. Via modelling analysis, a strong association was identified between visceral adiposity and plasma diacylglycerol (DAG) and EAT and triacylglycerol (TAG) (both DAG and TAG are composed of saturated fatty acids) [44]. In this study, EAT is also correlated with increased levels of phosphatidylglycerol (PG) species including PG 20:3/20:3 and PG 22:5/18:1 and with decreased levels of ether phosphatidylethanolamine (PE-O) lipid species that are mainly composed of plasmalogens [44]. Additionally, Perreault and colleagues set out to determine the ability of lipidomics performed in the serum to predict ectopic lipid accumulation in skeletal muscle, in particular, the ability to predict TAG, DAG and ceramide. After analysis of 215 serum lipids, they found that in obese individuals, ganglioside C22:0 and lactosylceramide C14:0 levels in the serum predicted muscle TAG levels while serum DAG C36:1 and free fatty acid (FFA) C18:4 could predict muscle TAG levels. Furthermore, serum TAG C58:5, cholesterol ester C24:1, phosphatidylcholine C38:1 and FFA C14:2 were good predictors of the ceramide levels in muscle. Moving forward, confirmation of such findings could allow for a panel of plasma lipids to accurately depict the state of ectopic lipid deposition in peripheral tissues such as skeletal muscle and prove useful in the clinical setting [45].

6.2. Tissue lipidomics in human obesity

While plasma is an obvious location to identify a prognostic marker, studying the lipidomic profile in adipose tissue itself or in other metabolic organs is of great interest to understand the biology of the condition. In a study of 20 obese, but otherwise healthy women, lipidomics was carried out on subcutaneous adipose tissue samples. Participants were divided into those with high content of liver fat or those with a low content of liver fat to determine if adipose tissue is altered in those discordant for intrahepatic lipid content. Analysis of 154 lipid species revealed increased concentrations of TAGs particularly long chain, and ceramides, specifically Cer (d18:1/24:1) in the group with more liver fat [46]. In another study carried out in obese insulin-resistant women compared to obese women with normal insulin levels, lipid profiling revealed an increase in G_{M3} ganglioside and phosphatidylethanolamine (PE) lipid species in omental adipose tissue [47]. These findings corresponded to an increase in ST3GAL5, the synthesis enzyme for G_{M3} ganglioside, and a decrease in phosphatidylethanolamine methyl transferase (PEMT), the degradation enzyme of PEs [47]. Thus, these changes may contribute to the obesity-induced insulin-resistant state.

In a human lipidomics screening of plasma and skeletal muscle samples comparing lean individuals with those who were obese or overweight but insulin sensitive (as defined by glucose infusion rate during a hyperinsulinemic-euglycemic clamp) and those who were obese and overweight but insulin resistant, demonstrated that there was no defining difference in the skeletal muscle of those who were lean as compared to those that were overweight or obese [48]. The plasma samples did demonstrate a higher quantity of TAG and lower plasmalogen species in those who were overweight or obese compared to lean. However, in individuals who were overweight or had obesity but were discordant for insulin resistance those who were insulin-resistant had higher levels of C18:0 sphingolipids in skeletal muscle and higher levels of DAG and cholesterol ester (CE) and a decrease in LPC and lysoalklphosphatidycholine in the plasma [48]. This suggested that insulin resistance has a greater impact within the obese setting on the lipidomic profile than what obesity has on the profile in comparison to those that are lean.

6.3. Plasma lipidomics in obese rodent models

Plasma lipidomics has been assessed in various rodent models of obesity and to investigate the effect on the lipidome of various intervention studies. Barber and colleagues performed lipidomics in plasma samples from mice fed a high-fat diet for 12 weeks. Compared to low-fat diet control mice, these mice had increased levels of TAG, DAG and sphingolipid species, while there was a reduction in LPC levels [43]. To describe these LPC effects further, a high-fat feeding time course study was completed which noted an increase in LPC 18:0 and 20:0 after just 1 week of high-fat feeding. However, LPC 15:0, 16:1, 18:1, 18:2, 20:1 and 20:5 were all significantly decreased from baseline at 1 week and continued to be decreased out to 6 weeks of high-fat feeding [43]. While most of the LPC species were decreased some species such as 18:0 were elevated. Also utilising a high-fat diet to induce obesity, Li and colleagues identified LPC 18:0 as a potential biomarker of obesity [49] confirming the findings of Barber and authors.

6.4. Lipidomic analysis in tissues from rodents

Gaining access to rodent organ samples is far more convenient than human tissues and thus can be used more readily to access intra-tissue lipid content. Sixteen-week old wild type (WT) and the leptin-deficient *ob/ob* mice, a genetic model of obesity that becomes overweight due to hyperphagia, were studied for their hepatic lipidomic profiles using non-targeted analysis via ultra-performance liquid chromatography (UPLC) coupled to quadrupole mass spectrometry (MS). The obese mice had an increased level of TAG and DAG lipid species in the liver as well as diacylphosphoglycerols and ceramide species, while there was a decrease in the sphingomyelins [50]. Using high-fat feeding to induce obesity, Turner et al. performed a tissue lipid profiling study over a course of time of the high-fat dietary intervention [51]. Liver TAG was increased after 1 week of high-fat feeding and peaked at 16 weeks of high-fat feeding whilst numerous DAG species were elevated in the liver at 1, 3 and 16 weeks of feeding. Hepatic ceramide content was unchanged after 1 week of high-fat feeding, the 20:0 and 22:0 species elevated at 3 weeks of feeding and the 18:0 and 20:0 species increased at 16 weeks of high-fat feeding. Whilst these species were increased with high-fat feeding, the 24:1 and 24:0 species were significantly decreased at both 3 and 16 weeks of high-fat feeding [51]. In the epididymal adipose tissue, TAG levels and numerous DAG species were elevated at 16 weeks of high-fat feeding. Ceramide and sphingomyelin species were increased at both 1 and 16 weeks of high-fat feeding. Analysis of the skeletal muscle revealed an increase in TAG and DAG levels at 3 and 16 weeks post-high-fat feeding, whilst in terms of ceramide levels, only the 18:0 ceramide species was increased at 3 and 16 weeks [51]. These studies have highlighted the lipid changes that occur in tissues during obesity induced by different means.

The use of metabolomics and lipidomics is set to continue as they may prove useful in providing indications of metabolic health in the obese setting. Identification of metabolites as"biomarkers" may make it possible to identify individuals at risk of developing obesity, which could be useful as a way of tracking disease progression and provide a predictive tool for diseases associated with obesity. These measures could also theoretically be used to give an indication of the effectiveness of new weight-loss therapies and their impact on metabolism. Studies have already taken place investigating bariatric surgery, in particular, Roux-en-Y gastric bypass surgery. How this type of surgery impacts the metabolome was not very well described so Arora et al. analysed the plasma metabolome and lipidome of morbidly obese individuals prior to and after surgery to describe the effects of surgery [52]. From 96 metabolites and 192 molecular lipid species compared, the factors that were most different at 42 days post-surgery were decanoic acid and octanoic acid whose levels increased and the sphingomyelins 18:1, 21:0 and 18:1, 22:3 whose levels decreased [52]. Moving forward, it is likely that a greater understanding of fluxomics will be utilised. Fluxomics is an analytical method that describes the rates of metabolic reactions within a sample. This is important as metabolism is a dynamic process, and metabolomics and lipidomics analysis will only provide a snapshot or static picture of the metabolic reactions in the cell. It could be stated well that it is not the quantity of metabolites that is important in the obese setting but the rates at which they undergo metabolic reactions.

7. Microbiomics

Metagenomics is a broad term used for the study of genetic material collected from environmental samples including but not limited to soil, sediment and water and in particular relevance to obesity, the gut. The gut microbiota contains all the organisms within the gut and the gut microbiome contains the genome that is within these organisms. Measuring the microbiomic status of the gut environment allows for the study of the composition of all microbes in that ecosystem. Whilst the microbiota consists of all bacteria, fungi, archea, viruses and other microbes, most of the research effort in relation to gut microbiota has been focused on the bacteria portion. This is no surprise given the widespread dominance of bacteria in and on the human body and indeed throughout all ecosystems on Earth. Also no surprise given the location of this ecosystem is the findings over the last decade that the composition of the gut microbiota is altered with obesity and is impacted by the diet of the host. The relationship between the composition and activity of the resident gut microbiota and the effect that this has on the metabolism of the host is currently being delicately teased out and it is an area that has really benefitted from the modern sequencing methods and analytical techniques. By identifying the microbiome and comparing results to electronic databases, an understanding can be formed on the species of bacteria that compose a microbiota community. Like other"omes" mentioned throughout this discussion, modern advances in technology regarding sequencing has allowed further insight into the precise make-up of the gut microbiota and how it is altered under different pathological conditions. At the forefront of these, analysis has been the use of highly conserved 16S sRNA genes as a molecular marker for microbial diversity (proxies for different species). With the development of sequencing technologies it has become possible to analyse all 16S rRNA genes in a sample and compare it with relevant databases that have been complied [53].

7.1. Gut microbiota and obesity in humans

Human gut microbiota composition is formed in early life with colonisation occurring over the first 3–5 years until it reaches a more stable, adult-like microbiota configuration [54]. However, in adulthood, alterations in this composition of bacteria can be observed in individuals with varying degrees of adiposity or metabolic health. Differences in the distal gut microbiota of obese versus lean humans has been demonstrated with the relative proportion of the phylum of bacteria named bacteroidetes found to be decreased in obese individuals compared to lean individuals, along with the finding that the bacteroidetes abundance increase as obese individuals lose weight [55]. These findings must be noted as somewhat controversial given other studies have shown no difference between obese and non-obese groups in relation to the proportion of bacteroidetes nor any change in the proportion of bacteroidetes measured in faeces once obese individuals lose weight [56]. These observed differences could come down to the way in which the samples were obtained, the methods involved in measuring the bacteria or the differing diets that the obese individuals recruited to the study were consuming. In this latter study, it was observed that the phylum of bacteria called Firmicutes was reduced in faecal samples from obese subjects on weight-loss diets, correlating changes in gut bacteria species to changes in adiposity [56]. It is difficult to distinguish whether changes in gut microbiota are just a response to obesity or weight loss are actually a causative factor.

One way to test whether human gut microbiota composition is causative in inducing an obesity-associated phenotype is to take gut microbiota from humans and populate the gut of germ-free mice (mice raised in an isolator so as to never be exposed to microorganisms) who have no gut microbiota. Although there are of course some species differences, on a whole, mice and humans share most of the same genes (~99%) and similar microbiota profiles making this type of experimental setup relevant for the evaluation of microbiota-induced physiological effects on the host [57]. Utilising faecal samples obtained from adult human female twins that were discordant for obesity, Ridaura et al. were able to demonstrate that an obesity phenotype is transmissible from human to rodent [58]. In these studies, germ-free mice were transplanted with the faecal matter of either the lean or obese human twin resulting in an increase in total body weight and fat mass in the mice receiving the microbiota from the obese twin. Intriguingly, if mice with the lean twin's microbiota and mice with the obese twin's microbiota were housed together (mice are coprophagic so will eat their cage mates' faeces), a recolonisation process occurred where bacteroidetes species from the lean microbiota invaded into the obese microbiota and this correlated with a protective metabolic phenotype where obesity-related traits were no longer observed. This raises the possibility of a potential protective effect on obesity of these bacteroidetes species [58].

7.2. Gut microbiota and obesity in animal models

Other studies utilising germ-free mice have demonstrated that microorganisms may have a role to play in dictating body weight. Germ-free mice have less body fat than regularly raised mice despite the fact they actually eat more and take in more calories which should oppose this affect [59]. Further studies in germ-free mice have demonstrated that an obese pheno-type is transmissible from mouse to mouse via the gut microbiota. Germ-free mice receiving microbiota transplants by oral gavage with microbiota either sourced from genetically obese *ob/ob* mice or lean mice have demonstrated that recipients of the *ob/ob* microbiota put on more body fat in the weeks after being inoculated as compared to those who received the "lean" microbiota transplant [60]. 16S-rRNA-gene-sequence-based analysis of samples obtained in this study demonstrated that the *ob/ob* donor microbiota samples had a greater abundance of firmicutes bacteria compared with that of the lean donor microbiota samples [60] indicating the possibility that enriching the gut with firmicutes may drive the body weight phenotype. Indeed a number of rodent studies have raised the possibility that the ratio of the phyla bac-teroidetes to that of the phyla firmicutes is associated with obesity. In comparison with lean mice, *ob/ob* mice have a ~50% reduction in the abundance of bacteroidetes and an increase in firmicutes [61]. High-fat feeding studies utilised to induce obesity via a dietary means also have found an increase in the firmicutes species [62] indicating that both obesity induced by hyperphagia (*ob/ob* mice) and obesity induced by energy dense food (high-fat diet) is associ-ated with an increase in firmicutes. As differences in gut microbiota communities may impact obesity and the metabolism of the host mouse, this should be considered a confounding factor when comparing different mouse strains, or the same mouse strain but from different mouse vendors or animal facilities as each facility is likely to harbour its own unique microbiota signature.

7.3. How would the gut microbiota cause obesity or contribute to obesity progression?

There are many possible reasons as to why the gut microbiota composition may impact the host and result in the development of obesity. First, certain types of gut microbiota may be more efficient in extracting energy out of food that passes through the gut and therefore make available more energy for the host in which they reside. Bomb calorimetry analysis measuring the energy content of faeces revealed that *ob/ob* mice have significantly less energy remain-ing in their faeces relative to their lean littermates suggestive that the microbiota within *ob/ob* mice are better at harvesting and extracting energy from the food within their digestive tract [60]. Other possibilities include the role of inflammation. Obesity has been associated with a type of chronic low-grade inflammation and modification of the gut microbiota has been suggested to increase the leakiness of the gut barrier resulting in the increased appearance of microbial products such as lipopolysaccharide (LPS) (endotoxin) in the circulation [63, 64]. These products could potential cause peripheral tissue inflammation and impede normal metabolism. Yet another possibility is the fact that the gut microbiota is responsible for the production of metabolites such as short-chain fatty acids (SCFAs) that are produced by the fermentation of dietary fibres by the bacteria in the gut [65]. SCFAs are organic acids with an aliphatic tail of less than six carbons and comprise of acetate, propionate, butyrate and valerate and are used by the host as an energy source. It is hypothesised that alterations in the production of these SCFAs with obesity could adversely affect satiety, hepatic glucose and lipid production as well as inflammatory processes and contribute to the progression of obesity and related conditions [66]. Thus, the microbiome composition can have an impact on another one of the"omes" the metabolome of the host and alter physiological processes via this mechanism. An interaction between the microbiome and the lipidome may also be at play. This is evident in a study of 893 individuals which identified 34 bacterial taxa associated with body mass index and blood lipids [67]. Cross-validation analysis revealed that the microbiota present explains 4.5% of the variance in body mass index observed and 6% of the plasma triglycerides variance and this was independent of factors such as age and sex that were taken into consideration in the analysis [67].

The gut microbiota may play an important role in the balance between metabolic health and disease. If a characteristic microbiota signature can be described and confirmed in obesity (or in specific types of obesity) then the potential exists to modify this composition and improve health. Whilst the simplest solution to restore the composition of the microbiota would be a change in diet, other avenues such as prebiotic, probiotics and microbiota transplants are also being explored.

8. Conclusion

Herein, we have provided a review of the information that has been sourced from the study of the various"omes" in relation to obesity—from the genome and epigenome that provided the initial coding information regarding body weight regulation right through to the functional"omes" the proteome and metabolome that carry out the physiological cellular functions of these codes. As further investment is made in technologies to increase the capability and detection of these"omic" molecules, a multi-disciplinary team approach will be required to extract the most information and perhaps more importantly, the most relevant physiological information in relation to obesity. A systems biology approach is needed to understand the complexity of the physiology of all the reactions that take place due to the interaction between all of the genetic, proteomic and metabolomic information. Engineers are vitally important in furthering the technological capacities of machinery and bioinformaticians in developing ways to explore these complicated data sets to ensure that the data are collected and analysed in a meaningful way. Graphical representation of the data in a digestible fashion is essential to foster understanding of these findings of scientists of different fields. Cell biologists, biochemists and physiologists will play an important role in characterising these findings in proof-of-concept experiments in laboratory, and health and medical practitioners armed with these findings will ultimately deliver knowledge and hopefully personalised treatment strategies to the obese patients in the clinic.

Author details

Darren Henstridge and Kiymet Bozaoglu*

*Address all correspondence to: Kiymet.bozaoglu@bakeridi.edu.au

Baker IDI Heart and Diabetes Institute, Melbourne, VIC, Australia

References

[1] NCDRF Collaboration, Trends in adult body-mass index in 200 countries from 1975 to 2014: a pooled analysis of 1698 population-based measurement studies with 19.2 million participants. Lancet, 2016. **387**(10026): pp. 1377–96.

[2] Lozano, R., et al., Global and regional mortality from 235 causes of death for 20 age groups in 1990 and 2010: a systematic analysis for the Global Burden of Disease Study 2010. Lancet, 2012. **380**(9859): pp. 2095–128.

[3] Malis, C., et al., Total and regional fat distribution is strongly influenced by genetic factors in young and elderly twins. Obes Res, 2005. **13**(12): pp. 2139–45.

[4] International Human Genome Sequencing Consortium, Finishing the euchromatic sequence of the human genome. Nature, 2004. **431**(7011): pp. 931–45.

[5] International HapMap Consortium, The International HapMap project. Nature, 2003. **426**(6968): pp. 789–96.

[6] Genomes Project Consortium, A map of human genome variation from population-scale sequencing. Nature, 2010. **467**(7319): pp. 1061–73.

[7] Wellcome Trust Case Control Consortium, Genome-wide association study of 14,000 cases of seven common diseases and 3,000 shared controls. Nature, 2007. **447**(7145): pp. 661–78.

[8] Frayling, T.M., et al., A common variant in the FTO gene is associated with body mass index and predisposes to childhood and adult obesity. Science, 2007. **316**(5826): pp. 889–94.

[9] Loos, R.J., et al., Common variants near MC4R are associated with fat mass, weight and risk of obesity. Nat Genet, 2008. **40**(6): pp. 768–75.

[10] Hagg, S., et al., Gene-based meta-analysis of genome-wide association studies implicates new loci involved in obesity. Hum Mol Genet, 2015. **24**(23): pp. 6849–60.

[11] Locke, A.E., et al., Genetic studies of body mass index yield new insights for obesity biology. Nature, 2015. **518**(7538): pp. 197–206.

[12] Shungin, D., et al., New genetic loci link adipose and insulin biology to body fat distribution. Nature, 2015. **518**(7538): pp. 187–96.

[13] Felix, J.F., et al., Genome-wide association analysis identifies three new susceptibility loci for childhood body mass index. Hum Mol Genet, 2016. **25**(2): pp. 389–403.

[14] Kilpelainen, T.O., et al., Genome-wide meta-analysis uncovers novel loci influencing circulating leptin levels. Nat Commun, 2016. **7**: p. 10494.

[15] Lu, Y., et al., New loci for body fat percentage reveal link between adiposity and cardiometabolic disease risk. Nat Commun, 2016. **7**: p. 10495.

[16] Manolio, T.A., et al., Finding the missing heritability of complex diseases. Nature, 2009. **461**(7265): pp. 747–53.

[17] Zuk, O., et al., The mystery of missing heritability: Genetic interactions create phantom heritability. Proc Natl Acad Sci U S A, 2012. **109**(4): pp. 1193–8.

[18] Zuk, O., et al., Searching for missing heritability: designing rare variant association studies. Proc Natl Acad Sci U S A, 2014. **111**(4): pp. E455–64.

[19] Barker, D.J. and C. Osmond, Infant mortality, childhood nutrition, and ischaemic heart disease in England and Wales. Lancet, 1986. **1**(8489): pp. 1077–81.

[20] McMillen, I.C., et al., The early origins of later obesity: pathways and mechanisms. Adv Exp Med Biol, 2009. **646**: pp. 71–81.

[21] Bouret, S., B.E. Levin, and S.E. Ozanne, Gene-environment interactions controlling energy and glucose homeostasis and the developmental origins of obesity. Physiol Rev, 2015. **95**(1): pp. 47–82.

[22] Dominguez-Salas, P., et al., Maternal nutrition at conception modulates DNA methylation of human metastable epialleles. Nat Commun, 2014. **5**: p. 3746.

[23] Williams-Wyss, O., et al., Embryo number and periconceptional undernutrition in the sheep have differential effects on adrenal epigenotype, growth, and development. Am J Physiol Endocrinol Metab, 2014. **307**(2): pp. E141–50.

[24] Li, C.C., et al., Maternal obesity and diabetes induces latent metabolic defects and widespread epigenetic changes in isogenic mice. Epigenetics, 2013. **8**(6): pp. 602–11.

[25] Suter, M.A., et al., In utero exposure to a maternal high-fat diet alters the epigenetic histone code in a murine model. Am J Obstet Gynecol, 2014. **210**(5): pp. 463e1–e11.

[26] Gluckman, P.D., et al., Metabolic plasticity during mammalian development is directionally dependent on early nutritional status. Proc Natl Acad Sci U S A, 2007. **104**(31): pp. 12796–800.

[27] Borengasser, S.J., et al., Maternal obesity enhances white adipose tissue differentiation and alters genome-scale DNA methylation in male rat offspring. Endocrinology, 2013. **154**(11): pp. 4113–25.

[28] Suter, M., et al., Epigenomics: maternal high-fat diet exposure in utero disrupts peripheral circadian gene expression in nonhuman primates. FASEB J, 2011. **25**(2): pp. 714–26.

[29] Ost, A., et al., Paternal diet defines offspring chromatin state and intergenerational obesity. Cell, 2014. **159**(6): pp. 1352–64.

[30] Begum, G., et al., Epigenetic changes in fetal hypothalamic energy regulating pathways are associated with maternal undernutrition and twinning. FASEB J, 2012. **26**(4): pp. 1694-703.

[31] Lan, X., et al., Maternal diet during pregnancy induces gene expression and DNA methylation changes in fetal tissues in sheep. Front Genet, 2013. **4**: p. 49.

[32] Tobi, E.W., et al., DNA methylation signatures link prenatal famine exposure to growth and metabolism. Nat Commun, 2014. **5**: p. 5592.

[33] Cooper, W.N., et al., DNA methylation profiling at imprinted loci after periconceptional micronutrient supplementation in humans: results of a pilot randomized controlled trial. FASEB J, 2012. **26**(5): pp. 1782–90.

[34] Sharp, G.C., et al., Maternal pre-pregnancy BMI and gestational weight gain, offspring DNA methylation and later offspring adiposity: findings from the Avon Longitudinal Study of parents and children. Int J Epidemiol, 2015. **44**(4): pp. 1288–304.

[35] Portela, A. and M. Esteller, Epigenetic modifications and human disease. Nat Biotechnol, 2010. **28**(10): pp. 1057–68.

[36] Aslibekyan, S., et al., Epigenome-wide study identifies novel methylation loci associated with body mass index and waist circumference. Obesity (Silver Spring), 2015. **23**(7): pp. 1493–501.

[37] Demerath, E.W., et al., Epigenome-wide association study (EWAS) of BMI, BMI change and waist circumference in African American adults identifies multiple replicated loci. Hum Mol Genet, 2015. **24**(15): pp. 4464–79.

[38] Crujeiras, A.B., et al., Genome-wide DNA methylation pattern in visceral adipose tissue differentiates insulin-resistant from insulin-sensitive obese subjects. Transl Res, 2016.

[39] Ali, O., et al., Methylation of SOCS3 is inversely associated with metabolic syndrome in an epigenome-wide association study of obesity. Epigenetics, 2016: pp. 1–9.

[40] Laird, P.W., The power and the promise of DNA methylation markers. Nat Rev Cancer, 2003. **3**(4): pp. 253–66.

[41] Campion, J., et al., TNF-alpha promoter methylation as a predictive biomarker for weight-loss response. Obesity (Silver Spring), 2009. **17**(6): pp. 1293–7.

[42] Arner, P., et al., The epigenetic signature of systemic insulin resistance in obese women. Diabetologia, 2016.

[43] Ronn, T., et al., A six months exercise intervention influences the genome-wide DNA methylation pattern in human adipose tissue. PLoS Genet, 2013. **9**(6): p. e1003572.

[44] Barres, R., et al., Weight loss after gastric bypass surgery in human obesity remodels promoter methylation. Cell Rep, 2013. **3**(4): pp. 1020–7.

[45] Huang, Y.T., et al., Epigenetic patterns in successful weight loss maintainers: a pilot study. Int J Obes (Lond), 2015. **39**(5): pp. 865–8.

[46] Vogel, C. and E.M. Marcotte, Insights into the regulation of protein abundance from proteomic and transcriptomic analyses. Nat Rev Genet, 2012. **13**(4): pp. 227–32.

[47] Humphrey, S.J., et al., Dynamic adipocyte phosphoproteome reveals that Akt directly regulates mTORC2. Cell Metab, 2013. **17**(6): pp. 1009–20.

[48] Wilson-Fritch, L., et al., Mitochondrial biogenesis and remodeling during adipogenesis and in response to the insulin sensitizer rosiglitazone. Mol Cell Biol, 2003. **23**(3): pp. 1085–94.

[49] Perez-Perez, R., et al., Differential proteomics of omental and subcutaneous adipose tissue reflects their unalike biochemical and metabolic properties. J Proteome Res, 2009. **8**(4): pp. 1682–93.

[50] Abu-Farha, M., et al., Proteomics analysis of human obesity reveals the epigenetic factor HDAC4 as a potential target for obesity. PLoS One, 2013. **8**(9): p. e75342.

[51] Zvonic, S., et al., Secretome of primary cultures of human adipose-derived stem cells: modulation of serpins by adipogenesis. Mol Cell Proteomics, 2007. **6**(1): pp. 18–28.

[52] Asfa, A.S., et al., Phosphoprotein network analysis of white adipose tissues unveils deregulated pathways in response to high-fat diet. Sci Rep, 2016. **6**: p. 25844.

[53] Xie, W.D., et al., Proteomic profile of visceral adipose tissues between low-fat diet-fed obesity-resistant and obesity-prone C57BL/6 mice. Mol Med Rep, 2010. **3**(6): pp. 1047–52.

[54] Baiges, I., et al., Lipogenesis is decreased by grape seed proanthocyanidins according to liver proteomics of rats fed a high fat diet. Mol Cell Proteomics, 2010. **9**(7): pp. 1499–513.

[55] Nesteruk, M., et al., Mitochondrial-related proteomic changes during obesity and fasting in mice are greater in the liver than skeletal muscles. Funct Integr Genomics, 2014. **14**(1): pp. 245–59.

[56] Hochberg, Z., Metabolomics of the obese. Int J Obes (Lond), 2006. **30**(Suppl 2): p. S4.

[57] Park, S., K.C. Sadanala, and E.K. Kim, A metabolomic approach to understanding the metabolic link between obesity and diabetes. Mol Cells, 2015. **38**(7): pp. 587–96.

[58] Felig, P., et al., Splanchnic glucose and amino acid metabolism in obesity. J Clin Invest, 1974. **53**(2): pp. 582–90.

[59] Martin, F.P., et al., Topographical body fat distribution links to amino acid and lipid metabolism in healthy obese women [corrected]. PLoS One, 2013. **8**(9): p. e73445.

[60] Yamakado, M., et al., Plasma amino acid profile is associated with visceral fat accumulation in obese Japanese subjects. Clin Obes, 2012. **2**(1-2): pp. 29–40.

[61] Newgard, C.B., et al., A branched-chain amino acid-related metabolic signature that differentiates obese and lean humans and contributes to insulin resistance. Cell Metab, 2009. **9**(4): pp. 311–26.

[62] Gao, X., et al., Serum metabolic biomarkers distinguish metabolically healthy peripherally obese from unhealthy centrally obese individuals. Nutr Metab (Lond), 2016. **13**: p. 33.

[63] Chen, H.H., et al., The metabolome profiling and pathway analysis in metabolic healthy and abnormal obesity. Int J Obes (Lond), 2015. **39**(8): pp. 1241–8.

[64] Dina, C., et al., Variation in FTO contributes to childhood obesity and severe adult obesity. Nat Genet, 2007. **39**(6): pp. 724–6.

[65] Kim, Y.J., et al., Association of metabolites with obesity and type 2 diabetes based on FTO genotype. PLoS One, 2016. **11**(6): p. e0156612.

[66] Kim, I.Y., et al., 1H NMR-based metabolomic study on resistance to diet-induced obesity in AHNAK knock-out mice. Biochem Biophys Res Commun, 2010. **403**(3-4): pp. 428–34.

[67] Kiehl, T.R., et al., Generation and characterization of Sca2 (ataxin-2) knockout mice. Biochem Biophys Res Commun, 2006. **339**(1): pp. 17–24.

[68] Meierhofer, D., et al., Ataxin-2 (Atxn2)-knock-out mice show branched chain amino acids and fatty acids pathway alterations. Mol Cell Proteomics, 2016. **15**(5): pp. 1728–39.

[69] Meikle, P.J. and M.J. Christopher, Lipidomics is providing new insight into the metabolic syndrome and its sequelae. Curr Opin Lipidol, 2011. **22**(3): pp. 210–5.

[70] Pietilainen, K.H., et al., Acquired obesity is associated with changes in the serum lipidomic profile independent of genetic effects--a monozygotic twin study. PLoS One, 2007. **2**(2): p. e218.

[71] Mamtani, M., et al., Plasma dihydroceramide species associate with waist circumference in Mexican American families. Obesity (Silver Spring), 2014. **22**(3): pp. 950–6.

[72] Rauschert, S., et al., Lipidomics reveals associations of phospholipids with obesity and insulin resistance in young adults. J Clin Endocrinol Metab, 2016. **101**(3): pp. 871–9.

[73] Barber, M.N., et al., Plasma lysophosphatidylcholine levels are reduced in obesity and type 2 diabetes. PLoS One, 2012. **7**(7): p. e41456.

[74] Scherer, M., et al., Blood plasma lipidomic signature of epicardial fat in healthy obese women. Obesity (Silver Spring), 2015. **23**(1): pp. 130–7.

[75] Perreault, L., et al., Biomarkers of ectopic fat deposition: The next frontier in serum lipidomics. J Clin Endocrinol Metab, 2016. **101**(1): pp. 176–82.

[76] Kolak, M., et al., Adipose tissue inflammation and increased ceramide content characterize subjects with high liver fat content independent of obesity. Diabetes, 2007. **56**(8): pp. 1960–8.

[77] Wentworth, J.M., et al., GM3 ganglioside and phosphatidylethanolamine-containing lipids are adipose tissue markers of insulin resistance in obese women. Int J Obes (Lond), 2016. **40**(4): pp. 706–13.

[78] Tonks, K.T., et al., Skeletal muscle and plasma lipidomic signatures of insulin resistance and overweight/obesity in humans. Obesity (Silver Spring), 2016. **24**(4): pp. 908–16.

[79] Li, F., et al., Lipidomics reveals a link between CYP1B1 and SCD1 in promoting obesity. J Proteome Res, 2014. **13**(5): pp. 2679–87.

[80] Yetukuri, L., et al., Bioinformatics strategies for lipidomics analysis: characterization of obesity related hepatic steatosis. BMC Syst Biol, 2007. **1**: p. 12.

[81] Turner, N., et al., Distinct patterns of tissue-specific lipid accumulation during the induction of insulin resistance in mice by high-fat feeding. Diabetologia, 2013. **56**(7): pp. 1638–48.

[82] Arora, T., et al., Roux-en-Y gastric bypass surgery induces early plasma metabolomic and lipidomic alterations in humans associated with diabetes remission. PLoS One, 2015. **10**(5): p. e0126401.

[83] Foster, J.A., et al., Measuring the microbiome: perspectives on advances in DNA-based techniques for exploring microbial life. Brief Bioinform, 2012. **13**(4): pp. 420–9.

[84] Rodriguez, J.M., et al., The composition of the gut microbiota throughout life, with an emphasis on early life. Microb Ecol Health Dis, 2015. **26**: p. 26050.

[85] Ley, R.E., et al., Microbial ecology: human gut microbes associated with obesity. Nature, 2006. **444**(7122): pp. 1022–3.

[86] Duncan, S.H., et al., Human colonic microbiota associated with diet, obesity and weight loss. Int J Obes (Lond), 2008. **32**(11): pp. 1720–4.

[87] Kostic, A.D., M.R. Howitt, and W.S. Garrett, Exploring host-microbiota interactions in animal models and humans. Genes Dev, 2013. **27**(7): pp. 701–18.

[88] Ridaura, V.K., et al., Gut microbiota from twins discordant for obesity modulate metabolism in mice. Science, 2013. **341**(6150): p. 1241214.

[89] Backhed, F., et al., The gut microbiota as an environmental factor that regulates fat storage. Proc Natl Acad Sci U S A, 2004. **101**(44): pp. 15718–23.

[90] Turnbaugh, P.J., et al., An obesity-associated gut microbiome with increased capacity for energy harvest. Nature, 2006. **444**(7122): pp. 1027–31.

[91] Ley, R.E., et al., Obesity alters gut microbial ecology. Proc Natl Acad Sci U S A, 2005. **102**(31): pp. 11070–5.

[92] Murphy, E.F., et al., Composition and energy harvesting capacity of the gut microbiota: relationship to diet, obesity and time in mouse models. Gut, 2010. **59**(12): pp. 1635–42.

[93] Lam, Y.Y., et al., Increased gut permeability and microbiota change associate with mesenteric fat inflammation and metabolic dysfunction in diet-induced obese mice. PLoS One, 2012. **7**(3): p. e34233.

[94] Cani, P.D., et al., Changes in gut microbiota control metabolic endotoxemia-induced inflammation in high-fat diet-induced obesity and diabetes in mice. Diabetes, 2008. **57**(6): pp. 1470–81.

[95] Boulange, C.L., et al., Impact of the gut microbiota on inflammation, obesity, and metabolic disease. Genome Med, 2016. **8**(1): p. 42.

[96] Hartstra, A.V., et al., Insights into the role of the microbiome in obesity and type 2 diabetes. Diabetes Care, 2015. **38**(1): pp. 159–65.

[97] Fu, J., et al., The gut microbiome contributes to a substantial proportion of the variation in blood lipids. Circ Res, 2015. **117**(9): pp. 817–24.

9

New Thoughts on Pediatric Genetic Obesity: Pathogenesis, Clinical Characteristics and Treatment Approach

Stefano Stagi, Martina Bianconi,

Maria Amina Sammarco, Rosangela Artuso,

Sabrina Giglio and Maurizio de Martino

Abstract

Historically, some genetic syndromes and monogenic forms of obesity have been identified by clinical features and by sequencing candidate genes in patients with severe obesity. The phenotypic expression of genetic factors involved in obesity is variable, thereby allowing to distinguish several clinical pictures of obesity. Monogenic obesity is described as rare and severe early-onset obesity with abnormal feeding behavior and endocrine disorders. Many of the findings emerged from studying families who displayed a classical Mendelian pattern of inheritance. On the contrary, patients with syndromic obesity show a various degree of intellectual disability, different dysmorphic features, and organ-specific abnormalities. But to date, not all involved genes have been identified so far. New diagnostic tools, such as genome-wide studies, array CGH, and whole-exome sequencing, have highlighted more complex models of inheritance, and even more candidate genes were identified. This increase of knowledge may provide insights into the mechanisms involved in the regulation of body weight and finally lead to specific treatments. In these patients, hyperphagia is often a primary phenotypic component. Substantial gaps in understanding the molecular basis of inherited hyperphagia syndromes are present today with a lack of mechanistic targets that can serve as a basis for pharmacologic and behavioral treatments. We have evaluated retrospectively the literature data on weight, body mass index (BMI), clinical features, treatments, and treatment response in pediatric patients with forms of genetic obesity. However, this chapter provides an updated picture of emerging knowledge outlined by the more comprehensive genetic approaches, trying to outline more candidate genes for these forms of genetic obesity. Relevant papers will be identified through systematic searches of the PubMed, EMBASE and Cochrane databases. All published studies in the English language concerning these disorders will be evaluated. Keywords in the literature search will be entered in all combinations. Searches will be augmented by manually reviewing the reference lists of all original articles and all systematic review articles, with each study being evaluated for inclusion.

Keywords: obesity, children, adolescence, next-generation sequencing, array CGH, pediatrics, diabetes, hyperphagia

1. Introduction

The World Health Organization defines being overweight and obesity as a "clinical condition characterized by an abnormal or excessive fat accumulation that may impair health" [1]. In 2014, an estimated 41 million children under the age of 5 were overweight or obese [1]. Once considered a problem only in high-income countries, being overweight and obesity are now dramatically on the rise in low- and middle-income countries, particularly in urban settings [1].

Therefore, obesity is considered a global epidemic and can cause serious health repercussions. In fact, in addition to causing a significant morbidity and premature mortality and to have psychological and social consequences, it is associated with medical conditions, such as type II diabetes (non-insulin-dependent diabetes mellitus or NIDDM), hypertension, coronary artery disease and many forms of cancer [2].

In order to create the best management programs and to determine novel therapeutic targets, it has become essential to understand the factors causing today's rising epidemic of childhood obesity [3].

Obesity is a complex condition, caused by multiple factors. It is characterized by an altered energy system, determined by the interaction of biological, social, and behavioral factors that cause an increase in food intake and a reduction in energy expenditure [4].

This global epidemic and the increase of its prevalence show that this condition is the result not only of genetic causes, but also of environmental factors (high availability of palatable and energy dense foods) [4]. However, some individuals manage to maintain a healthy body weight in an "obesogenic" environment, but the weight gain may be determined by their genetic susceptibility [4].

Recently, major advances in obesity research emerged concerning the molecular mechanisms contributing to the obese condition. However, several studies and data concerning the genetics and other important factors in the susceptibility risk of developing obesity are became increasingly evident [5]; in fact, available data suggest that 40–77% of the observed variance in human body weight can be accounted for, by inherited factors [6–8].

The strongest risk factor for childhood and adolescent obesity is parental obesity [9]. The risk becomes especially elevated if both parents are obese [10]. On the contrary, the pattern of inheritance of monogenic obesity is different (which may or may not be related to specific syndromes). In fact, they are attributable to a Mendelian model which recognizes a rare causative mutation to load a single gene that can be expressed in the heterozygous and homozygous state [11].

Patients can be affected by monogenic forms, in which obesity is the predominant feature but it is not associated with malformations, or by syndromic obesity: in the latter case, they show also a pattern of clinical features, including developmental delay, dysmorphic features, and/or other developmental abnormalities [12].

Furthermore, historically, some genetic syndromes and monogenic forms of obesity have been identified by clinical features and by sequencing candidate genes in patients with severe obesity. Many of the initial findings emerged from studying families who displayed a classical Mendelian pattern of inheritance; however, more comprehensive genetic approaches, such as genome-wide studies, array CGH, and next-generation sequencing examinations, have highlighted more complex models of inheritance, and ever more candidate genes were identified [13]. In broad terms, most cases of patients with genetic forms of obesity are oligogenic, determined by interaction between genetic and environmental factors. In these cases, the genetic make-up influences weight and the individual responses to nutrition and physical activity. In addition to this form of obesity, there are others caused by a single gene or it appears to be related to a specific syndrome. Monogenic obesity typically is caused by a single gene mutation with severe obesity as the main symptom; syndromic obesity, on the other hand, has many characteristics, of which obesity is one symptom [13].

The increase of knowledge about the functional and physiological features of these different obesity forms may provide insights into the mechanisms involved in the regulation of body weight and finally lead to specific treatments. In these patients, hyperphagia is frequently a primary phenotypic component. Substantial gaps in understanding the molecular basis of inherited hyperphagia syndromes are present today with a lack of mechanistic targets that can serve as a basis for pharmacologic and behavioral treatments.

The comprehension of the molecular mechanisms of obesity progressed enormously in the last years thanks to the development of faster and more precise genetic screening tools applied in cohort studies or in examinations with focus on subjects and their families.

Several clinical presentations in obesity depend on the genes involved:

1. Monogenic obesity, described as rare and severe early-onset obesity, associated with endocrine disorders. The impact of genetics is high and only little dependent on environmental factors.

2. Syndromic obesity that corresponds to severe obesity associated with additional phenotypes (mental retardation, dysmorphic features, and organ-specific developmental abnormalities). Prader-Willi (PWS) and Bardet-Biedl (BBS) syndromes are the two most frequently linked to obesity, but more than 100 syndromes are now associated with obesity.

3. Oligogenic obesity, characterized by a variable severity, partly dependent on environmental factors and the absence of a specific phenotype. This type of obesity is responsible for 2–3% in adults and children.

Rare genetic forms of obesity are important to be detected clinically because it allows to progress in understanding the physiopathology of obesity. On the other hand, there is a specific management of these forms of obesity provided by specialized and multidisciplinary teams.

2. Monogenic obesity

A "monogene" is by textbook definition, a gene with a strong effect on the phenotype (Mendelian traits or Mendelian—single gene conditions), giving rise to a one-on-one relationship between genotype and phenotype.

So, monogenic and not syndromic obesity is caused by a single mutation of a gene.

This form of obesity occurs in infancy and is often associated with additional behavior, developmental or endocrinological disabilities, such as hyperphagia and hypogonadism; however, significant developmental delays are not visible, and the obesity is often not associated with other clinical manifestations [3, 6, 8, 13–17].

The types of monogenic obesity are summarized in **Table 1** [10–12, 18].

Monogenic obesity	Gene name	Main distinguishing features in addition to obesity
LEP deficiency	*LEP*	Hypogonadism, absent or delayed puberty, frequent infections, undetectable serum leptin
LEPR deficiency	*LEPR*	Hypogonadism, absent or delayed puberty
SH2B2 deficiency	*SH2B1*	Severe insulin resistance and disproportionate to degree of obesity; in rare cases presence of developmental delay
POMC deficiency	*POMC*	Hypogonadism, absent or delayed puberty, hair and cute hypopigmentation, isolated ACTH deficiency
MC4-R deficiency	*MC4-R*	Accelerated growth, increased final height
PCSK1 deficiency	*PCSK1*	Hypogonadism, absent or delayed puberty, postprandial hypoglycemia, elevated plasma proinsulin, severe malabsorption in the neonatal period
SIM1 deficiency	*SIM 1*	Spectrum of developmental delay
BDNF/trkB deficiency	*BDNF o NTRK2*	Developmental delay, hyperactivity, impaired memory, impaired pain sensation
CART deficiency	*CART*	Anxiety and depression

Adapted with permission from Ramachandrappa and Farooqi [19].

Table 1. Main features of monogenic not syndromic obesity.

These types of monogenic obesity are caused by mutations in leptin–melanocortin hypothalamic pathway genes. These genes regulate the sense of appetite and hunger (**Figure 1**).

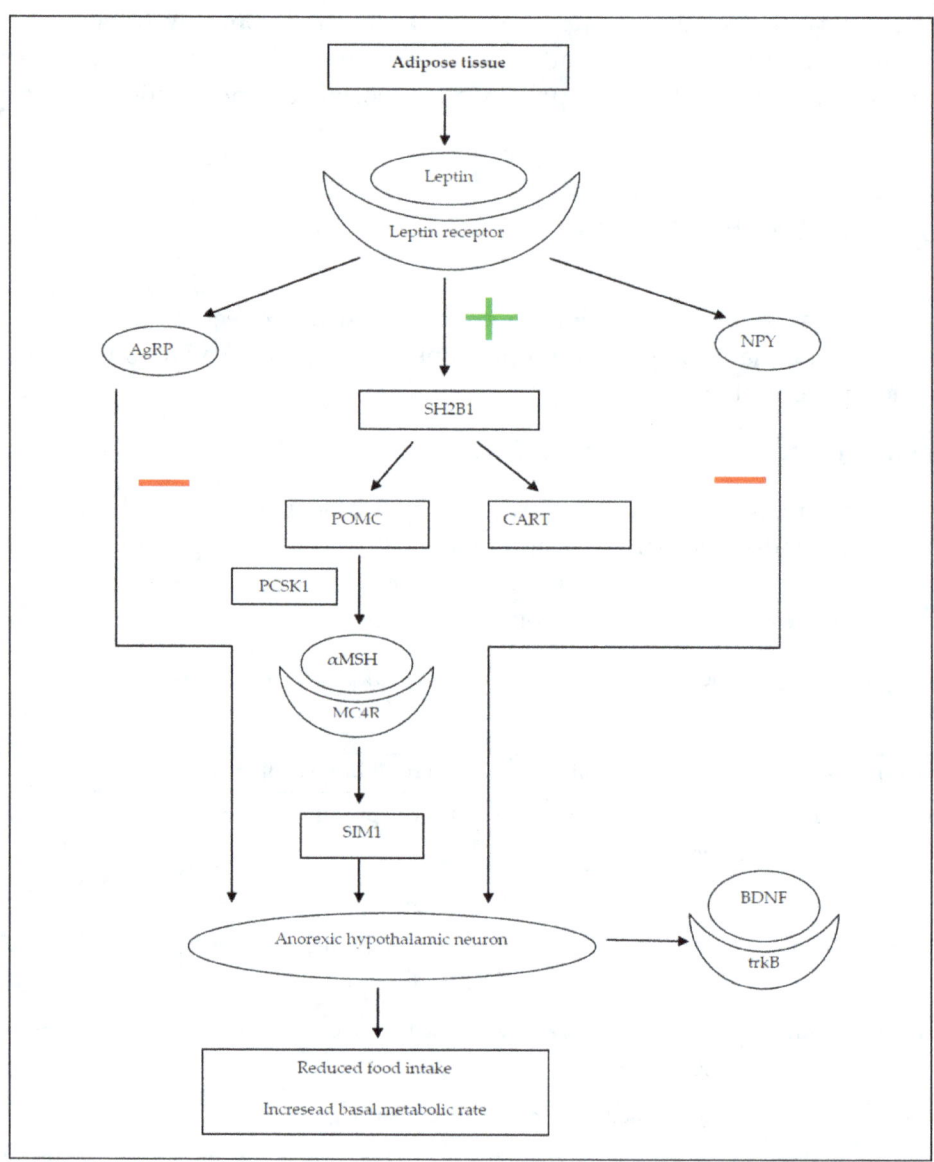

Figure 1. Appetite regulation: inhibitory (-) and favoring (+) mechanisms. Adapted with permission from Perrone et al. [11].

2.1. Congenital leptin deficiency (OMIM #614962)

In 1997, two severely obese cousins (an 8-year-old female child with a weight of 86 kg and a 2-year-old male child with a weight of 29 kg) were reported from a highly consanguineous family of Pakistani origin [20]. Despite their severe obesity, both children had undetectable levels of serum leptin and a mutation in the gene encoding leptin mapped at 7q32.1. The disease is caused by mutations in the *LEP* gene (OMIM *164160) typically leading to defects in protein synthesis or secretion, and therefore to the absence or very low blood levels of this hormone [21–23].

However, recently the first cases of functional leptin deficiency have been described [23, 24]. This entity is characterized by detectable immunoreactive levels of circulating leptin, but bioinactivity of the hormone due to defective receptor binding [23, 24].

So, serum leptin may be a useful marker in patients with severe early-onset obesity as an undetectable serum leptin is highly suggestive of a diagnosis of congenital leptin deficiency due to homozygous loss of function mutations in the *LEP* gene [12]. Leptin-deficient subjects are born of normal birth weight but exhibit rapid weight gain in the first few months of life resulting in severe obesity [25].

Leptin deficiency causes the loss of appetite control, so it is associated with hyperphagia, increased energy intake and aggressive behavior when food is denied. Other phenotypic features include hypothalamic hypothyroidism, hypogonadotropic hypogonadism (because leptin stimulates hypothalamic gonadotropin-releasing hormone [GnRH] production), elevated plasma insulin, T-cell abnormalities (because leptin also stimulates the inflammatory response and proliferation of T cells and cytokines Th1 mediated), and advanced bone age [26]. Currently, the prevalence of mutations in leptin is about 1% [12].

Leptin deficiency is entirely treatable with daily subcutaneous injections of recombinant human leptin with beneficial effects on the degree of hyperphagia, reversal of the immune defects and infection risk and permissive effects on the development of puberty [25]. The major effect of leptin administration is the normalization of hyperphagia and enhanced satiety [25, 27].

2.2. Congenital leptin-receptor deficiency (OMIM #614963)

In 1998 (1 year after the discovery of the congenital leptin deficiency), patients with similar phenotypic characteristic of leptin deficiency, but with a high blood level of leptin, were reported [28]. In these patients, a mutation in the leptin receptor (*LEPR*, OMIM *601007), mapped at 1p31.3, has been described [28].

One subsequent study has demonstrated that 3% of a group of patients with severe, early-onset obesity had a pathogenic *LEPR* mutation, but blood levels of leptin were not very high, suggesting that blood leptin levels cannot be used as a marker for leptin-receptor deficiency [29].

In literature, many mutations of the leptin receptor are described. Most recently, three novel mutations have been reported in the *LEPR* in two unrelated affected obese girls when latest genetic analysis techniques like whole-exome sequencing and targeted sequencing have been used for the mutational analysis in this gene [30, 31].

The clinical phenotypes associated with congenital leptin-receptor deficiency are similar to those of leptin deficiency, with severe obesity from the first few months of the life, hypothalamic hypothyroidism and hypogonadotropic hypogonadism [12, 26].

On the contrary, in these patients, because of a non-functional LEPR, leptin treatment is ineffective. Other factors could possibly bypass normal leptin delivery systems, but these are not yet currently available for the treatment of these patients [32].

2.3. SH2B1 deficiency

The Src-homology-2 B adaptor protein 1 (*SH2B1*, OMIM *608937) is a key intermediary in leptin signaling, promoting the activation of the leptin signaling pathway downstream of Janus kinase 2 (*JAK2*, OMIM *147796) [15]. So, leptin-stimulated activation of hypothalamic JAK2 is dramatically attenuated in *SH2B1* knockout mice [33].

In 2010, it was described that the 220-kb 16p11.2 deletion (28.73–28.95 Mb) seen in three patients co-segregated with severe early-onset obesity alone [14]. This deletion includes a small number of genes, one of which was *SH2B1*, known to be involved in leptin and insulin signaling [12]. However, several mutations in the *SH2B1* gene have also been reported in association with early-onset obesity, severe insulin resistance and behavioral abnormalities in some patients [34].

The phenotype of the children with *SH2B1*-containing deletions is characterized by extreme hyperphagia and fasting insulin levels disproportionately elevated compared to age and obesity-matched controls [15]. As expected, obese *SH2B1* KO mice develop hyperglycemia, hyperinsulinemia, glucose intolerance, and insulin resistance and NIDDM [35]. Interestingly, central and peripheral SH2B1 seem to regulate insulin sensitivity and glucose metabolism independently of its action on body weight in man and mice [36].

In these patients, there is no specific treatment, but care must be taken in starting a specific follow-up on the hyperphagia, obesity and alteration of gluco-insulinemic metabolism.

2.4. POMC deficiency (OMIM #609734)

In 1997, a role of central melanocortin signaling in the control of energy homeostasis was known [37]. Proopiomelanocortin (POMC) acts on anorectic targets of leptin in the brain [38]. The POMC, through to proconvertase 1 (PCSK1), is the precursor of a-melanocyte-stimulating-hormone anorectic peptide (a-MSH); the latter acts on melanocortin 4 receptor (MC4-R) anorectic neurons and suppresses the appetite and food intake [39].

Monogenic obesity from POMC deficiency manifests itself when there are homozygous null mutations. Heterozygous carriers of null *POMC* gene mutations have a significantly higher risk of being obese or overweight but are not invariably associated with obesity [19].

Since POMC is the precursor of adrenocorticotropic hormone (ACTH) and melanocyte-stimulating-hormone anorectic peptide (MSH), POMC-deficient newborns have adrenal crisis and pale skin and hair. Also, POMC deficiency causes hyperphagia and childhood obesity [3, 40]. The clinical features are comparable to those reported in patients with mutations in the receptor for POMC-derived ligands, MC4R (see below in the next chapter) [12].

Two important *POMC* mutations have been described in literature: the first is the rare mutation *R236G* that disrupts a di-basic cleavage site between β-MSH and β-endorphin, resulting in a β-MSH/β-endorphin fusion protein that binds to MC4R but has reduced ability to activate the receptor [38, 41]. The second is a rare missense mutation in the region encoding β-MSH, *Tyr221Cys* that cannot bind to and activate signaling from the MC4R, and obese children carrying the *Tyr221Cys* variant are hyperphagic and showed increased linear growth, features of MC4R deficiency [42].

Specific treatment was not available until January 2016, when the US Food and Drug Administration awarded orphan drug status to the first α-MSH-based therapy for obesity. The α-MSH analog RM-493 [43, 44], also known as setmelanotide, was awarded orphan drug status for POMC deficiency and Prader-Willi syndrome [37].

2.5. Melanocortin-4 receptor deficiency (MC4R)

Among all forms of monogenic obesity, the most common is caused by MC4-R deficiency. Heterozygous mutations have been reported in many ethnic groups of obese patients and prevalence varies from 0.5 to 1.0% in obese adults, up to 6% in individuals with severe infantile onset obesity [45]. In 2014, a case of childhood obesity associated with compound heterozygosity for two mutations of *MC4R* gene (OMIM *155541), mapped at 18q21.32, was described [46]. In the same year, another new inactivating homozygous mutation of the *MC4R* gene in a girl with the severe obesity and hyperphagia was reported [47].

Mutations of this gene are codominant with variable penetrance and expressivity in heterozygous carriers [48]. Both heterozygous and homozygous mutations in *MC4R* have been implicated in obesity, but extreme obesity is incompletely penetrant in heterozygous patients [3]. Also, in these patients, genetic and environmental factors influence the severity of obesity associated with mutations of *MC4-R*.

The main clinical features include hyperphagia in early appearance (but not as severe as that seen in leptin deficiency) and an increase in fat mass, lean mass and bone mineral density [45]. These patients also have an accelerated growth that seems to be a consequence of hyperinsulinemia which such patients present from the earliest periods of life. It is apparently not related to a dysfunction of the GH axis [3, 49]. Despite this early hyperinsulinemia, obese adult subjects who are heterozygous for mutations in the *MC4R* gene are not at increased risk of developing glucose intolerance and NIDDM compared to controls of similar age and adiposity [12, 45].

Currently, there are no specific therapies for the MC4-R deficiency, but these individuals may benefit from surgical therapies, which could be taken into consideration in adults [12].

2.6. PCSK1 deficiency (OMIM #600955)

Pro-protein convertases (PCs) are a family of serine endoproteases that cleave inactive pro-peptides into biologically active peptides [50]. Two of these pro-protein, proprotein convertase, subtilisin/kexin-type 1 (PCSK1) and PCSK2 are selectively expressed in neuroendocrine tissues and cleave pro-hormones such as POMC, thyrotropin-releasing hormone (TRH), GnRH, proinsulin, proglucagon [12].

Patients with heterozygous or homozygous mutations in the *PCSK1* gene (OMIM *162150), mapped at 5q15, present small bowel enteropathy, early-onset obesity and complex neuroendocrine effects due to a failure to process the pro-hormones such as diabetes insipidus, glucocorticoid deficiency, hypogonadism, and altered glucose homeostasis [51, 52].

A typical characteristic of these patients is a history of severe intestinal malabsorption in the neonatal period, probably due to altered cleavage of intestinal peptides in the enteroendocrine cells [51].

Over the past few years, two meta-analysis about *PCSK1* mutations have been published: the first in 2014 confirmed the association of *PCSK1* SNPs with obesity and provides the first evidence that the association between *PCSK1 rs6232* and obesity is stronger for childhood obesity than for adult obesity; the second meta-analysis tried to study the association of *PCSK1* variants *rs6232* and *rs6234/rs6235* with quantitative BMI variation and common obesity risk in subjects from diverse ethnic groups. In this study, cohort age-group significantly modulated the association between *rs6232*, *rs6234/rs6235* and obesity with the effect sizes for both SNPs being stronger in children/adolescents than in adults.

It is thought also that the most common PCSK1 variants predispose to obesity especially in an "obesogenic" environment with free access to high-caloric food [53].

Currently, there are no specific therapies for the PCSK1 deficiency, but these individuals frequently required a prolonged course of parenteral nutrition therapy, particularly in the first year of life [54]. However, exogenous administration of several hormone may be necessary in relation to the hormonal deficiencies diagnosed [54].

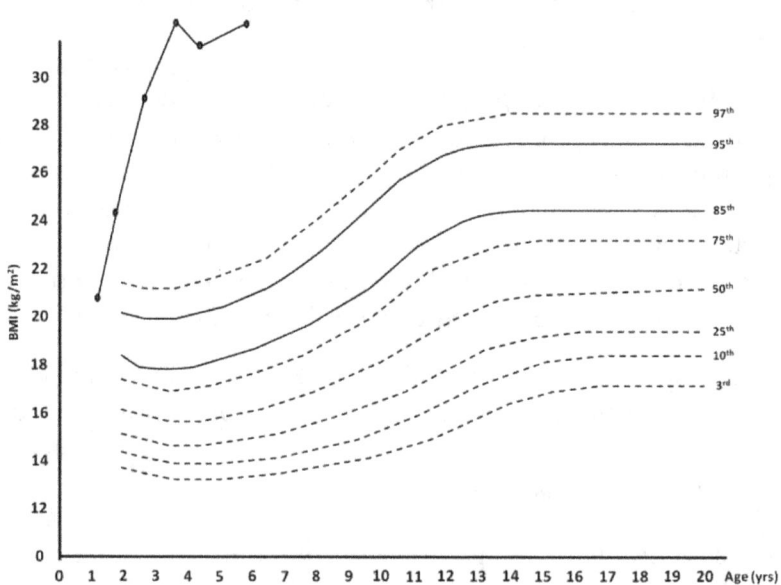

Figure 2. Girl with 6q16.3 deletion involving *SIM1* gene. It is evident that the extreme increase of the BMI of the patient and the reduction after the interdisciplinary approach.

2.7. SIM1 deficiency

Single-minded 1 (SIM1) is a transcription factor involved in the development of the supraoptic and paraventricular nuclei, acting downstream signal cascade of MC4-R. Obesity and hyperphagia have been reported in a patient with a balanced translocation disrupting *SIM1* [55] and multiple heterozygous missense mutations (6q16.3; OMIM *603128) [56]. However, some mutations of *SIM1* have incomplete penetrance and variable phenotype [57]. The similar phenotype between patients with SMI1 and MC4-R deficiency suggests that some effects of SIM1 are mediated by altered melanocortin signaling. On the other hand, some children with *SIM1* mutations have neuro-behavioral disorders including autism spectrum and "Prader-Willi-like" phenotype (**Figure 2**) [3, 12].

In mice, hyperphagia associated with SIM1 deficit can be improved by the administration of oxytocin, a neurotransmitter involved in the modulation of emotion (impaired oxytocinergic signaling is also one possible mechanism implicated in the obesity) [58].

2.8. Other types of non-syndromic genetic obesity

Mutations of the *BDNF* (*brain-derived neurotrophic factor*, OMIM *113505, mapped at 11p14.1) and its receptor TrKb (*tyrosin kinase B receptor*, OMIM *600456, mapped at 9q21.33) are rare causes of monogenic obesity acting downstream signal cascade of MC4-R and blocking translation [59].

BDNF's role in energy homeostasis emerged in the 1990s with the observation that intracerebroventricular BDNF administration suppresses appetite and induces weight loss in rodents, and *Bdnf* heterozygous knockout mice exhibit hyperphagia and obesity [60]. Complete lack of BDNF during embryologic development is perinatally lethal, but haploinsufficiency for BDNF or inactivating mutations of the BDNF receptor was associated with increased ad libitum food intake, severe early-onset obesity, hyperactivity, and cognitive impairment [60, 61]. Multiple genome-wide association studies of obesity in children and adults of different racial and ethnic populations have found associations for single-nucleotide polymorphisms (SNPs) at the BDNF locus and BMI, in particular for *G196A* variant (*rs6265*), which leads to a valine to methionine substitution at the 66th amino acid position (*Val66Met*) of the N-terminal prodomain of pro-BDNF. Furthermore, modifying factors—particularly sex, lifestyle behaviors, and psychotropic medication use—appear to be important confounders for the association between rs6265 and BMI [60–62]. In addition, the minor C allele of intronic *rs12291063* SNP was associated with lower BDNF expression and higher BMI [63].

NTRK2 (*TrkB*) mutation (which interferes with receptor autophosphorylation) causes the same symptoms of BDNF deficiency such as hyperphagia, obesity, impaired nociception, and intellectual disability [64, 65]. Recently, a *de novo* mutations in *TrkB* was found in a boy with severe obesity and impairment in learning, memory and nociception, and in a girl with hyperphagia and severe obesity [66].

Another cause of non-syndromic monogenic obesity is due to a gene mutation of *CART* (*cocaine- and amphetamine-regulated transcript*, OMIM *602606), mapped at 5q13.2. CART is an anorexigenic peptide produced by specific hypotalamic neurons in response to the stimulus of leptin. It would appear to mediate the termogenetic effects and energy expenditures characteristic of leptin. It has been shown that mutations in the *CART* gene are associated with reduced levels of the peptide encoded by it. Adolescents carrying a missense mutation in the *CART* gene exhibit severe obesity associated with anxiety and depression [11, 67, 68].

Other recent forms of monogenic obesity, still being defined, are associated with *MRAP2* (*melanocortin 2 receptor accessory protein 2*, OMIM *615410, mapped at 6q14.2) mutation encoding a *MC4-R* co-receptor, and with *KSR2* (*Kinase suppressor of Ras 2*. OMIM *610737, mapped at 12q24.22-q24.23) mutation, a protein involved in intracellular signal with a role in energy homeostasis [69–72].

3. Syndromic obesity

To date have been identified syndromic forms (e.g., Prader-Willi Syndrome) in which obesity can be associated with other signs and symptoms, such as intellectual disability, dysmorfic features and unusual behaviors.

In these syndromes, obesity can be caused by hyperphagia because are involved genes related to central nervous system appetite control centers.

Recently, the genetic bases for some of these syndromes have been elucidated and are beginning to provide insights into the pathogenesis of the derangements of energy homeostasis.

Table 2 reports the main syndromic forms of obesity. High-throughput technologies, and in particular copy number variants (CNVs) detection, are likely to result in the identification and recognition of multiple new syndromes where obesity and developmental delay are closely associated [12].

Syndrome	Clinical features in addition to obesity	Prevalence	Genetic
Bardet-Biedl	Mental retardation, retinal dystrophy or pigmentary retinopathy, dysmorphic extremities, hypogonadism, kidney anomalies	1/125,000 to 1/175,000 births	BBS1 (11q13); BBS2 (16q12.2); BBS3 (*ARL6*, 3q11); BBS4 (15q24.1); BBS5 (2q31.1); BBS6 (*MKKS*, 20p12); BBS7 (4q27); BBS8 (*TTC8*, 14q31); BBS9 (*PTHB1*, 7p14); BBS10 (*C12ORF58*, 12q21.2); BBS 11 (*TRIM32*, 9q33.1); BBS12 (*FLJ35630*, 4q27); BBS13 (*MKS1*, 17q23); BBS14 (*CEP290*, 12q21.3); BBS15 (*WDPCP*, 2p15); BBS16 (*SDCCAG8*, 1q43); BBS17 (*LZTFL1*, 3p21); BBS18 (*BBIP1*, 10q25); BBS19 (*IFT27*, 22q12)
Prader-Willi	Neonatal hypotonia, mental retardation, hyperphagia,	1/25,000 births	Lack of the paternal segment 15q11-q13 (microdeletion, maternal disomy, imprinting

Syndrome	Clinical features in addition to obesity	Prevalence	Genetic
	facial dysmorphy, hypogonadotrophic hypogonadism, short stature		defect or reciprocal translocation)
Cohen	Retinal dystrophy, prominent central incisors, dysmorphic extremities, microcephaly, cyclic neutropenia	Diagnosed in fewer than 1000 patients worldwide	Autosomal recessive *COH1* gene (chr 8q22-q23)
Alström	Retinal dystrophy, neurosensory deafness, diabetes, dilated cardiomyopathy	Diagnosed in about 950 patients worldwide	Autosomal recessive *ALMS1* gene (chr 2p13-p14)
X fragile	Mental retardation, hyperkinetic behavior, macroorchidism, large ears, prominent jaw	1/2500 births	X-linked *FMR1* gene (Xq27.3)
Borjeson-Forssman-Lehmann	Mental retardation, hypotonia, hypogonadism, facial dysmorphy with large ears, epilepsy	Approximately 50 reported patients	X-linked *PHF6* gene (Xq26-q27)
Albright hereditary osteodystrophy	Short stature, skeletal defects, facial dysmorphy, endocrine anomalies	1/1,000,000 births	Autosomal dominant *GNAS1* gene (20q13.2)
Ulnar–mammary	Upper limb malformation (from hypoplasia of the terminal phalanx of the fifth digit to aplasia of hand and upper limbs on the ulnar side), abnormal development of mammary glands and nipples, teeth, genitalia, and of apocrine glands		Autosomal dominant *TBX3* gene (12q24.21)
Simpson-Golabi-Behmel	Multiple congenital abnormalities, pre-/post-natal overgrowth, distinctive craniofacial features, macrocephaly, and organomegaly.		X-linked *GPC4* gene (Xq26)
MEHMO syndrome	Mental retardation, epileptic seizures, hypogenitalism, microcephaly and obesity	Approximately <1/1,000,000 births	X-linked locus MEHMO (Xp22.13-p21.1)
1p36 deletion syndrome	Delayed growth, malformations, moderate to severe intellectual disability, seizures, hearing and vision impairment, and certain particular facial features.	1/5000 to 1/10,000 live births	Autosomal dominant microdeletion of 1p36
16p11.2 deletion syndrome	Developmental delay, intellectual disability, autism spectrum disorders, impaired communication, socialization skills	Approximately 3/10,000 births	Autosomal dominant microdeletion of 16p11.2
ACP1, TMEM18, MYT1L deletion	Hyperphagia, intellectual deficiency, severe behavioral difficulties	Approximately 13 reported patients	Paternal deletion encompassing the *ACP1, TMEM18, MYT1L* genes (2p25)

Table 2. Main forms of syndromic obesity.

3.1. Developmental obesity syndromes involving ciliary dysfunction

Some genes linked to obesity have been associated with the function or formation of primary cilia, subcellular organelles, which serve a sensory function for most cell types. The ciliopathies form a class of genetic disease whose etiology lies with primary ciliary dysfunction. Some peculiar features can be found, such as retinal degeneration. This feature is of particular interest for its clinical relevance, rarity, and diagnostic power. Between these groups of diseases, we can include the Bardet-Biedl syndrome (BBS) and Alström syndrome (ALMS).

BBS has become a model ciliopathy because it became the first disease whose etiology lay in primary ciliary disorder [73]. It is a rare autosomal recessive genetic disorder with severe multiorgan impairment [74]. Its frequency in Europe and North America falls below 1:100,000 [75]. The disease symptoms may significantly vary between the patients; therefore, the diagnosis relies on the number of primary and secondary features of BBS [74]. Multiple articles summarize the data on frequencies of various symptoms in BBS patients [75, 76]. However, it is very important to realize that almost all clinical studies analyzed patients of various ages. Many individuals with BBS look virtually healthy at birth unless they were born with a polydactyly. Other symptoms of BBS tend to gradually emerge during or after the first decade of life; thus, patients diagnosed at early childhood tend to have fewer clinical features of the disease [74]. There are six primary features of BBS, that is, rod-cone dystrophy, polydactyly, obesity, genital abnormalities, renal defects, and learning difficulties. Secondary features include developmental delay, speech deficit, brachydactyly or syndactyly, dental defects, ataxia or poor coordination, olfactory deficit, diabetes mellitus, and congenital heart disease [75]. Some authors also mention hypertension, liver abnormalities, bronchial asthma, otitis, rhinitis, craniofacial dysmorphism, etc. [75–78].

However, the phenotype can be different: generally, obesity occurs early in life of patients affected by BBS, but the literature shows that 52% of post-pubertal BBS patients are obese [79]. It is recommended to assign BBS diagnosis to patients bearing at least 4 out of 6 primary features of the disease. If only three primary features are detected, two secondary features are required to confirm the presence of BBS.

These criteria describe BBS mainly as a clinical entity; they do not fully account to the existence of patients with attenuated forms of the disease as well as to possible gene-specific manifestations of BBS [80, 81].

At least 20 BBS genes have already been identified, and all of them are involved in primary cilia functioning. Genetic diagnosis of BBS is complicated due to lack of gene-specific disease symptoms; however, it is gradually becoming more accessible with the invention of multigene sequencing technologies [74].

The first five BBS loci were identified via linkage analysis of large BBS pedigrees [82–86] with corresponding genes cloned some years later [87–92]. The first gene assigned to BBS was *MKKS* (*MKS*; OMIM *604896) already known to induce McKusick-Kaufman syndrome; given that it did not belong to previously identified BBS loci, it was named *BBS6*. At present, there are already 21 known BBS genes (*BBS1–BBS20* and *NPHP1*), and their number is likely to increase due to the invention of exome sequencing and analysis of previously unstudied populations

[74]. Strikingly, all BBS genes participate in cilia functioning, being a part of BBSome (*BBS1* [11q13.2; OMIM *209901], *BBS2* [16q13; OMIM *606151], *BBS4* [15q24.1; OMIM *600374], *BBS5* [2q31.1; OMIM *603650], *BBS7* [4q27; OMIM *607590], *BBS8* [14q31.3; OMIM *608132], *BBS9* [7p14.3; OMIM *607968], *BBS17* [3p21.31; OMIM *606568], and *BBS18* [10q25.2; OMIM *613605]); chaperonin complex (*BBS6* [20p12.2; OMIM *604896], *BBS10* [12q21.2; OMIM *610148], and *BBS12* [4q27; OMIM *610683]); basal body (*BBS13* [17q22; OMIM *609883], *BBS14* [12q21.32; OMIM *610142], *BBS15* [2p15; OMIM *613580], and *BBS16* [1q43-q44; OMIM *613524]) or having some related biological function (*BBS3* [3q11.2; OMIM *608845], *BBS11* [9q33.1; OMIM *602290], *BBS19* [22q12.3; OMIM *615870], *BBS20,* and *NPHP1* [2q13; OMIM *607100]) [74].

Many of these genes appear to affect proteins localized to the basal body, a key element of the monocilium thought to be important for intercellular sensing in mammalian cells including neurons [73]. The literature shows that ciliary function is associated with leptin signaling [93]. As evidenced by some studies in mice, hyperphagia and obesity are caused by conditional post-natal knockout of proteins involved in intraflagellar transport [94], but they occur also when the loss of cilia affects the neurons, in particular POMC neurons [94].

Alström syndrome (ALMS; OMIM #203800) is a rare genetic disorder that has been included in the ciliopathies group, in the last few years [95].

The estimated prevalence for ALMS is one to nine cases per 1,000,000 individuals with nearly 900 cases described worldwide to date. Symptoms first appear in infancy and progressive development of multi-organ pathology lead to a reduced life expectancy. Variability in age of

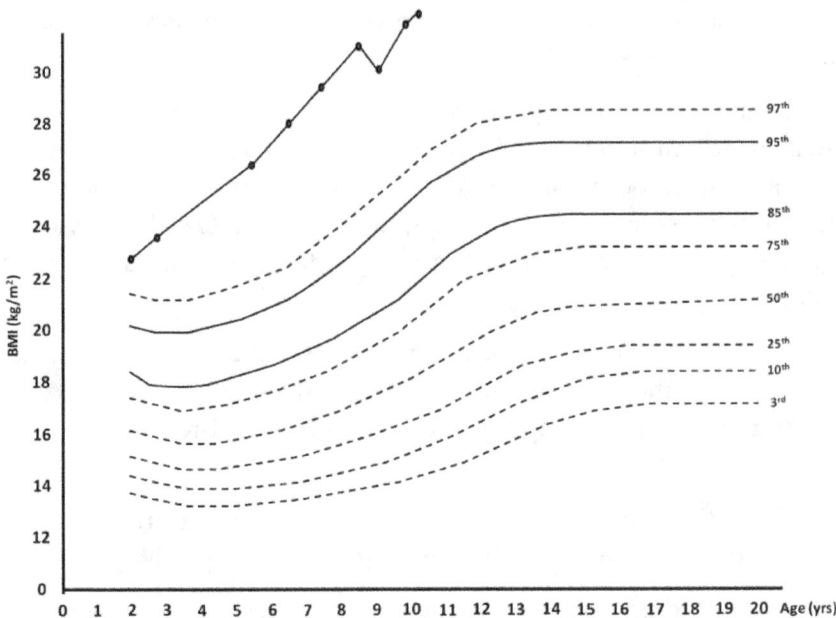

Figure 3. BMI growth chart in a girl with Alström syndrome.

onset and severity of clinical symptoms, even within families, are likely due to genetic background [95].

Children typically develop obesity by age 5 years, associated with hyperinsulinemia, chronic hyperglycemia and neurosensory deficits (**Figure 3**) [6]. Children affected by ALMS, like children with BBS, have visual impairment and deafness that occurs early in life but its incidence is higher in these patients as well as NIDDM, found in up to 70% of individuals by age 20 years [96, 97].

In addition, ALMS is also associated with cardiomyopathy, renal anomalies and endocrinopathies such as hypertriglyceridemia, pubertal delay, and hyperandrogenism and growth hormone deficiency [97].

Until now, disease-causing mutations in the *ALMS1* (2p13.1; OMIM *606844) gene have been involved in this disorder.

The diagnosis is based on the phenotype of the patient, and it is confirmed when two mutations in *ALMS1* gene are identifies through molecular analysis.

However, it is difficult to diagnose early ALMS first of all because symptoms arise gradually and secondly because the phenotypes overlap, in particular with BBS in the case of ALMS [98].

In recent times, thanks to the discovery of new genetic tools, in particular next-generation sequencing (NGS) technology, a large number of patients have been diagnosed. The advent of these new techniques allows early diagnosis also in those patients who do not have a characteristic phenotype, thus preventing long-term complications that can be caused by a delay in diagnosis [99].

Today, the most used genetic techniques are whole-exome sequencing (WES) and whole-genome sequencing, thanks to their low cost. However, they are also important because they allow to exclude the mutations in other genes [99, 100].

The WES is a rapid and easier technique because it analyzes all coding regions in the genome [100]. Thanks to it, in fact, mutations in *ALMS1* gene have been identified in individuals, whose phenotype did not seem to be typical of ALMS; therefore, it is fundamental to identifying pathogenic mutations in compound heterozygous state in *ALMS1* gene, overcoming also limitation of genetic panels in patient suffering from familial dilated cardiomyopathy and severe heart failure [101].

In fact, as reported in literature, the association of WES and a previous linkage analysis has allowed to identify the pathogenic mutations in *ALMS1* gene in a consanguineous Turkish family with severe dilated cardiomyopathy although it did not present the typical phenotype of ALMS [102].

Moreover, these mutations have been shown also in consanguineous Leber congenital amaurosis families through homozygosity mapping followed by WES [103].

As evidenced by these studies, the simultaneous use of different genetic techniques is fundamental both in the case of consanguineous families that in patients without the typical ALMS phenotype [95].

For management of the disease and to identify an accurate treatment, it is important for both the present of typical clinical features that an appropriate genetic diagnosis, which may be carried out by NGS techniques, thanks to its low cost compared with traditional polymerase chain reaction and direct Sanger sequencing [103].

4. Imprinted genetic syndromes

Prader-Willi syndrome (PWS, OMIM #176270) is a disorder caused by errors in genomic imprinting, which generally occur during both male and female gametogenesis. In particular, there is the loss of expression of paternal genes normally active and located in the chromosome 15q11-q13 region [104–108]. Conversely, a loss of expression of the preferentially maternally expressed *UBE3A* (OMIM *601623) gene in this region leads to Angelman syndrome (AS; OMIM #105830), an entirely different clinical disorder that causes developmental disabilities and neurological problems, such as difficulty speaking, balancing and walking, and, in some cases, seizures [109, 110].

According to several studies, most individuals with PWS (about two-thirds) have a de novo paternally inherited deletion of the chromosome 15q11-q13 region; about 25% of cases have maternal disomy 15 (chromosome 15 is inherited from the mother) [111]; less than 3% of patients have defects in the genomic imprinting center due to microdeletions or epimutations [104, 106, 112, 113], while rearrangements of the 15q11-q13 region or chromosomal translocations are rare [104, 114].

However, this syndrome, whose prevalence is around of 1/10,000–1/30,000, is considered the most common cause of syndomic obesity [115].

The cardinal features of PWS include infantile hypotonia, feeding difficulties due to a poor suck and failure to thrive (FTT), followed in later infancy or early childhood by excessive appetite with gradual development of obesity, short stature and/or decreased growth velocity due to growth hormone (GH) deficiency, intellectual disabilities (average IQ of 65), behavioral problems (e.g., temper tantrums, outburst and skin picking) and particular facial appearance (e.g., a small upturned nose, narrow bifrontal diameter with almond-shaped eyes, down-turned corners of the mouth with sticky salivary secretions and generally lighter skin, hair and eye color than other family members) [105, 106]. Hypothalamic dysfunction has been implicated in many manifestations of this syndrome including hyperphagia, temperature instability, high pain threshold, sleep-disordered breathing and multiple endocrine abnormalities [105, 107, 108].

Initially, two nutritional phases have been described in children with PWS:

• phase 1: the individual often presents FTT; he exhibits hypotonia with difficult feeding;

• phase 2: the individual is hyperphagic, and this condition will lead to obesity [105, 108].

To date, instead, seven different nutritional phases (five main phases and sub-phases in phases 1 and 2) have been identified.

As following, focusing on nutrition, although in the early phases, the child has poor appetite, the latter increases in phase 2b and leads progressively to hyperphagia, evident in phase 3 (**Table 3**).

Phases	Median ages	Clinical characteristics
0	Prenatal to birth	Decreased fetal movements and lower birth weight than sibs
1a	0–9 months	Hypotonia with difficulty feeding and decreased appetite. Needs assistance with feeding either through feeding tubes [nasal/oral gastric tube or gastrostomy tube] or orally with special, widened nipples
1b	9–25 months	Improved feeding and appetite and normal growth
2a	2.1–4.5 years	Weight increasing without appetite increase or excess calories. Will become obese if given the recommended daily allowance [RDA] for calories. Typically needs to be restricted to 60–80% of RDA to prevent obesity
2b	4.5–8 years	Weight and appetite are increased but can feel full
3	8 years to adulthood	Hyperphagic, rarely feels full
4	Adulthood	Appetite is no longer insatiable

Adapted with permission from Cassidy et al. [107].

Table 3. Clinical characteristics of the nutritional phases seen in Prader-Willi syndrome.

Analyzing the seven phases, we highlight the following:

• phase 0: the infant has growth restriction and decreased fetal movements;

• sub-phase 1a: the infant is hypotonic with difficulty feeding and with or without FTT;

• sub-phase 1b: the infant grows normally, and he improves appetite, also if weight gain is normal;

• sub-phase 2a: the child has a weight gain although there is not an increased appetite or caloric intake;

• sub-phase 2b: in addition to weight gain, there is an increased appetite;

• phase 3: the individual is hyperphagic; he seeks foods and presents the loss of sense of satiety;

• phase 4: it is typical of adults, who have an insatiable appetite and are able to feel full [107].

As said previously, individuals with PWS present an appetite that gradually increases and leads to obesity. In recent years, some studies have been conducted to understand the mechanisms controlling appetitive behavior, energy expenditure and body composition.

The central nervous system, in particular the hypothalamus that determines changes in energy balance, is involved in these processes.

One of the determining factors for the development of obesity in these patients is ghrelin, a 28 amino acid peptide produced in the stomach, that transmit satiety signal and whose level in obese PWS individuals is high [116, 117]. Circulating ghrelin levels are elevated in young children with PWS long before the onset of hyperphagia, especially during the early phase of poor appetite and feeding [118].

The literature reports that about 25% of the adults with PWS presents NIDDM (non-insulin-dependent diabetes mellitus) [119]; however, some studies show that in PWS, children fasting insulin concentrations and homeostasis model assessment insulin resistance index are lower than in obese control [120].

This syndrome, as mentioned, represents an human disorder related to genomic imprinting.

Although the DNA sequence of the imprinted maternally and paternally inherited alleles is the same, multiple epigenetic factors (such as DNA methylation, histone modifications and chromatin conformation) ultimately will determine whether the imprinted allele is expressed or repressed [121, 122].

DNA methylation analysis is the most efficient way to start the genetic workup if PWS is suspected clinically, but it cannot distinguish the molecular class (i.e., deletion; uniparental disomy, UPD; or imprinting defect, ID). Therefore, once the diagnosis of PWS is established by DNA methylation analysis, determination of the molecular class is the next step.

There are different genetic testing used in PWS: CMA-SNP array or FISH (fluorescence in situ hybridization) for deletion of 15q11.2-q13, DNA polymorphism analysis for UPD or ID or testing with MS-MLPA analysis for an IC deletion, important for the diagnosis of both of these individuals who do not have sufficient features because they are too young than of those who do not exhibit the typical phenotype [107].

4.1. Cohen syndrome

Cohen syndrome (CS) is an inherited disorder characterized by developmental delay, intellectual disability, microcephaly and hypotonia. Other features include progressive myopia, retinal dystrophy, hypermobility and distinctive facial features [6, 12]. Characteristic facial features include thick hair and eyebrows, long eyelashes, down-slanting and wave-shaped, a bulbous nasal tip, a smooth or shortened philtrum, and prominent upper central teeth [6, 12]. Children with CS tend to manifest failure to thrive in infancy and early childhood but subsequently become significantly overweight in the late childhood and adolescence. The obesity tends to be truncal in nature [6, 12]. In contrast to PWS, appetite and food intake are not increased during this time period, and activity is not noticeably decreased. Among individuals with CS, the prevalence of short stature is approximately 65% and delayed puberty 74%; clinical endocrinologic evaluations did not identify explanations for these findings [6, 12].

4.2. 1p36 deletion syndrome

1p36 deletion syndrome is a disorder characterized by severe intellectual disability, hypotonia, heart defects, hearing impairment and typical craniofacial features. In fact, patients with this syndrome show straight eyebrows, deeply set eyes, midface hypoplasia, broad and flat nasal root/bridge, long philtrum, pointed chin, large, late-closing anterior fontanel, microbrachyce-phaly, epicanthal folds and posteriorly rotated, low-set, abnormal ears. Other typical findings include brachy/camptodactyly and short feet. Developmental delay and intellectual disability of variable degree are present in all, and hypotonia in 95%. Seizures occur in 44–58% of affected individuals. Other findings include prenatal-onset growth deficiency, structural brain abnor-malities, congenital heart defects, vision problems, deafness, skeletal anomalies, abnormalities of the external genitalia and renal abnormalities. Obesity, which occurs as the consequence of hyperphagia, is also frequently observed in patients with the 1p36 deletion syndrome [123]. In this recent report [124], 40% of patients had obesity and hypercholesterolemia, and 1 patient developed NIDDM. Some authors suggested candidate regions for hyperphagia and obesity, such as *PRKCZ*, that may be associated with obesity because this gene is involved in carbo-hydrate or lipid metabolism, or insulin signaling [123]. It is suggested that genetic or environ-mental factors more likely contribute to the development of obesity and DM. However, a subset of patients may become overweight and obese with hyperphagia and NIDDM [125]. Previous studies observed that obesity was found exclusively in female patients with 1p36 deletion who showed growth restriction during the fetal period [126]. Because patients with 1p36 deletion show hypotonia and hyperphagia with obesity and NIDDM, which are also characteristic features of patients with PWS, some patients with 1p36 deletion may be misdiagnosed as having PWS.

4.3. 16p11.2 deletion syndrome

16p11.2 microdeletion syndrome is a chromosomal anomaly characterized by developmental and language delays, intellectual disability, social impairments represented by autism spectrum disorders, variable dysmorphisms and predisposition to obesity. In fact, in a screening cohort of patients with extreme obesity, enriched for patients with birth defects and/ or neurocognitive deficiencies using method to detect copy number variations, recurrent, *de novo* deletions of 16p11.2 were identified in approximately 3% of cases. In these patients, durable weight loss has not been reported. So durable weight control is recommended although no data are available on the efficacy of early intervention in deletion carriers. However, impaired cognition may also result in abnormal eating behavior contributing to the obesity [127, 128]. Some data seem to hypothesize that this deletion may affect the neural circuitry involved in the energy balance. The early increase in head circumference seems to precede the onset of obesity [129]. The 16p11.2 deletion includes the *SH2B1* gene, an adaptor protein involved in leptin and insulin signaling which may be involved in the pathogenesis of the obesity and insulin resistance observed in this deletion [130].

Additionally, deficiencies of *SIM1* (single minded), *BDNF* (brain-derived neurotrophic factor) and *NTRK2* (neurotrophic tyrosine receptor kinase encoding the TrK protein, the receptor for BDNF) genes are associated with syndromic conditions involved in the functioning of the hypothalamus downstream of MC4R-expressing neurons and leading severe hyperphagic obesity. For example, haplodeficiency of *BDNF* has also been implicated in the obesity occurring in a subset of patients with WAGR (Wilms tumor, aniridia, genitourinary malformations and retardation) syndrome [62].

4.4. Oligogenic obesity

Oligogenic obesity or common obesity is the result of the set of behavioral, environmental and genetic factors that may influence individual responses to diet and physical activity [131] (**Figure 4**).

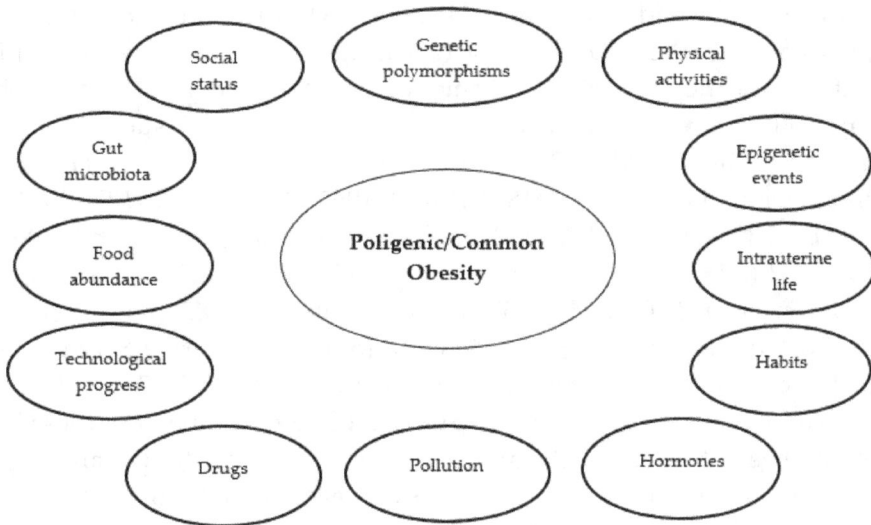

Figure 4. Gene–environment interactions in common obesity. Adapted with permission from Mutch and Clément [131].

The obesogenic changes of our environment in recent decades, especially the unlimited supply of cheap food with high palatability and high energy density, associated with genetic susceptibility are the causes of the current obesity epidemic [132].

The recent rapid rise in prevalence of childhood obesity suggests that, probably, environmental factors have a large impact on body weight in patients with common obesity although individual responses to these environmental factors are influenced by genetic factors called susceptibility genes [3].

Any of a group of alleles, at distinct gene loci that collectively control the inheritance of a quantitative phenotype or modify the expression of a qualitative character, are termed "polygenic" variants. A polygenic variant by itself has a small effect on the phenotype; only in combination with other predisposing variants does a sizeable phenotypic effect arise. Potentially, many such polygenic variants play a role in body weight regulation. It is estimated that the total number of genes with a small effect most likely exceeds [133]. These genes are involved in a variety of biological functions such as the regulation of food intake, energy expenditure, carbohydrate and lipid metabolism and adipose tissue development [131].

Therefore, unlike monogenic obesity, many genes and chromosome regions contribute to common obesity phenotype.

Genome-wide association studies have identified genetic risks for obesity. In less than 4 years, 52 genetic loci have been identified to be unequivocally associated with obesity-related traits [134]. However, these loci have only small effects on obesity susceptibility and explain just a fraction of the total variance. As such, their accuracy to predict obesity is poor and not competitive with the predictive ability of traditional risk factors such as parental and childhood obesity. The first convincing GWAS discovery for any obesity-related trait was made in 2007 for BMI when the *FTO* locus was found to be associated with obesity-related traits and specifically with extreme and early-onset obesity in children and adolescents [134–136]. Following the discovery of the *FTO* locus, one new locus near the *MC4R* was identified, a gene in which mutations are known to be the commonest cause of extreme childhood obesity. Also in recent years, other new BMI-associated loci were discovered such as near *TMEM18* (*transmembrane protein 18*, OMIM *613220, 2p25.3), near *KCTD15* (*potassium channel tetramerization domain-containing protein 15*, OMIM *615240, 19q13.11), near *GNPDA2* (*glucosamine-6-phosphate deaminase 2*, OMIM *613222, 4p12), in *SH2B1* (*SH2B adaptor protein 1*, OMIM *608937, 16q11.2), in *MTCH2* (*mitochondrial carrier homolog 2*, OMIM *613221, 11p11.2), near *NEGR1* (*neuronal growth regulator 1*, OMIM *613173, 1p31.1), near *FAIM2* (*FAS apoptotic inhibitory molecule 2*, OMIM *604306, 12q13.12), near *SEC16B* (*SEC16, homolog of S. cerevisiae B*, OMIM *612855, 1q25.2), near *ETV5* (*ETS variant gene 5*, OMIM *601600, 3q27.2) and in *BDNF* (*brain-derived neurotrophic factor*, OMIM *113505, 11p14.1). Although for many of these loci, association with BMI has been observed in children and in adolescents [64, 137], and in populations of non-white origin, their replication has been less consistent than for the *FTO* and near-*MC4R* loci for relatively small sample size of the replication studies [134].

Furthermore, longitudinal studies have been published in recent years that have followed up children over time; these studies indicated that GWAS-discovered risk variants influence the development of obesity in part by accelerating weight gain during infancy and childhood [138–140], but the mechanisms by which this occurs are not yet fully elucidated. One of the mechanisms involved may be the different sense of appetite, but the results of the studies are controversial [141, 142].

5. Epigenetics and obesity

Heritability estimates of BMI from twin studies range from 50 to 90% [143], so it plays a fundamental role in determining body weight. However, this latest figure appears in contradiction to the evidence of an epidemic increase in pediatric obesity over the last 20 years, time totally inadequate to record permanent changes in the genome. Only the reprogramming of gene expression through epigenetic modifications resulting from relevant environmental changes that have taken place mostly in the early periods of life may partially justify this phenomenon [11]. Epigenetic regulation of gene expression emerged in the last few years as a potential factor that might explain individual differences in obesity risk

[144]. Epigenetics can be defined as heritable changes that are mitotically stable (and potentially meiotically) and affect gene function but do not involve changes in the DNA sequence [145].

Currently, there is a growing interest in the study of the relationship between genetic variation, epigenetic variation and disease simultaneously. The two main mechanisms that lead to epigenetic changes are DNA methylation, and the alterations to histone proteins that alter the likelihood that specific genes are transcribed [146, 147].

Interindividual variations in epigenetic changes like CpG methylation can potentially alter gene function and predispose to obesity. The variation in the degree of methylation, in fact, is able to modulate the expression of genes involved in controlling hypothalamic appetite [148]. Using a genome-wide approach, obesity has been related to changes in DNA methylation status in peripheral blood leukocytes of lean and obese adolescents for two genes: in the UBASH3A (*ubiquitin-associated and SH3 domain-containing protein A*, OMIM *605736, 21q22.3) gene, a CpG site showed higher methylation levels in obese cases, and one CpG site in the promoter region TRIM3 (*tripartite motif-containing protein 3*, OMIM *605493, 11p15.4) gene, showed lower methylation levels in the obese cases [149]. Also the obesity risk allele of FTO has been associated with higher methylation of sites within the first intron of the FTO gene, suggesting an interaction between genetic and epigenetic factors [150]. In addition, the obesity risk allele of FTO affects the methylation status of sites related to other genes (KARS [16q23.1; OMIM *601421], TERF2IP [16q23.1; OMIM *605061], MSI1 [12q24.31; OMIM *603328], STON1 [2p16.3; OMIM *605357] and BCAS3 [OMIM *607470]), showing that the FTO gene may influence the methylation level of other genes [151]. Finally, a recent work has demonstrated that hypermethylation of the POMC gene plays an important role in preparing to obesity by reducing the expression of the gene itself [148].

Epigenetic changes usually occur during prenatal development or the early post-natal period. Already *in utero*, in fact, there may be a switch of energy balance resulting from exposure to specific environmental factors, resulting in epigenetic changes that can affect the potential of the fat mass of offspring. For example in a recent work, the methylation status of CpG from five candidate genes in umbilical cord tissue DNA from healthy neonates was measured, and it was found that higher methylation levels within promoter region of RXRA (*retinoid X receptor, alpha*, OMIM *180245, 9q34.2) gene, measured at birth, were strongly correlated with greater adiposity in later childhood [152]. Maternal nutrition is a major factor leading to epigenetic changes. Thus, the levels of vitamins consumed in pregnancy such as folate, methionine and vitamin B12, which affect methylation, become very important [147]. One study showed that prenatal exposure to malnutrition can determine abnormal DNA methylation resulting in epigenetic modifications that remain for the whole existence and that predispose to obesity and metabolic and cardiovascular risk in later life [153]. On the other hand also glycemic status during pregnancy is an important factor; in fact, hyperglycemia, as well as having a strong impact on the child's weight, can increase the risk of developing insulin resistance and obesity [147].

6. Steatosis and genetic of steatosis

Non-alcoholic fatty liver disease (NAFLD) actually represents the most frequent cause of chronic liver disease in industrialized countries in children and adolescents, as a direct consequence of the rise in childhood obesity [154]. Italian epidemiological data indicate that NAFLD affects approximately 3–10% of general pediatric population. This percentage increases up to >70%, with a male-to-female ratio of 2:1, in obese children [155]. NAFLD is defined by hepatic fat infiltration >5% hepatocytes, in the absence of other causes of liver pathology (such as daily alcohol utilization and either viral, autoimmune or drug-induced liver disease). It includes a spectrum of disease ranging from intrahepatic fat accumulation (steatosis) to various degrees of necrotic inflammation and fibrosis (non-alcoholic steatohepatatis [NASH]); simple steatosis has generally a benign course, but, rarely in children, NASH may progress to advanced and severe liver damage like cirrhosis and its complications (hepatocellular carcinoma and portal hypertension) [154, 156].

The pathogenesis of NAFLD appears to be multifactorial. The principal risk factor for fatty liver in childhood is obesity, but several other factors contribute to NAFLD development, including race/ethnicity, genetic factors, environmental exposures and alterations in the gut microbiome [157]. The dramatic rise in the prevalence of pediatric NAFLD is closely associated with the epidemic of obesity and metabolic syndrome; as in adulthood, pediatric NAFLD is associated with severe metabolic impairments such as insulin resistance, hypertension and abdominal obesity, determining an increased risk of developing type 2 diabetes mellitus, the metabolic syndrome and cardiovascular diseases [157, 158]. In addition, unhealthy food choices and the excessive fructose consumption in particular the fructose contained in the most common soda can promote the development of fatty liver [159].

The prevalence of hepatic steatosis varies among different ethnic groups. The ethnic group with the highest prevalence is the American Hispanic one (45%) followed by the Caucasian (33%) and the African-American (24%). The fatty liver prevalence in Europe, Australia and Middle East encompasses from 20 to 30%. In India, the fatty liver prevalence in urban populations encompasses from 16 to 32%; but in rural India, where there are traditional diets and lifestyles, the prevalence is lower (about 9%); this evidence suggests that a sedentary lifestyle and globalization of Western diet could be associated with an increase in the fatty liver prevalence in developing nations. In all the ethnicity, NAFLD is more prevalent in boys than in girls with a male to female ratio of 2:1 [160, 161].

Regarding to genetic factors, one of the most important gene involved in determining hepatic steatosis is the *patatin-like phospholipase-containing domain 3* gene (*PNPLA3*). Genome-wide association studies and other pediatric studies have revealed that the *rs738409* (I148M) variant for *PNPLA3* confers susceptibility to NAFLD-promoting hepatic accumulation of triglycerides and cholesterol by inhibition of triglyceride hydrolysis [162]. In addition, a recent case-control study has demonstrated that the *rs9939609A* allele of the fat mass and obesity-associated gene (*FTO*) increases the risk of NAFLD [157].

Another gene that acts together with *PNPLA3* in determining hepatic steatosis is the glucokinase regulatory protein (*GCKR*) gene which encodes for the glucokinase regulatory protein

(GCKRP) that inhibits the glucokinase (GCK) activity competing with the glucose, substrate of GCK. It has been demonstrated that the GCKRP L466 variant encodes for a protein that indirectly increased GCK activity. This increase in GCK hepatic activity promotes hepatic glucose metabolism, raises the concentrations of malonyl coenzyme A, a substrate for de novo lipogenesis, and contributes in liver fat accumulation [160, 163]. In addition, a study conducted in Chinese children has shown that that the polymorphism *rs11235972* of the *uncoupling protein 3* (*UCP3*) gene is associated with the occurrence of NAFLD. *UCP3* is a mitochondrial protein with a highly selective expression in skeletal muscle, a major site of thermogenesis in humans. Genetic variants of *UCP3* have been associated with NIDDM and obesity [164].

Apolipoprotein C3 gene (*APOC3*) *rs2854117* and *rs2854116* variants and *farnesyl-diphosphate farnesyltransferase 1* (*FDFT1*) gene *rs2645424* variant have been also associated with NAFLD in adult [160]. Also in the recent years, genetic studies have demonstrated that single-nucleotide polymorphisms (SNPs) in genes involved in lipid metabolism (*Lipin 1, LPIN1*), oxidative stress (*superoxide dismutase 2, −SOD2*), insulin signaling (*insulin receptor substrate-1, IRS-1*) and fibrogenesis (*Kruppel-like factor 6, KLF6*) have been associated with a high risk for NAFLD development and progression [154]. Finally, a recent study evaluated the combined effect of four-polymorphisms genetic risk score in predicting NASH in NAFLD obese children with increased liver enzymes to help NASH diagnosis with the other non-invasive diagnostic tests [165].

In conclusion, obesity and fatty liver disease often go hand in hand even in the pediatric population, and both are pathologies related to genetic and environmental factors.

7. Genetic approach to obesity

Recognizing the monogenic syndromic and not syndromic obesity is really very important for at least two reasons: firstly, because it is hoped that, in the near future, making use of the results of other research in the field of obesity, obese patients can benefit from specific treatment (such as leptin administration and MC4R receptor agonists); secondly, because it is hoped that they will benefit from a multidisciplinary approach to the management of the symptoms, however, the clinical features of patients with genetic obesity are often very blurred, so that diagnosis can escape at first. **Figure 5** shows a diagnostic classification algorithm which can be useful in territorial pediatrics to suspect monogenic obesity and in the second and third levels in hospitals to orientate themselves in the execution of all the diagnostic tests in order to confirm the final diagnosis [12].

The genetic contribution to common obesity has been established initially through family, twin and adoption studies. Twin studies have shown a relatively high heritability ranging from 40 to 77% [6]. Gene identification for the last 15 years has been based on two genetic epidemiological approaches (candidate gene and genome-wide linkage methods). Recently, genome-wide association studies have brought great information on obesity-related genes.

Candidate-gene studies: The design of the candidate gene approach is simple; candidate genes are genes that, according to their characteristics, can be considered causally related to the

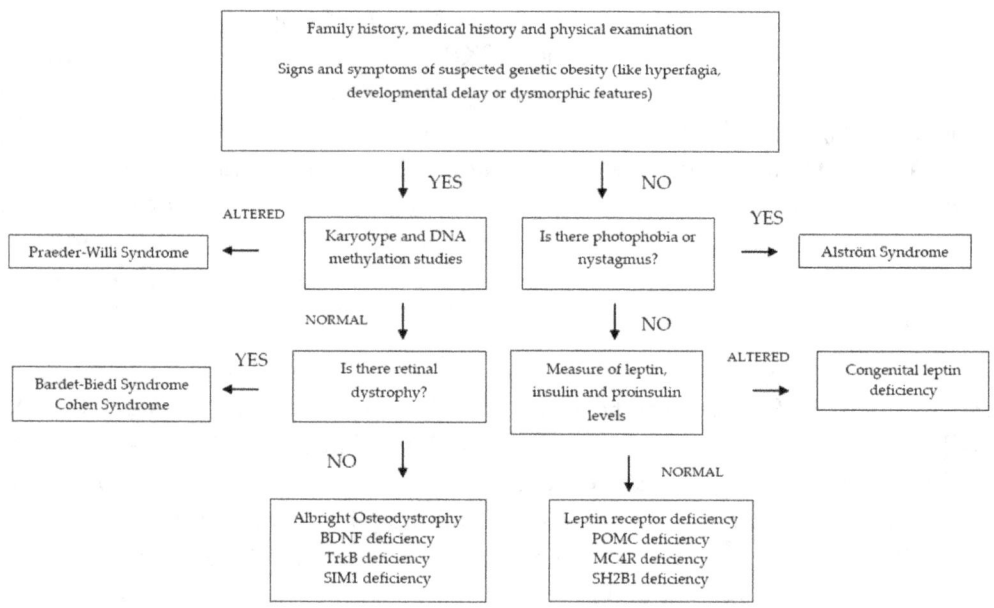

Figure 5. Diagnostic approach to genetic obesity. Adapted with permission from Farooqi and O'Rahilly [12].

disease. This method is based on the following resources: animal models using gene knockout and transgenic approaches and cellular model systems showing their role in metabolic pathways involved in glucose metabolism. There are two main types of candidates that are generally considered in such studies: functional and positional. Functional candidates are genes with products that are in some way involved in the pathogenesis of the disease. Positional candidates are genes that are identified because they lie within genomic regions that have been shown to be genetically important in linkage or association studies, or by the detection of chromosomal translocations that disrupt the gene [2, 3]. The latest update of the Human Obesity GeneMap reported 127 candidate genes for obesity-related traits. Results of large-scale studies suggest that obesity is strongly associated with genetic variants in the *MC4R* gene, *adrenergic β3 receptor* (*ADRB3*) gene, *PCSK1* gene, *BDNF* gene and *endocannabinoid receptor 1* (*CNR1*) gene [16].

Genome-wide linkage studies: Genome-wide linkage studies (GWLS) identify new, unforeseen genetic variants associated with a disease or a feature of interest. They rely on kinship of study participants and seek to identify chromosomal regions that tend to be co-inherited by individuals. The limit of genome-wide linkage studies is that they have a rather coarse resolution and typically identify broad intervals that require follow-up genotyping to pinpoint the genes that underlie the linkage signal [17]. The latest Human Obesity Gene Map update reported 253 loci from 61 genome-wide linkage scans, of which 15 loci have been replicated in at least three studies [16].

Genome-wide association studies: Genome-wide association studies (GWAS) are used in genetic research to look for associations between many (typically hundreds of thousands) specific genetic variations (more commonly, single-nucleotide polymorphisms, SNP) and particular diseases or traits. Genome-wide association studies have a higher resolution levels and are able to narrow down the locus associated with greater accuracy, so this approach took place in the genome-wide linkage studies for common disease [3]. This new approach has found about 30 loci associated with obesity and high BMI. The strongest association is with FTO gene (the fat-mass and obesity-related gene) mutations. Also BDNF, SH2B1 e NEGR1 mutations are associated with obesity and support that obesity is a disorder of hypothalamic function [17].

Since the beginning of the genome-wide association study (GWAS) era in 2005, a number of large GWASs have been conducted on obesity-related traits in humans. A large meta-analysis from 46 studies conducted by the Genetic Investigation of Anthropometric Traits (GIANT) [166] consortium identified 32 SNPs robustly associated with adult BMI. The majority of these SNPs demonstrated directionally consistent effects in age- and sex-adjusted BMI in children and adolescents. However, even in combination, the 32 established SNPs explain <2% of the variation in BMI in either adults or children. The mismatch between the high heritability estimates from twin and other family studies (40–70%) and the small percentage of variation explained through GWAS (<2%) is called the problem of "missing heritability" [167, 168]. A portion of the missing heritability appears to be due to rare genetic variants and some non-additive genetic effects that are not found in analyses GWAS that showed only additional effects of common SNPs with minor allele frequencies (MAF) of >5%. Another part of the missing heritability can be explained by the fact that multiple additional common genetic mutations contribute to obesity, but they have a small effect that cannot be found by GWAS analyses [168].

New types of analyses, such as genome-wide complex trait analysis (GCTA), analysis of uncommon (MAF 0.5–1%) or rare (MAF 0.5%) variants and structural variants not detected by GWAS arrays, epigenetic analysis and gene–gene interactions (epistasis), are helping to fill that gap [167]. The purpose of the novel approach called genome-wide complex trait analysis (GCTA) is not to identify specific SNPs related to the target phenotype, but rather to estimate the total additive genetic effect of the common SNPs used on currently available DNA arrays [168].

The rare variant—common disease hypothesis—suggests that rare variants contribute significantly to complex traits. Probably, the obese phenotype is the consequence of additive effects and interactions among multiple alleles with varying magnitude of effect. Actually, we know that only 1% of the human genome is transcribed into mRNA and translated into proteins. An additional 0.5% is regulatory regions that control gene expression. Functions of the remaining 98.5% of the genome remain unknown. Rare variants might be identified by massive genotyping or deep sequencing in large families thanks to novel techniques that sequence millions of DNA strands in parallel and at low cost such as next-generation sequencing techniques [169].

Copy number variants (CNVs) represent another source of the heritability that is missed by GWAS studies. Copy number variants (CNVs) are products of genomic rearrangements, resulting in deletions, duplications, inversions and translocations [167, 170]. The most established CNV in the obesity field is a large, rare chromosomal deletion at 16p11.2; this deletion includes a small number of genes, one of which is SH2B1, known to be involved in leptin and insulin signaling. The search for CNVs in the context of obesity has proved fruitful, and it has become quite clear they play a role in the missing heritability that still needs to be explained for the disease [19, 170].

8. Treatment options in patients with genetic obesity

The use of pharmacologic treatment for obesity is recommended by the American Academy of Pediatrics (AAP) as an adjunct to lifestyle changes when obesity-related health risks exist and lifestyle changes have not been effective for an individual. In addition, the AAP recommends pharmacotherapy only for children with BMI ≥99th percentile [171]. On the other hand, the Endocrine Society has suggested limiting pharmacotherapy to patients with a BMI over the 95th percentile who have failed diet and lifestyle intervention, or in limited cases with a BMI over the 85th percentile and severe comorbidities [147]. Overweight children should not be treated with pharmacotherapeutic agents unless significant, severe comorbidities persist despite intensive lifestyle modification. In these children, a strong family history of NIDDM or cardiovascular risk factors strengthens the case for pharmacotherapy [172].

There are currently only a few drugs approved for the treatment of obesity; such drugs belong to different pharmacologic categories with different mechanisms of action. A major class of medications used in weight treatment is appetite suppressants also called anorexigenic agents. These drugs increase hypotalamic levels of norepinephrine, dopamine and serotonin-promoting satiety and decreasing hunger [173]. Among the appetite suppressant drugs, sibutramine was used to treat obesity in children until recently. In 2010, sibutramine was withdrawn by the United States Federal Drug Administration (US FDA) and European Medicine Agency (EMA) for increased cardiovascular risk for individuals taking the medication [174]. As well, other drugs of the same class like ephedrine and fenfluramine were withdrawn from the market for their adverse effects [147]. With the withdrawal of sibutramine, orlistat and metformin are now the only available drugs for the treatment of pediatric obesity.

Orlistat, an inhibitor of pancreatic lipases, prevents the breakdown of triglycerides into absorbable fatty acids and monoglycerols. Thus, about one-third of the dietary intake, triglycerides is not absorbed. It reduces body weight, total cholesterol and LDL cholesterol, and the risk of NIDDM in adults with abnormal carbohydrate metabolism. In USA, orlistat is approved by the FDA in adolescents older than 12 years [175]. It is associated with a significant fall in BMI of $0.7\,kg/m^2$, but treatment is associated with increased rates of side effects including abdominal discomfort, pain, steatorrhoea and decreased absorption of the fat-soluble vitamins A, D, E and K. So, it is important to take those fat-soluble vitamins supplementation 2-h distance from orlistat administration [147]. Side effects are usually mild to moderate and generally decrease in frequency with continued treatment; this decrease may result from patients learning to consume less dietary fat to avoid these side effects. Typically, doses of 120 mg by mouth three times daily are needed for effectiveness [176, 177].

Although metformin has not been approved by the US FDA for the treatment of obesity, it may be effective as a weight loss agent in addition to its effects as a hypoglycemic agent. Its major site of action is the liver: the drug increases glucose uptake, decreases hepatic gluconeogenesis and reduces hepatic glucose production; also, metformin inhibits lipogenesis and increases insulin sensitivity and may have an effect as an appetite suppressant. The major benefits of the medication are reduction of food intake, weight loss, visceral fat reduction, improvement of the lipid profile and of the carbohydrate intolerance [172, 175, 178]. A systematic assessed five randomized controlled trials all with follow-up of at least 6 months; compared to placebo, metformin reduced BMI by 1.42 kg/m^2 in obese children [179]. Patients treated with metformin report abdominal discomfort, which improves when the drug is taken with food. There is also a risk of vitamin B12 deficiency; therefore, a multivitamin is recommended. The risk of lactic acidosis has been observed in adults but not seen in pediatric patients [147].

Octreotide, a somatostatin analogue, has been investigated as a treatment for hypothalamic obesity. It binds receptors on the beta cells of the pancreas and inhibits insulin release [147]. A study comparing octreotide with placebo has demonstrated statistically significant weight loss and statistically significant mean decreases in BMI among those treated with octreotide for 6 months [180]. Octreotide works better in patients with insulin hypersecretion and insulin resistance. A study has demonstrated that greater weight loss correlated with a greater degree of insulin hypersecretion [181]. The high cost of the drug and the various side effects (gastrointestinal problems, gallstones, GH and TSH suppression, cardiac dysfunction) limit currently use [175].

In the case of monogenic obesity, subcutaneous injection of recombinant human leptin in children and adults with *LEP* mutations resulted in weight loss, mainly of fat mass, with a major effect on reducing food and hyperphagia, induction of puberty (even in adults) and improvement in T-cell responsiveness [24, 25, 27, 182]. Leptin treatment works in patients with leptin deficiency or with bioinactive leptin, but on the other hand, leptin treatment is useless in LEPR-deficient subjects, because the receptor mutations make it inactive [24, 183].

In the case of children with PWS, GH therapy can improve growth, body composition, muscle thickness, physical strength and agility, motor performance, fat utilization, and lipid metabolism [184–186]. The best response to GH in PWS patients is observed in the first 12 months of treatment. Although early treatment is important for the improvement in body composition, generally, in practice, it is possible to start treatment only after 2 years of age. Treatment can be started in a dose of 0.034 mg/kg/day (0.24 mg/kg/week) in infants, and toddlers and IGF-1 and IGFBP-3 levels are used to specify the dose of GH therapy. Benefits of continuing GH therapy in adulthood remain unclear although an improvement has been observed in body composition and cognitive functions in patients who received treatment only in adulthood. Contraindications for GH therapy in PWS patients are severe obesity, uncontrolled diabetes mellitus, untreated severe OSA, active cancer and psychosis [108].

A number of the PWS features, such as hyperphagia, obesity and behavioral anomalies, may be due to consequent hypothalamic hyposecretion of oxytocin for the reduction of paraventricular nucleus neurons. A few studies have investigated the capacity of exogenous oxytocin to improve these PWS features, but other research is necessary [183].

For MC4R-deficient obese patients, currently, there are no specific treatments. Different MC4R agonists were studied in vivo in animal and human studies, and almost all studies are currently in the preclinical phase. These pharmacological MC4R agonists can restore normal activity in mutated receptors, and in obese animal, models cause decreased food intake, increased total energy expenditure, weight loss and weight-independent improvement of insulin sensitivity after 8 weeks of treatment [43, 187].

Finally, most recent studies on the treatment of obesity have focused on the potential role of plants used for obesity and its metabolic disorders treatments, exerting a positive effect on lipid and glucose metabolism, and anti-inflammatory activity [188]. For example, green tea disclosed anti-obesity effects in both *in vitro* and *in vivo*, decreasing adipose tissue through the reduction of adipocytes differentiation and proliferation, showing a positive effect in lipid profile, and lipid and carbohydrates metabolisms, and anti-inflammatory activity [188].

However, in literature, the anti-obesity properties and the mechanisms of action of some plants such as *Camellia sinensis, Hibiscus sabdariffa, Hypericum perforatum, Persea americana, Phaseolus vulgaris, Capsicum annuum, Rosmarinus officinalis, Ilex paraguariensis, Citrus paradisi, Citrus limon, Punica granatum, Aloe vera, Taraxacum officinale* and *Arachis hypogea* have been described [188]. However, polysaccharide macromolecules slowing the rate of carbohydrate and fat absorption have been also described reduce insulinemic peaks, enhancing β-cell function and potentially restoring the insulin secretory reserve in patients with impaired glucose tolerance or NIDDM and genetic obesity history [189].

Another possible therapy for childhood obesity is bariatric surgery. There are 3 types of bariatric procedures: malabsorptive, restrictive and combination procedures. The first procedures are the jejunoileal bypass and the biliopancreatic diversion with duodenal switch that manage to lose weight by reducing nutrient absorption through the gut anatomical rearrangements; however, these procedures are not approved in children for their high morbidity and mortality. The Roux-en-Y gastric bypass (RYGB) is a combination procedure; it has become the most commonly performed bariatric surgical procedure, and it involves a reduction of stomach size and the reduction of intestinal absorptive capacity via the creation of a gastrojejunal anastomosis [171, 172, 190]. Laparoscopic adjustable gastric banding (LAGB) is a wholly restrictive procedure, and it has been used more recently. This bariatric procedure is to place a balloon around the esophagogastric junction and inflate it with saline until you get the desired effect of the stomach size reduction. This procedure is recommended in children because it is reversible and does not create permanent intestinal rearrangements [171, 172, 191]. Laparoscopic sleeve gastrectomy (LSG) is a new and attractive option for young patients. It is a new restrictive procedure without the malabsorptive component present in other bariatric procedures. This technique involves the removal of a large portion of the stomach through a vertical resection, and the remaining stomach has a volume drastically reduced, with a capacity of around 100/150 ml. Weight loss outcomes in some study were similar between pediatric and adult patients at all time points, suggesting that LSG is similarly safe and effective in young and adult patients through at least 1 year of follow-up [192].

The criteria for access to bariatric surgery in childhood are very restrictive: BMI >35 kg/m² with severe comorbidities or >40 kg/m² with comorbidities, Tanner stage 4 or 5, to achieve at least 95% of the growth estimate in the case of malabsorptive procedures, the ability to follow the post-operative diet and exercise, an adequate social support, ability to follow constantly medical indications and treatment and appropriate treatment of psychological problems [190]. Also it is recommended that bariatric surgery be done only in centers that can provide a multidisciplinary pre- and post-operative evaluation and psychological support both before and after the surgery [193].

Currently, data on bariatric surgery in children and adolescents with genetic obesity are limited and still controversial [183]. To date, bariatric surgery experience in treating children and adolescents with monogenic and syndromic forms of obesity is limited, and different bariatric procedures have been used with varying success [194]. Some studies have demonstrated the efficacy of bariatric surgery (in terms of weight loss and reduction of comorbidities such as obstructive sleep apnea, dyslipidemia, hypertension, diabetes mellitus and poor mobility) in patients with monogenic obesity (such as LEPR-deficient patients and patients with hetero-zygous *MC4R* mutations, but not in patients with homozygous *MC4R* mutation [195]) and syndromic obesity (such as PWS, BBS, Alström syndrome) but, due to the limited number of cases, the long-term efficacy and safety of bariatric surgery in genetic forms of obesity need further evaluation [183].

Even more in the early days are studies that try to correlate specific polymorphisms with response to bariatric surgery: For example, a study tried to find the presence of an association between several polymorphisms (including the *FTO* and *MC4R* genes) with post-operative weight loss [196]; another study found that a 15q26.1 locus is significantly associated with weight loss after Roux-en-Y gastric bypass surgery [197]. Thus, there is some evidence for the use of genomics to identify response to surgical procedures; the identification of genetic contributors could be useful to select those individuals who will obtain a greater benefit from a bariatric surgery. However, these results have yet to be confirmed.

9. Hyperphagia: etiopathogenesis and treatment

In the modern environment of plenty, obesity is favored by biological features that generally are advantageous in a restrictive environment, such as attraction to palatable and energy dense foods, slow satiety mechanisms and high metabolic efficiency [198].

The control of food intake and energy expenditure consists of a complex network of neural and hormonal systems that involving many genes [199]: in particular, the informations are collected at the peripheral level (intestine, stomach, adipose tissue); then, they are processed at the hypothalamic level and, finally, generate behavioral, endocrine and autonomic output [198].

In particular, much larger portions of the nervous system of animals and humans, including cortex, basal ganglia, and the limbic system, are concerned with the procurement of food as a basic and evolutionarily conserved survival mechanism to defend body weight [200]. These systems are directly and primarily involved in the interactions of the modern environment and lifestyle with the human body [198]. By focusing on the neural reward systems and the interaction between reward and homeostatic functions, it is possible to infer that the disturbance of this relationship determines obesity (**Figure 6**).

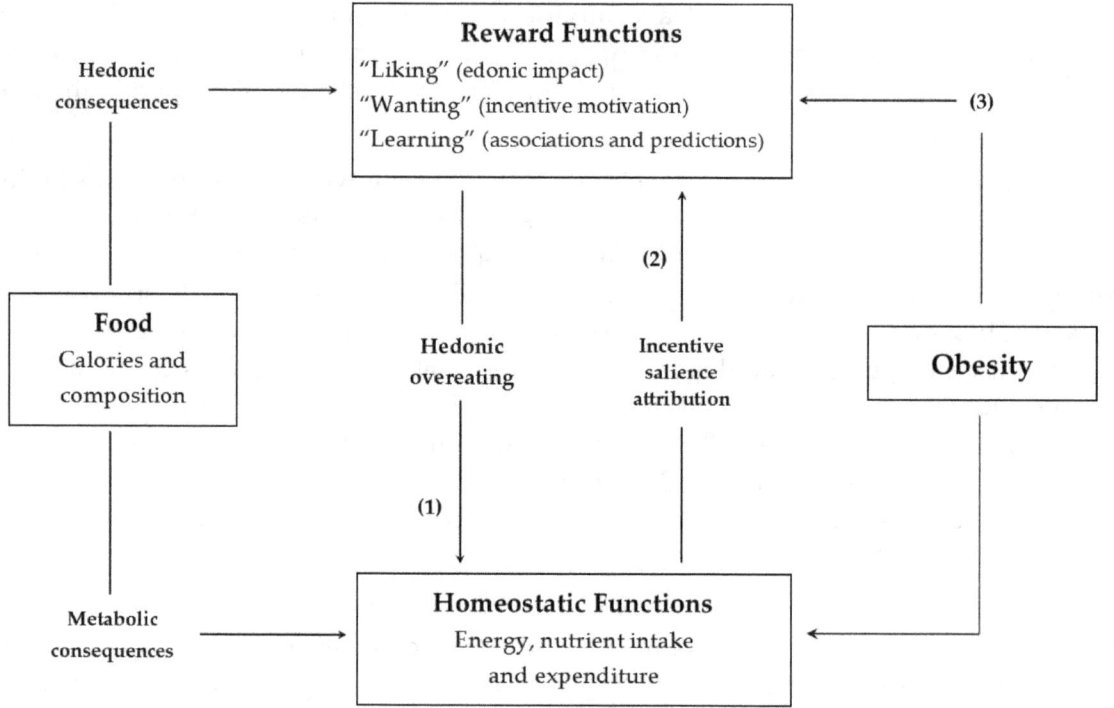

Figure 6. Relationship between metabolic and hedonic controls of food intake and energy balance. Adapted with permission from Berthoud et al. [198].

This process can generate hedonic and metabolic consequences, which are independent from each other: in particular, the hedonic consequences are regulated by reward functions while the metabolic consequences of food (defined in terms of their input of energy and their effects on body composition, particularly increased fat accretion as in obesity) are regulated by homeostatic functions.

The alteration of reward functions may be a cause (i.e., excessive caloric intake modulated by hedonic value of food (1)) and/or a consequence (induced by obese state (3)) of obesity [198].

As schematically depicted in **Figure 6**, several potential interactions exist between food reward and obesity.

In particular, there are three fundamental mechanisms involved in the development of obesity, which are not mutually exclusive, but a combination of all three is operative in most individuals: excessive intake of palatable and energy dense foods, differences (genetic and other preexistent) in reward functions and increase of obese state consequently to alterations of reward functions induced by obesity [198].

It is also important to realize that hyperphagia is not always necessary for obesity to develop, as the macronutrient composition of food can independently favor fat deposition.

In this regard, there is the *"gluttony hypothesis"* emerged from several studies in animals: in particular, although reward functions are not altered unlimited access to palatable food and food cues leads to excessive caloric intake (hedonic overeating) and, consequently, to obesity (defined as diet-induce obesity) [198].

However, it is important to underline that not all individuals exposed to environment of plenty show an increased food intake and weight gain; this means that there are genetic and epigenetic pre-existing alterations that make some individuals more vulnerable to the increased availability of palatable food and food cues [198].

One of the key questions is how the motivation to get a reward will translate into action. In most cases, the motivation for something comes from the pleasure that this has generated in the past, or in other words, to obtain what has been helpful. The dopamine signal seems to be a critical component in this process [198].

The limited information available suggests that repeated sucrose access can upregulate dopamine release [201] and dopamine transporter [202] and change dopamine D1 and D2 receptor availability [201] in the nucleus accumbens.

As demonstrated by some observations, such pleasing foods have a high potential for addiction for which the withdrawal from it can cause symptoms such as anxiety, stress, depression resulting behavior of relapse because of occurring neural and molecular changes. Therefore, it is critical for switching the cycle of addiction and the prevention of a further spiral of addiction [198].

An issue on which to focus is that excessive caloric intake, as part of a disease, can gradually worsen: in fact at the beginning, there is overeating; then, the individual eats also in the absence of physiological hunger. Subsequently, there will be loss of control over eating (binge eating), and finally, hyperphagia defined as a hallmark of inherited disorders, in which obesity is present [203].

The term "hyperphagia" includes a series of conditions, such as binge eating disorder, hormonal imbalances such as glucocorticoid excess, leptin signaling abnormalities, syndromes associated with obesity and cognitive impairment (e.g., PWS) [203] and can be used in different situations: for example, to evaluate hunger and satiety through appropriate scales for pathological individuals compared to healthy individuals [203], to evaluate excessive caloric intake and the impact on body size and body composition in pathological individuals [203] or to evaluate preoccupation and psychological symptoms such as anxiety, stress due to hyperphagic behavior and the consequences that it determines (e.g., continuous search for food, night eating, ingestion of inedible food, theft of food, etc.) [203].

A person with hyperphagia has an obsessive and compulsive behavior towards food and often continues to eat for a long time, even if he/she feels full. This excessive nutriment can cause abdominal pain, guilt or drowsiness.

In particular, obesity is associated with dysregulated signaling systems, such as leptin and insulin resistance, as well as increased signaling through proinflammatory cytokines and pathways activated by oxidative and endoplasmatic reticulum stress [204] (**Figure 7**).

As schematically depicted in **Figure 7**, obesity and, in turn, neurodegenerative diseases may be caused by leptin resistance, central insulin and altered regulation of energy balance, con-

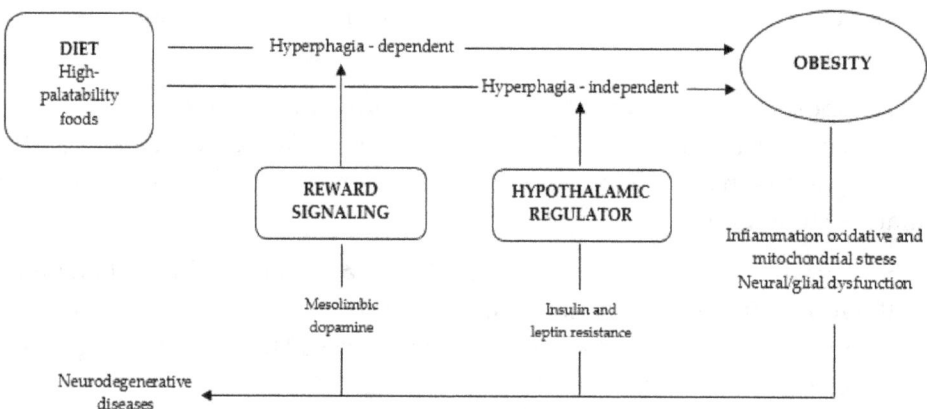

Figure 7. Secondary effects of obesity on reward circuitry and hypothalamic energy balance regulation. Adapted with permission from Berthoud et al. [198].

trolled by hypothalamus. About the latter, the literature shows that mitochondrial and oxidative stress increase due to high-fat diets leading to neural/glial dysfunction and, consequently, cytotoxic effects [198].

However, these toxic effects do not stop at the level of the hypothalamus but can also affect brain areas involved in reward processing [198].

10. Nutritional and behavioral approach to genetic obesity

The approach to the child with genetic obesity is very complex considering that obesity is associated with a number of complications that include the health of the child, and it must be focused on the entire family. Awareness about the problem by all family members and, in particular, changes in lifestyle and nutrition of the family are the most effective means both to ensure the compliance to the treatment, the success of the therapy and the maintenance of the long-term results.

The family, especially the parents, should be actively involved in the therapeutic program and become protagonists. The targeted intervention with "individual" programs only for the child, on the contrary, is often unsuccessful and frustrating for the child himself [205].

According to NICE guidelines on weight management in children dating from 2014 [206], it is important to:

- coordinate the care of children and young people around their individual and family needs [206];

- assess and intervene to improve child's health, considering his age and maturity. It is important to set goals based on needs and preferences both of the child that of the whole family [206];

- create an environment that promotes lifestyle changes within the family and in social settings. Parents (or carers) are responsible of these changes, especially if children are younger than 12 years old [206].

The initial assessment is important to collect data necessary for diagnosis and subsequent treatment. In particular, these informations regarding patient history (personal, familiar, healthy and social history), food/nutrition-related history (eating patterns, diet experience, physical activity, beliefs and attitudes about eating, etc.), anthropometric measures (current weight, weight history, etc.), biochemical data and medical tests (e.g., lipid profile, glucose profile, etc.); what the person has already tried and how successful this has been will be discussed, and what they learned from the experience; the person's readiness to adopt changes and their confidence in making changes will be assessed [206].

Multicomponent interventions are the treatment of choice. Weight management programs must include behavior change strategies to increase people's physical activity levels or decrease inactivity, improve eating behavior and the quality of the person's diet and reduce energy intake [206].

In particular, nutrition offered to obese children must also ensure the maintenance of adequate rhythms of growth and promote the maintenance of lean body mass (in particular of muscle mass), which represents the metabolically active compartment, and it is the large part of the total energy expenditure. Therefore, it must necessarily guarantee the macro- and micro-nutrients intake in relation to their age [205].

In overweight and obese children and young people, it is important a multidisciplinary intervention that includes dietary recommendations appropriate for age and complies with the principles for a healthy nutrition (in these patients, total energy intake should be below their energy expenditure) [206].

Dietary changes should be tailored to food preferences and allow for a flexible and individual approach to reducing calorie intake; it is important not to use unduly restrictive and nutritionally unbalanced diets because they are ineffective in the long term and can be harmful [206].

In these patients, it is also necessary that an intervention about physical activity is important not only for lose weight, but also for other health benefits, such as reduction risk of type 2 diabetes or heart diseases [206].

Therefore, obese and overweight children must be encouraged to become more active and to reduce inactive behaviors, such as sitting and watching television, using a computer or playing video games and to do at least 60 min of moderate or greater intensity physical activity each day. The activity can be in 1 session or several sessions lasting 10 min or more [206].

It is important to make the choice of activity with the child and ensure that it is appropriate to the child's ability and confidence, giving children the opportunity and support to do more exercise in their daily lives (e.g., walking, cycling, using the stairs and active play) or to do more regular, structured physical activity (e.g., football, swimming or dancing) [206].

Children affected by genetic obesity (e.g., PWS) often eat more than necessary for anxiety, sadness, boredom: in this case, it is important not only to reduce the amount of foods but also to search for reasons of suffering causing the overeating. It is important, therefore, to reconstruct the individual's self-esteem [206].

There are, however, barriers to parental involvement in the child's treatment: in some families, for cultural or psychological reasons, parents do not perceive their child as obese. In other families, parents may acknowledge that the child is obese but denies that this condition can have consequences.

Therefore, it is crucial to raise awareness among parents of the need to intervene, especially when behavioral changes are needed in the family [207].

Focusing on hyperphagic children, particularly those affected by Prader–Willi syndrome, parents must learn to celebrate each small goal, large or small, and to appreciate the acquisition of any new skill [208].

In these children, there are behavior changes that become more apparent and severe with age: in fact, they are concerned about food, hypersensitive, agitated, aggressive, impulsive, anxious. These behaviors are caused specially by their insatiable appetite that causes physical, emotional and social problems [209].

For these reasons, it is important to intervene to reduce stress not only for children, but also for the whole family.

However, to control the anxious behavior in children with PWS, the following information may be useful:

- having a regular daily routine, following appropriate food program;
- giving your child transitional warnings—that is, "after you finish that puzzle, it is time for bath" [209];
- preparing your child ahead of time if there is going to be a change in routine;
- re-directing your child to another activity;
- using positive reinforcement;
- speaking to your child in a calm, yet firm matter-of-fact tone [209].

In children with PWS, it is essential management food, based also on control food access, to ensure adequate nutrition, weight regulation and appropriate eating behaviors.

Crucial in this regard is the role of parents, who must support their children in these changes by adopting appropriate strategies.

However, each family will find the best way for them and for the specific need of their child.

First of all, it is important to follow an adequate food program that helps parents to monitor their food intake and reassures the child that the food will always be available: therefore, it represents the beginning for him to acquire the habit of eating healthy so that food can be controlled and could become a part of his daily routine [209].

This program is based on three main meals (breakfast, lunch, and dinner) and two or three snacks (mid-morning snack, afternoon snack, and perhaps evening snack) [209]. It is fundamental to respect scheduled times (food must be given every 2–3 h), avoiding giving food outside mealtimes. Whenever possible, all family members should eat at the same time and others should not eat in front of the child when it is not their scheduled meal/snack time [209].

Portion control is another adequate strategy: it must not be excessive, but appropriate for the child's age to ensure adequate growth [209].

However, food must be healthy considering that in children with PWS, calorie needs are lower due to reduced metabolism. Food must be given only by parents/caregivers and served on the plate prior to being eaten, avoiding other platters/bowls of food visible on the table and to share or offer them other food [209].

At the end of the meal, it is important to remove the empty plate from the table and encourage the child to play away from the table or from the kitchenette until all food has been taken away. It is important to keep food out of sight and reach of children, keeping it under lock and key if necessary [209] (**Figure 8**).

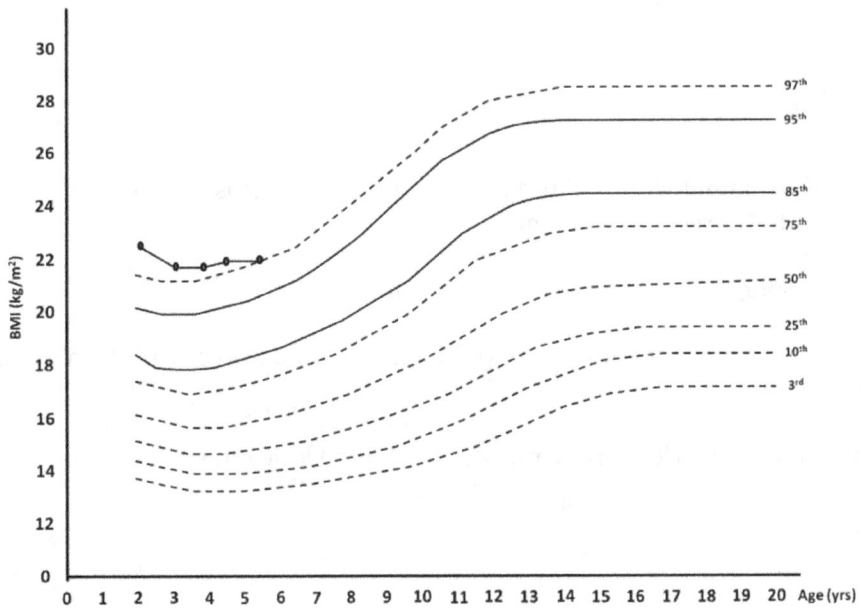

Figure 8. Girl with Bardet-Biedl syndrome. You can see the amelioration of the BMI after the interdisciplinary approach to hyperphagia.

11. Conclusions

This chapter may bring a significant contribution to the updating of knowledge of the genetic susceptibility and provide a better clarification of which variants are truly associated with the predisposition to develop an obese phenotype. This chapter may also help to understand better the genetic diversity that could be associated in subjects with genetic forms of obesity. However, this chapter may help to understand this complex problem and the different approaches to treatment. In these forms of genetic obesity, the team approach to therapy (nurse educators, nutritionists, exercise physiologists, and counsellors) is the basis for treatment. Dramatic reductions in BMI are difficult to achieve and sustain, so counselling and therapy should start with realistic goals that emphasize gradual reductions of body fat and BMI and maintenance of weight loss. Finally, this chapter may provide news on the need for new therapeutic approaches in the field of childhood obesity as the basis of the hyperphagia treatment, a typical feature of these syndromes.

Acknowledgements

Conflicting interests: The authors declare that they have no conflicting interests.

Financial conflicting interests: The authors do not have any financial and non-financial conflicting interests in relation to this manuscript.

Author details

Stefano Stagi[1*], Martina Bianconi[1], Maria Amina Sammarco[1], Rosangela Artuso[2], Sabrina Giglio[2] and Maurizio de Martino[1]

*Address all correspondence to: stefano.stagi@yahoo.it

1 Health Sciences Department, University of Florence, Anna Meyer Children's University Hospital, Florence, Italy

2 Genetics and Molecular Medicine Unit, Anna Meyer Children's University Hospital, Florence, Italy

References

[1] WHO. Obesity and overweight. Fact sheet no. 311 [Internet]. 2016. Available from: http://www.who.int/mediacentre/factsheets/fs311/en/ [Accessed: 2016-07-06].

[2] Bell CG, Walley AJ, Froguel P. The genetics of human obesity. *Nature Reviews. Genetics* 2005;6:221–234.

[3] Puiu M, Emandi AC, Arghirescu S. Genetics and Obesity. In: Genetic Disorders, Puiu M Ed., InTech Edition 2013, pp 271–292.

[4] Aston LM, Kroese M, editors. Genomics of obesity. The application of public health genomics to the prevention of management of obesity in the UK. 2 Worts Causeway Cambridge: PHG Foundation; 2013. 2 p.

[5] Albuquerque D, Stice E, Rodríguez-López R et al. Current review of genetics of human obesity: from molecular mechanisms to an evolutionary perspective. *Molecular Genetics and Genomics* 2015;290:1191–1221.

[6] Farooqi IS. Genetic and hereditary aspects of childhood obesity. *Best Practice & Research. Clinical Endocrinology & Metabolism* 2005;19:359–374.

[7] O'Rahilly S, Farooqi IS. Human obesity as a heritable disorder of the central control of energy balance. *International Journal of Obesity (London)* 2008;32:S55–61.

[8] Llewellyn CH, Van Jaarsveld CHM, Boniface D et al. Eating rate is a heritable phenotype related to weight in children. *American Journal of Clinical Nutrition* 2008;88:1560–1566.

[9] Reilly JJ, Armstrong J, Dorosty AR et al. Early life risk factors for obesity in childhood: cohort study. *BMJ* 2005;330:1357.

[10] Magnusson PKE, Rasmussen F. Familial resemblance of body mass index and familial risk of high and low body mass index. A study of young men in Sweden. *International Journal of Obesity and Related Metabolic Disorders* 2002;26:1225–1231.

[11] Perrone L, Marzuillo P, Miraglia Del Giudice E. [From "genetic" obesity to epigenetics in obesity.] *Prospettive in Pediatria* 2015;45:123–130.

[12] Farooqi S, O'Rahilly S. Genetic obesity syndromes. In: Grant SFA, editor. The genetics of obesity. New York: Springer Science+Business Media; 2014. p. 23–32.

[13] Stein QP, Mroch AR, De Berg KL et al. The influential role of genes in obesity. *South Dakota Journal of Medicine* 2011;12–5:17.

[14] Bochukova EG, Huang N, Keogh J et al. Large, rare chromosomal deletions associated with severe early-onset obesity. *Nature* 2010;436:666–670.

[15] Perrone L, Marzuillo P, Grandone A et al. Chromosome 16p11.2 deletions: another piece in the genetic puzzle of childhood obesity. *Italian Journal of Pediatrics* 2010;36:43.

[16] Rankinen T, Zuberi A, Chagnon YC et al. The human obesity gene map: the 2005 update. *Obesity (Silver Spring)* 2006;14:529–644.

[17] Cheung WW, Mao P. Recent advances in obesity: genetics and beyond. *ISRN Endocrinology* 2012;2012:536905.

[18] Morandi A, Maffeis C. [Monogenic obesity.] *L'Endocrinologo* 2014;15:280–285.

[19] Ramachandrappa S, Farooqi IS. Genetic approaches to understanding human obesity. *The Journal of Clinical Investigation* 2011;121:2080–2086.

[20] Montague CT, Farooqi IS, Whitehead JP et al. Congenital leptin deficiency is associated with severe early-onset obesity in humans. *Nature* 1997;387:903–908.

[21] Farooqi IS, O'Rahilly S. 20 years of leptin: human disorders of leptin action. *The Journal of Endocrinology* 2014;223:T63–T70.

[22] Funcke JB, von Schnurbein J, Lennerz B et al. Monogenic forms of childhood obesity due to mutations in the leptin gene. *Molecular and Cellular Pediatrics* 2014;1:3.

[23] Wabitsch M, Funcke JB, von Schnurbein J et al. Severe early-onset obesity due to bioinactive leptin caused by a p.N103K mutation in the leptin gene. *The Journal of Clinical Endocrinology and Metabolism* 2015;100:3227–3230.

[24] Wabitsch M, Funcke JB, Lennerz B et al. Biologically inactive leptin and early-onset extreme obesity. *The New England Journal of Medicine* 2015;372:48–54.

[25] Farooqi IS, Matarese G, Lord GM et al. Beneficial effects of leptin on obesity, T cell hyporesponsiveness, and neuroendocrine/metabolic dysfunction of human congenital leptin deficiency. *The Journal of Clinical Investigation* 2002;110:1093–1103.

[26] Farooqi I, O'Rahilly S. Monogenic human obesity syndromes. *Recent Progress in Hormone Research* 2004;59:409–424.

[27] Farooqi IS, Jebb SA, Langmack G et al. Effects of recombinant leptin therapy in a child with congenital leptin deficiency. *The New England Journal of Medicine* 1999;341:879–884.

[28] Clement K, Vaisse C, Lahlou N et al. A mutation in the human leptin receptor gene causes obesity and pituitary dysfunction. *Nature* 1998; 392:398–401.

[29] Farooqi IS, Wangensteen T, Collins S et al. Clinical and molecular genetic spectrum of congenital deficiency of the leptin receptor. *The New England Journal of Medicine* 2007;356:237–247.

[30] Hannema SE, Wit JM, Houdijk ME et al. Novel leptin receptor mutations identified in two girls with severe obesity are associated with increased bone mineral density. *Hormone Research in Paediatrics* 2016;85:412–420.

[31] Wasim M, Awan FR, Najam SS et al. Role of leptin deficiency, inefficiency, and leptin receptors in obesity. *Biochemical Genetics* 2016;54(5):565–72.

[32] Dubern B, Clement K. Leptin and leptin receptor-related monogenic obesity. *Biochimie* 2012;94:2111–2115.

[33] Ren D, Li M, Duan C, Rui L. Identification of SH2-B as a key regulator of leptin sensitivity, energy balance, and body weight in mice. *Cell Metabolism* 2005;2:95–104.

[34] Doche ME, Bochukova EG, Su HW et al. Human SH2B1 mutations are associated with maladaptive behaviors and obesity. *The Journal of Clinical Investigation* 2012;122:4732–4736.

[35] Duan C, Yang H, White MF, Rui L. Disruption of the SH2-B gene causes age-dependent insulin resistance and glucose intolerance. *Molecular and Cellular Biology* 2004;24: 7435–7443.

[36] Rui L. SH2B1 regulation of energy balance, body weight, and glucose metabolism. *World Journal of Diabetes* 2014;5:511–526.

[37] Anderson EJ, Çakir I, Carrington SJ et al. 60 years of POMC: regulation of feeding and energy homeostasis by α-MSH. *Journal of Molecular Endocrinology* 2016;56:T157–T174.

[38] Shabana, Hasnain S. Prevalence of POMC R236G mutation in Pakistan. *Obesity Research & Clinical Practice* 2015;31. pii:S1871-403X(15)00166-0.

[39] Kim JH, Choi JH. Pathophysiology and clinical characteristics of hypothalamic obesity in children and adolescents. *Annals of Pediatrics Endocrinology & Metabolism* 2013;18:161–167.

[40] Krude H, Biebermann H, Luck W et al. A severe early-onset obesity, adrenal insufficiency and red hair pigmentation caused by POMC mutations in humans. *Nature Genetics* 1998;19:155–157.

[41] Challis BG, Pritchard LE, Creemers JW et al. A missense mutation disrupting a dibasic prohormone processing site in pro-opiomelanocortin (POMC) increases susceptibility to early-onset obesity through a novel molecular mechanism. *Human Molecular Genetics* 2002;11:1997–2004.

[42] Lee YS, Challis BG, Thompson DA et al. A POMC variant implicates beta-melanocytestimulating hormone in the control of human energy balance. *Cell Metabolism* 2006;3:135–140.

[43] Kievit P, Halem H, Marks DL, et al. Chronic treatment with a melanocortin-4 receptor agonist causes weight loss, reduces insulin resistance, and improves cardiovascular function in diet-induced obese rhesus macaques. *Diabetes* 2013;62:490–497.

[44] Chen KY, Muniyappa R, Abel BS, et al. RM-493, a melanocortin-4 receptor (MC4R) agonist, increases resting energy expenditure in obese individuals. *The Journal of Clinical Endocrinology and Metabolism* 2015;100:1639–1645.

[45] Farooqi IS, Keogh JM, Yeo GS, et al. Clinical spectrum of obesity and mutations in the melanocortin 4 receptor gene. *The New England Journal of Medicine* 2003; 348:1085–1095.

[46] Doulla M, McIntyre AD, Hegele RA et al. A novel MC4R mutation associated with childhood-onset obesity: a case report. *Paediatrics & Child Health* 2014;19:515–518.

[47] Delhanty PJ, Bouw E, Huisman M et al. Functional characterization of a new human melanocortin-4 receptor homozygous mutation (N72K) that is associated with early-onset obesity. *Molecular Biology Reports* 2014;41:7967–7972.

[48] Stutzmann F, Tan K, Vatin V, et al. Prevalence of melanocortin-4 receptor deficiency in Europeans and their age-dependent penetrance in multigenerational pedigrees. *Diabetes* 2008; 57:2511–2518.

[49] Martinelli CE, Keogh JM, Greenfield JR, et al. Obesity due to melanocortin 4 receptor (MC4R) deficiency is associated with increased linear growth and final height, fasting hyperinsulinemia, and incompletely suppressed growth hormone secretion. *The Journal of Clinical Endocrinology and Metabolism* 2011;96:E181–E188.

[50] Seidah NG. The proprotein convertases, 20 years later. *Methods in Molecular Biology* 2011;768:23–57.

[51] Jackson RS, Creemers JW, Ohagi S et al. Obesity and impaired prohormone processing associated with mutations in the human prohormone convertase 1 gene. *Nature Genetics* 1997;16:303–306.

[52] Jackson RS, Creemers JW, Farooqi IS et al. Small-intestinal dysfunction accompanies the complex endocrinopathy of human proprotein convertase 1 deficiency. *The Journal of Clinical Investigation* 2003;112:1550–1560.

[53] Nead KT, Li A, Wehner MR et al. Contribution of common non-synonymous variants in PCSK1 to body mass index variation and risk of obesity: a systematic review and meta-analysis with evidence from up to 331 175 individuals. *Human Molecular Genetics* 2015;24:3582–3594.

[54] Martín MG, Lindberg I, Solorzano-Vargas RS et al. Congenital proprotein convertase 1/3 deficiency causes malabsorptive diarrhea and other endocrinopathies in a pediatric cohort. *Gastroenterology* 2013;145:138–148.

[55] Stijnen P, Tuand K, Varga TV et al. The association of common variants in PCSK1 with obesity: a HuGE review and meta-analysis. *American Journal of Epidemiology* 2014;180: 1051–1065.

[56] Holder JL Jr, Butte NF, Zinn AR. Profound obesity associated with a balanced translocation that disrupts the SIM1 gene. *Human Molecular Genetics* 2000;9:101–108.

[57] El Khattabi L, Guimiot F, Pipiras E et al. Incomplete penetrance and phenotypic variability of 6q16 deletions including SIM1. *European Journal of Human Genetics:EJHG* 2015;23:1010–1018.

[58] Kublaoui BM, Gemelli T, Tolson KP et al. Oxytocin deficiency mediates hyperphagic obesity of Sim1 haploinsufficient mice. *Molecular Endocrinology* 2008;22:1723–1734.

[59] Xu B, Goulding EH, Zang K, et al. Brain-derived neurotrophic factor regulates energy balance downstream of melanocortin-4 receptor. *Nature Neuroscience* 2003;6:736–742.

[60] Han JC. Rare syndromes and common variants of the brain-derived neurotrophic factor gene in human obesity. *Progress in Molecular Biology and Translational Science* 2016;140: 75–95.

[61] Gray J, Yeo GS, Cox JJ et al. Hyperphagia, severe obesity, impaired cognitive function, and hyperactivity associated with functional loss of one copy of the brain-derived neurotrophic factor (BDNF) gene. *Diabetes* 2006;55:3366–3371

[62] Zhao J, Bradfield JP, Li M, et al. The role of obesity-associated loci identified in genome-wide association studies in the determination of pediatric BMI. *Obesity* 2009;17:2254–2257.

[63] Mou Z, Hyde TM, Lipska BK, et al. Human obesity associated with an intronic SNP in the brain-derived neurotrophic factor locus. *Cell Reports* 2015;13:1073–1080.

[64] Yeo GS, Connie Hung CC, Rochford J et al. A de novo mutation affecting human TrkB associated with severe obesity and developmental delay. *Nature Neuroscience* 2004;7: 1187–1189.

[65] Gray J, Yeo G, Hung C et al. Functional characterization of human NTRK2 mutations identified in patients with severe early-onset obesity. *International Journal of Obesity* 2007;31:359–364.

[66] Xu B, Xie X. Neurotrophic factor control of satiety and body weight. *Nature Reviews. Neuroscience* 2016;17:282–292.

[67] Miraglia del Giudice E, Santoro N, Cirillo G et al. Mutational screening of the CART gene in obese children: identifying a mutation (Leu34Phe) associated with reduced resting energy expenditure and cosegregating with obesity phenotype in a large family. *Diabetes* 2001;50:2157–2160.

[68] Miraglia del Giudice E, Santoro N, Fiumani P et al. Adolescents carrying a missense mutation in the CART gene exhibit increased anxiety and depression. *Depression and Anxiety* 2006;23:90–92.

[69] Asai M, Ramachandrappa S, Joachim M, et al. Loss of function of the melanocortin 2 receptor accessory protein 2 is associated with mammalian obesity. *Science* 2013;341: 275–278.

[70] Geets E, Zegers D, Beckers S et al. Copy number variation (CNV) analysis and mutation analysis of the 6q14.1-6q16.3 genes SIM1 and MRAP2 in Prader Willi like patients. *Molecular Genetics and Metabolism* 2016;117:383–388.

[71] Pearce LR, Atanassova N, Banton MC et al. KSR2 mutations are associated with obesity, insulin resistance, and impaired cellular fuel oxidation. *Cell* 2013;155:765–777.

[72] Pilbrow AP. Discovery of an obesity susceptibility gene, KSR2, provides new insight into energy homeostasis pathways. *Circulation Cardiovascolar Genetics* 2014;7:218–219.

[73] Ansley SJ, Badano JL, Blacque OE et al. Basal body dysfunction is a likely cause of pleiotropic Bardet-Biedl syndrome. *Nature* 2003;425:628–633.

[74] Suspitsin EN, Imyanitov EN. Bardet-Biedl syndrome. *Molecular Syndromology* 2016;7: 62–71.

[75] Forsythe E, Beales PL. Bardet-Biedl syndrome. *European Journal of Human Genetics* 2013;21:8–13.

[76] M'hamdi O, Ouertani I, Chaabouni-Bouhamed H. Update on the genetics of Bardet-Biedl syndrome. *Molecular Syndromology* 2014;5:51–56.

[77] Shoemark A, Dixon M, Beales PL et al. Bardet Biedl syndrome: motile ciliary phenotype. *Chest* 2015;147:764–770.

[78] Khan SA, Muhammad N, Khan MA et al. Genetics of human Bardet-Biedl syndrome, an updates. *Clinical Genetics* 2016;90:3–15.

[79] Ristow M. Neurodegenerative disorders associated with diabetes mellitus. *Journal of Molecular Medicine* 2004;82:510–529.

[80] Pawlik B, Mir A, Iqbal H et al. Novel familial BBS12 mutation associated with a mild phenotype: implications for clinical and molecular diagnostic strategies. *Molecular Syndromology* 2010;1:27–34.

[81] Estrada-Cuzcano A, Koenekoop RK, Senechal A et al. BBS1 mutations in a wide spectrum of phenotypes ranging from nonsyndromic retinitis pigmentosa to Bardet-Biedl syndrome. *Archives of Ophthalmology* 2012;130:1425–1432.

[82] Kwitek-Black AE, Carmi R, Duyk GM et al. Linkage of Bardet-Biedl syndrome to chromosome 16q and evidence for non-allelic genetic heterogeneity. *Nature Genetics* 1993;5:392–396.

[83] Leppert M, Baird L, Anderson KL et al. Bardet-Biedl syndrome is linked to DNA markers on chromosome 11q and is genetically heterogeneous. *Nature Genetics* 1994;7:108–112.

[84] Sheffield VC, Carmi R, Kwitek-Black A et al. Identification of a Bardet-Biedl syndrome locus on chromosome 3 and evaluation of an efficient approach to homozygosity mapping. *Human Molecular Genetics* 1994;3:1331–1335.

[85] Carmi R, Rokhlina T, Kwitek-Black AE et al. Use of a DNA pooling strategy to identify a human obesity syndrome locus on chromosome 15. *Human Molecular Genetics* 1995;4:9–13.

[86] Young TL, Woods MO, Parfrey PS et al. A founder effect in the Newfoundland population reduces the Bardet-Biedl syndrome I (BBS1) interval to 1 cM. *American Journal of Human Genetics* 1999;65:1680–1687.

[87] Mykytyn K, Braun T, Carmi R et al. Identification of the gene that, when mutated, causes the human obesity syndrome BBS4. *Nature Genetics* 2001;28:188–191.

[88] Mykytyn K, Nishimura DY, Searby CC et al. Identification of the gene (BBS1) most commonly involved in Bardet-Biedl syndrome, a complex human obesity syndrome. *Nature Genetics* 2002;31:435–438.

[89] Nishimura DY, Searby CC, Carmi R et al. Positional cloning of a novel gene on chromosome 16q causing Bardet-Biedl syndrome (BBS2). *Human Molecular Genetics* 2001;10:865–874.

[90] Chiang AP, Nishimura D, Searby C et al. Comparative genomic analysis identifies an ADP-ribosylation factor-like gene as the cause of Bardet-Biedl syndrome (BBS3). *American Journal of Human Genetics* 2004;75:475–484.

[91] Fan Y, Esmail MA, Ansley SJ et al. Mutations in a member of the Ras superfamily of small GTP-binding proteins causes Bardet-Biedl syndrome. *Nature Genetics* 2004;36: 989–993.

[92] Li JB, Gerdes JM, Haycraft CJ et al. Comparative genomics identifies a flagellar and basal body proteome that includes the BBS5 human disease gene. *Cell* 2004;117:541–552.

[93] Seo S, Guo DF, Bugge K et al. Requirement of Bardet-Biedl syndrome proteins for leptin receptor signaling. *Human Molecular Genetics* 2009;18:1323–1331.

[94] Davenport JR, Watts AJ, Roper VC et al. Disruption of intraflagellar transport in adult mice leads to obesity and slow-onset cystic kidney disease. *Current Biology* 2007;17:1586–1594.

[95] Álvarez Satta M, Castro-Sánchez S, Valverde D. Alström syndrome: current perspectives. *The Application of Clinical Genetics* 2015;8:171–179.

[96] Mason K, Page L, Balikcioglu PG. Screening for hormonal, monogenic, and syndromic disorders in obese infants and children. *Pediatric Annals* 2014;43:e218–e224.

[97] Girard D, Petrovsky N. Alström syndrome: insights into the pathogenesis of metabolic disorders. *Nature Reviews. Endocrinology* 2011;7:77–88.

[98] Marshall JD, Maffei P, Collin GB et al. Alström syndrome: genetics and clinical overview. *Current Genomics* 2011;12:225–235.

[99] Marshall JD, Maffei P, Beck S et al. Clinical utility gene card for: Alström syndrome—update 2013. *European Journal of Human Genetics* 2013; 21(11).

[100] Katagiri S, Yoshitake K, Akahori M et al. Whole-exome sequencing identifies a novel ALMS1 mutation (p.Q2051X) in two Japanese brothers with Alström syndrome. *Molecular Vision* 2013;19:2393–2406.

[101] Long PA, Evans JM, Olson TM. Exome sequencing establishes diagnosis of Alström syndrome in an infant presenting with non-syndromic dilated cardiomyopathy. *American Journal of Medical Genetics. Part A.* 2015;167A:886–890.

[102] Louw JL, Corveleyn A, Jia Y et al. Homozygous loss-of-function mutation in ALMS1 causes the lethal disorder mitogenic cardiomyopathy in two siblings. *European Journal of Medical Genetics* 2014;57:532–535.

[103] Wang X, Wang H, Cao M et al. Whole-exome sequencing identifies ALMS1, IQCB1, CNGA3, and MYO7A mutations in patients with Leber congenital amaurosis. *Human Mutation* 2011;32:1450–1459.

[104] Bittel DC, Butler MG. Prader-Willi syndrome: clinical genetics, cytogenetics and molecular biology. *Expert Reviews in Molecular Medicine* 2005;7:1–20.

[105] Butler M, Lee PDK, Whitman BY, editors. Management of Prader-Willi syndrome. 3rd ed. New York: Springer-Verlag; 2006.

[106] Butler MG. Prader-Willi syndrome: obesity due to genomic imprinting. *Current Genomics* 2011;12:204–215.

[107] Cassidy SB, Schwartz S, Miller JL et al. Prader-Willi syndrome. *Genetics in Medicine* 2012;14:10–26.

[108] Aycan Z, Bas VN. Prader-Willi syndrome and growth hormone deficiency. *Journal of Clinical Research in Pediatric Endocrinology* 2014;6:62–67.

[109] Buiting K. Prader-Willi syndrome and Angelman syndrome. *American Journal of Medical Genetics Part C: Seminars in Medical Genetics* 2010;154C:365–376.

[110] Williams CA, Driscoll DJ, Dagli AI. Clinical and genetic aspects of Angelman syndrome. *Genetics in Medicine* 2010;12:385–395.

[111] Angulo MA, Butler MG, Cataletto ME. Prader-Willi syndrome: a review of clinical, genetic, and endocrine findings. *Journal of Endocrinological Investigation* 2015;38:1249–1263.

[112] Nicholls RD, Knepper JL. Genome organization, function, and imprinting in Prader-Willi and Angelman syndromes. *Annual Review of Genomics and Human Genetics* 2001;2:153–175.

[113] Buiting K, Gross S, Lich C. Epimutations in Prader-Willi and Angelman syndromes: a molecular study of 136 patients with an imprinting defect. *American Journal of Human Genetics* 2003;72:571–577.

[114] Rocha CF, Paiva CL. Prader-Willi-like phenotypes: a systematic review of their chromosomal abnormalities. *Genetics and Molecular Research* 2014;13:2290–2298.

[115] Butler MG. Genomic imprinting disorders in humans: a mini-review. *Journal of Assisted Reproduction and Genetics* 2009;26:477–486.

[116] Cummings DE, Clement K, Purnell JQ et al. Elevated plasma ghrelin levels in Prader-Willi syndrome. *Nature Medicine* 2002;8:643–644.

[117] Del Parigi A, Tschöp M, Heiman ML et al. High circulating ghrelin: a potential cause for hyperphagia and obesity in Prader-Willi syndrome. *The Journal of Clinical Endocrinology and Metabolism* 2002;87:5461–5464.

[118] Kweh FA, Miller JL, Sulsona CR et al. Hyperghrelinemia in Prader-Willi syndrome begins in early infancy long before the onset of hyperphagia. *American Journal of Medical Genetics Part A* 2015;167A:69–79.

[119] Butler JV, Whittington JE, Holland AJ et al. Prevalence of, and risk factors for, physical ill-health in people with Prader-Willi syndrome: a population-based study. *Developmental Medicine and Child Neurology* 2002;44:248–255.

[120] Haqq AM, Muehlbauer MJ, Newgard CB et al. The metabolic phenotype of Prader-Willi syndrome (PWS) in childhood: heightened insulin sensitivity relative to body mass index. *The Journal of Clinical Endocrinology and Metabolism* 2011;96:E225–E232.

[121] Horsthemke B, Buiting K. Genomic imprinting and imprinting defects in humans. *Advances in Genetics* 2008;61:225–246.

[122] Horsthemke B. Mechanisms of imprint dysregulation. *American Journal of Medical Genetics Part C: Seminars in Medical Genetics* 2010;154C:321–328.

[123] D'Angelo CS, Kohl I, Varela MC, de Castro CI, Kim CA, Bertola DR et al. Extending the phenotype of monosomy 1p36 syndrome and mapping of a critical region for obesity and hyperphagia. *American Journal of Medical Genetics A.* 2010;152A:102–110

[124] Stagi S, Lapi E, Pantaleo M et al. Type II diabetes and impaired glucose tolerance due to severe hyperinsulinism in patients with 1p36 deletion syndrome and a Prader-Willi-like phenotype. *BMC Medical Genetics.* 2014;15:16.

[125] Bettiol H, Sabbag Filho D, Haeffner LS, Barbieri MA, Silva AA, Portela A et al. Do intrauterine growth restriction and overweight at primary school age increase the risk of elevated body mass index in young adults? *Brazilian Journal of Medical and Biological Research.* 2007;40:1237–1243.

[126] Shimada S, Shimojima K, Okamoto N, Sangu N, Hirasawa K, Matsuo M et al. Microarray analysis of 50 patients reveals the critical chromosomal regions responsible for 1p36 deletion syndrome-related complications. *Brain and Development.* 2015;37:515–526.

[127] Melville CA et al. The prevalence and determinants of obesity in adults with intellectual disabilities. *Obesity Reviews* 2007;8:223–30.

[128] Galioto R et al. Cognitive function in morbidly obese individuals with and without binge eating disorder. *Comprehensive Psychiatry* 2012;53:490–5

[129] Zufferey F, Sherr EH, Beckmann ND et al. A 600 kb deletion syndrome at 16p11.2 leads to energy imbalance and neuropsychiatric disorders. Journal of Medical Genetics 2012;49:660–668.

[130] Maillard AM. 16p11.2 Locus modulates response to satiety before the onset of obesity. *International Journal of Obesity (London).* 2016;40(5):870–876.

[131] Mutch DM, Clément K. Unraveling the genetics of human obesity. *PLoS Genetics* 2006;2:e188.

[132] Barsh GS, Farooqi IS, O'Rahilly S. Genetics of body-weight regulation. *Nature* 2000;404:644–651.

[133] Hinney A, Vogel CI, Hebebrand J. From monogenic to polygenic obesity: recent advances. *European Child & Adolescent Psychiatry* 2010;19:297–310.

[134] Loos RJ. Genetic determinants of common obesity and their value in prediction. *Best Practice & Research. Clinical Endocrinology & Metabolism* 2012;26:211–226.

[135] Fang H, Li Y, Du S et al. Variant rs9939609 in the FTO gene is associated with body mass index among Chinese children. *BMC Medical Genetics* 2010;11:136.

[136] Cecil JE, Tavendale R, Watt P et al. An obesity-associated FTO gene variant and increased energy intake in children. *New England Journal of Medicine* 2008;359:2558–2566.

[137] Willer CJ, Speliotes EK, Loos RJF et al. Six new loci associated with body mass index highlight a neuronal influence on body weight regulation. *Nature Genetics 2009*;41:25–34.

[138] Elks CE, Heude B, de Zegher F, et al. Associations between genetic obesity susceptibility and early postnatal fat and lean mass: an individual participant meta-analysis. *JAMA Pediatrics* 2014;168:1122–1130.

[139] Warrington NM, Howe LD, Wu YY, et al. Association of a body mass index genetic risk score with growth throughout childhood and adolescence. *PLoS One* 2013;8:e79547.

[140] Belsky DW, Moffitt TE, Houts R et al. Polygenic risk, rapid childhood growth, and the development of obesity: evidence from a 4-decade longitudinal study. *Archives of Pediatrics & Adolescent Medicine* 2012;166:515–521.

[141] Carnell S, Wardle J. Appetitive traits and child obesity: measurement, origins and implications for intervention. *The Proceedings of the Nutrition Society* 2008;67:343–355.

[142] Steinsbekk S, Belsky D, Guzey IC et al. Polygenic risk, appetite traits, and weight gain in middle childhood: a longitudinal study. *JAMA Pediatrics* 2016;170:e154472.

[143] Haworth CM, Plomin R, Carnell S et al. Childhood obesity: genetic and environmental overlap with normal-range BMI. *Obesity (Silver Spring)* 2008;16:1585–1590.

[144] Campion J, Milagro FI, Martinez J. Individuality and epigenetics in obesity. *Obesity Reviews: An Official Journal of the International Association for the Study of Obesity* 2009;10: 383–392.

[145] Bird A. DNA methylation patterns and epigenetic memory. *Genes and Development* 2002;16:6–21.

[146] Waterland RA. Epigenetic mechanisms affecting regulation of energy balance: many questions, few answers. *Annual Review of Nutrition* 2014;34:337–355.

[147] Crocker MK, Yanovski JA. Pediatric obesity: etiology and treatment. *Pediatrics Clinics of North America* 2011;58:1217–1240.

[148] Kuehnen P, Mischke M, Wiegand S et al. An Alu element-associated hypermethylation variant of the POMC gene is associated with childhood obesity. *PLoS Genetics* 2012;8:e1002543.

[149] Wang X, Zhu H, Snieder H et al. Obesity related methylation changes in DNA of peripheral blood leukocytes. *BMC Medicine* 2010;8:87.

[150] Gemma C, Sookoian S, Alvarinas J et al. Maternal pregestational BMI is associated with methylation of the PPARGC1A promoter in newborns. *Obesity (Silver Spring)* 2009;17:1032–1039.

[151] Almen MS, Jacobsson J, Moschonis G et al. Genome wide analysis reveals association of a FTO gene variant with epigenetic changes. *Genomics* 2012;99:132–137.

[152] Godfrey KM, Sheppard A, Gluckman PD et al. Epigenetic gene promoter methylation at birth is associated with child's later adiposity. *Diabetes* 2011;60:1528–1534.

[153] Tobi EW, Goeman JJ, Monajemi R et al. DNA methylation signatures link prenatal famine exposure to growth and metabolism. *Nature Communications* 2014;5:5592.

[154] Della Corte C, Vajro P, Socha P et al. Pediatric non-alcoholic fatty liver disease: recent advances. *Clinics and Research in Hepatology and Gastroenterology* 2014;38:419–422.

[155] Schwimmer JB, Deutsch R, Kahen T, Lavine JE, Stanley C, Behling C. Prevalence of fatty liver in children and adolescents. *Pediatrics* 2006;118:1388–1393.

[156] Giorgio V, Prono F, Graziano F et al. Pediatric non alcoholic fatty liver disease: old and new concepts on development, progression, metabolic insight and potential treatment targets. *BMC Pediatrics* 2013;13:40.

[157] Nobili V, Alkhouri N, Alisi A et al. Nonalcoholic fatty liver disease: a challenge for pediatricians. *JAMA Pediatrics* 2015;169:170–176.

[158] Nobili V, Svegliati-Baroni G, Alisi A et al. A 360-degree overview of paediatric NAFLD: recent insights. *Journal of Hepatology* 2013;58:1218—1229.

[159] Vos MB, Kimmons JE, Gillespie C et al. Dietary fructose consumption among US children and adults: the Third National Health and Nutrition Examination Survey. *Medscape Journal of Medicine* 2008;10:160.

[160] Marzuillo P, Miraglia del Giudice E, Santoro N. Pediatric fatty liver disease: role of ethnicity and genetics. *World Journal of Gastroenterology* 2014;20:7347–7355.

[161] Loomba R, Sanyal AJ. The global NAFLD epidemic. *Nature Reviews. Gastroenterology & Hepatology* 2013;10:686–690.

[162] Romeo S, Kozlitina J, Xing C, et al. Genetic variation in PNPLA3 confers susceptibility to nonalcoholic fatty liver disease. *Nature Genetics* 2008;40:1461–1465.

[163] Santoro N, Zhang CK, Zhao H et al. Variant in the glucokinase regulatory protein (GCKR) gene is associated with fatty liver in obese children and adolescents. *Hepatology* 2012;55:781–789.

[164] Xu YP, Liang L, Wang CL et al. Association between UCP3 gene polymorphisms and nonalcoholic fatty liver disease in Chinese children. *World Journal of Gastroenterology* 2013;19:5897–5903.

[165] Nobili V, Donati B, Panera N et al. A 4-polymorphism risk score predicts steatohepatitis in children with nonalcoholic fatty liver disease. *Journal of Pediatric Gastroenterology and Nutrition* 2014;58:632–636.

[166] Speliotes EK, Willer CJ, Berndt SI et al. Association analyses of 249 796 individuals reveal 18 new loci associated with body mass index. *Nature Genetics* 2010;42:937–948.

[167] Waalen J. The genetics of human obesity. *Translational Research: The Journal of Laboratory and Clinical Medicine* 2014;164:293–301.

[168] Llewellyn CH, Trzaskowski M, Plomin R et al. Finding the missing heritability in pediatric obesity: the contribution of genome-wide complex trait analysis. *International Journal of Obesity* 2013;37:1506–1509.

[169] Manco M, Dallapiccola B. Genetics of pediatric obesity. *Pediatrics* 2012;130:123–133.

[170] Xia Q, Grant SF. The genetics of human obesity. *Annals of the New York Academy of Sciences* 2013;1281:178–190.

[171] Dolinsky DH, Armstrong SC, Kinra S. The clinical treatment of childhood obesity. *Indian Journal of Pediatrics* 2013;80:Suppl1:S48–S54.

[172] August GP, Caprio S, Fennoy I et al. Prevention and treatment of pediatric obesity: an endocrine society clinical practice guideline based on expert opinion. *The Journal of Clinical Endocrinology and Metabolism* 2008;93:4576–4599.

[173] Freemark M. Pharmacotherapy of childhood obesity: an evidence-based, conceptual approach. *Diabetes Care* 2007;30:395–402.

[174] Pollack A. Abott labs withdraws meridia from the market. The New York Times. [Internet]. 2010 October 8; Sect. B3. Available from: http://www.nytimes.com/2010/10/09/health/09drug.html [Accessed: 06 Oct 2011].

[175] Chiarelli F, Capanna R. L'obesità in età pediatrica [Consensus development on childhood obesity]. *Medico e Bambino* 2005;24:513–525.

[176] Iughetti L, China M, Berri R et al. Pharmacological treatment of obesity in children and adolescents: present and future. *Journal of Obesity* 2011;2011:928165.

[177] Viner RM, Hsia Y, Tomsic T et al. Efficacy and safety of antiobesity drugs in children and adolescents: systematic review and meta-analysis. *Obesity Reviews: An Official Journal of the International Association for the Study of Obesity* 2010;11:593–602.

[178] Kay JP, Alemzadeh R, Langley G. Beneficial effects of metformin in normoglycemic morbidly obese adolescents. *Metabolism* 2001;50:1457–1461.

[179] Park MH, Kinra S, Ward KJ et al. Metformin for obesity in children and adolescents: a systematic review. *Diabetes Care* 2009;32:1743–1745.

[180] Lustig RH, Hinds PS, Ringwald-Smith K, et al. Octreotide therapy of pediatric hypothalamic obesity: a double-blind, placebo-controlled trial. *The Journal of Clinical Endocrinology and Metabolism* 2003;88:2586–2592.

[181] Lustig RH, Greenway F, Velasquez-Mieyer P et al. A multicenter, randomized, double-blind, placebocontrolled, dose-finding trial of a long-acting formulation of octreotide in promoting weight loss in obese adults with insulin hypersecretion. *International Journal of Obesity* 2006;30:331–341.

[182] Licinio J, Caglayan S, Ozata M et al. Phenotypic effects of leptin replacement on morbid obesity, diabetes mellitus, hypogonadism, and behavior in leptin-deficient adults. *Proceedings of the National Academy of Sciences of the United States of America* 2004;101:4531–4536.

[183] Huvenne H, Dubern B, Clément K et al. Rare genetic forms of obesity: clinical approach and current treatments in 2016. *Obesity Facts* 2016;9:158–173.

[184] Reus L, Pillen S, Pelzer BJ et al. Growth hormone therapy, muscle thickness, and motor development in Prader-Willi syndrome: an RCT. *Pediatrics* 2014;134:e1619–e1627.

[185] Carrel AL, Myers SE, Whitman BY et al. Long-term growth hormone therapy changes the natural history of body composition and motor function in children with Prader-Willi syndrome. *The Journal of Clinical Endocrinology and Metabolism* 2010;95:1131–1136.

[186] Sanchez-Ortiga R, Klibanski A, Tritos NA. Effects of recombinant human growth hormone therapy in adults with Prader-Willi syndrome: a meta-analysis. *Clinical Endocrinology* 2012;77:86–93.

[187] Fani L, Bak S, Delhanty P et al: The melanocortin-4 receptor as target for obesity treatment: a systematic review of emerging pharmacological therapeutic options. *International Journal of Obesity* 2014;38:163–169.

[188] Gamboa-Gómez CI, Rocha-Guzmán NE, Gallegos-Infante JA et al. Plants with potential use on obesity and its complications. *EXCLI J.* 2015;14:809–831.

[189] Stagi S, Lapi E, Seminara S et al: Policaptil gel retard significantly reduces body mass index and hyperinsulinism and may decrease the risk of type 2 diabetes mellitus (T2DM) in obese children and adolescents with family history of obesity and T2DM. *Italian Journal of Pediatrics.* 2015;41:10.

[190] Pratt JS, Lenders CM, Dionne EA, et al. Best practice updates for pediatric/adolescent weight loss surgery. *Obesity (Silver Spring)* 2009;17:901–910.

[191] Inge TH, Xanthakos SA, Zeller MH. Bariatric surgery for pediatric extreme obesity: now or later? *International Journal of Obesity* 2007;31:1–14.

[192] Alqahtani A, Alamri H, Elahmedi M et al. Laparoscopic sleeve gastrectomy in adult and pediatric obese patients: a comparative study. *Surgical Endoscopy* 2012;26:3094–3100.

[193] National Institute for Health and Clinical Excellence. Obesity: the prevention, identification, assessment and management of overweight and obesity in adults and children. [Internet]. London 2006. Available from: https://www.nice.org.uk/Guidance/cg43 [Accessed: 01 August 2016].

[194] Alqahtani AR, Elahmedi M, Alqahtani YA. Bariatric surgery in monogenic and syndromic forms of obesity. *Seminars in Pediatric Surgery* 2014;23:37–42.

[195] Elkhenini HF, New JP, Syed AA. Five-year outcome of bariatric surgery in a patient with melanocortin-4 receptor mutation. *Clinical Obesity* 2014;4:121–124.

[196] Still CD, Wood GC, Chu X et al. High allelic burden of four obesity SNPs is associated with poorer weight loss outcomes following gastric bypass surgery. *Obesity (Silver Spring)* 2011,19:1676–1683.

[197] Hatoum IJ, Greenawalt DM, Cotsapas C et al. Weight loss after gastric bypass is associated with a variant at 15q26.1. *American Journal of Human Genetics* 2013;92:827–834.

[198] Berthoud HR, Lenard NR, Andrew CS. Food reward, hyperphagia, and obesity. *American Journal of Physiology. Regulatory, Integrative and Comparative Physiology* 2011;300:R1266–R1277.

[199] Lenard NR, Berthoud HR. Central and peripheral regulation of food intake and physical activity: pathways and genes. *Obesity (Silver Spring)* 2008;16 *Suppl* 3:S11–S22.

[200] Saper CB, Chou TC, Elmquist JK. The need to feed: homeostatic and hedonic control of eating. *Neuron* 2002;36:199–211.

[201] Avena NM, Rada P, Hoebel BG. Evidence for sugar addiction: behavioral and neurochemical effects of intermittent, excessive sugar intake. *Neuroscience and Biobehavioral Reviews* 2008;32:20–39.

[202] Bello NT, Sweigart KL, Lakoski JM et al. Restricted feeding with scheduled sucrose access results in an upregulation of the rat dopamine transporter. *American Journal of Physiology (Regulatory, Integrative and Comparative Physiology)* 2003;284:R1260–R1268.

[203] Heymsfield SB, Avena NM, Baier L et al. Hyperphagia: current concepts and future directions. Proceedings of the 2nd International Conference on Hyperphagia. *Obesity (Silver Spring)* 2014;22 *Suppl* 1:S1–S17.

[204] Ahima RS, Qi Y, Singhal NS et al. Brain adipocytokine action and metabolic regulation. *Diabetes* 2006; 55 *Suppl* 2:S145–S154.

[205] Maffeis C, Silvagni D, Consolaro A et al. [Diagnostic assessment of the obesity]. *Area Pediatrica*, 2005; I–XV.

[206] NICE. Obesity: identification, assessment and management. Clinical Guideline CG189. London, UK: NICE; 2014. p. 10–24.

[207] Pitzalis G. [Obesity in children: education, diagnosis and treatment strategies]. Nestlè Nutrition Institute Prize 2008.

[208] Lobstein T, Baur L, Uuay R. for the IOTF Childhood Obesity Working Group. Obesity in children and young people: a crisis in public health. *Obesity Reviews* 2004;5 *Suppl 1*:4–85.

[209] Prader-Willi California Foundation. Supporting people with Prader-Willi syndrome [Internet]. Available from: www.pwcf.org/for-parents [Accessed: 2016-08-25].

10

Usefulness of Obese Animal Models in Antiobesity Drug Development

Takeshi Ohta, Yasutaka Murai and
Takahisa Yamada

Abstract

Obese animal models have played key roles to elucidate the etiology of obesity and develop antiobesity drugs. In the first half of the chapter, we introduce the characteristics of obese animal models. In the second half of the chapter, we show the results of pharmacological studies using obese animal models for new antiobesity drugs.

Keywords: animal model, diabetes, obesity

1. Introduction

The number of obese patients is rapidly increasing, due to the change of lifestyle, such as eating habits of high calorie-diet and sedentary life. Obesity and the obesity-related diseases, such as diabetes mellitus, dyslipidemia, and hypertension, are risk factors for several severe diseases, including cardiovascular disease and cancer, and deteriorate the quality of life (QOL) of patients and result in high medical expenses [1, 2]. Moreover, nonalcoholic fatty liver disease (NAFLD) is recently well recognized as the most common chronic liver disease, and the NAFLD is strongly associated with obesity and the related diseases [3, 4]. In Western countries, 4–22% of NAFLD patients lead to hepatocellular cartinoma [5]. Metabolic abnormalities based on obesity, such as hyperinsulinemia, dyslipidemia, and ectopic lipid accumulation, induce the various complications including microangiopathy and nonalcoholic steatohepatitis (NASH).

Obesity is considered to be caused by an imbalance in individual energy, and energy homeostasis in body is maintained by a balance between energy intake and energy expenditure. When the former exceeds the latter, overt energy is accumulated in adipose tissue and resulting in obesity [6]. The basic therapies for obesity are appropriate dietary restriction for the purpose of decreasing energy intake and effective exercise for the purpose of promoting energy expenditure. The life style modifications, such as diet therapy and exercise, mainly occupy the treatments for obesity; however, medical therapy is performed on patients who do not show weight loss effect by the life style modifications.

Medical therapy is a fundamental step in reducing the accumulation of excess fat. To reduce excess fat accumulation and excess body weight, antiobesity drugs that reduce lipid absorption in the intestine or appetite have been developed. In past years, centrally acting drugs, such as phentermine, mazindol, and fenfluramine, had been approved as antiobesity drugs, but the drugs have since been withdrawn in the USA and Europe [7, 8]. Mazindol is now available only in Japan [9]. In the 1990s, another type of antiobesity drug, orlistat, which inhibits lipid absorption in the intestine, was approved in the USA and Europe and is now also available [10]. Thereafter, sibutramine and rimonabant were developed; however, both drugs were withdrawn because of adverse effects [11]. Development of drug combinations, such as qsymia and contrave, has been recently promoted [12], and serotonin ($5HT_2c$)-R agonist lorcaserin was accepted by the FDA in 2012 [13]. In addition, a variety of drugs with various mechanisms, such as protein tyrosine phosphatase (PTP) 1B inhibitors, microsomal triglyceride transfer protein (MTP) inhibitors, diacylglycerol acyltransferase (DGAT) 1 inhibitors, and monoacylglycerol acyltransferase (MGAT) inhibitors, have been investigated in clinical and basic stages [14–19].

Animal models have played important roles in the development of these antiobesity drugs. Obese animal models are essential to elucidate the etiology for the drug development. In the first half of this chapter, we introduce the characteristics of obese animal models. Obese animal models are divided into two types: genetic and nongenetic models. An overview of the pathophysiological features, such as body weight, blood chemical parameters, and histopathology of microangiopathy, is presented for both types. Moreover, an obese model is expected to be used as a NASH model. An overview of the development of NASH-like hepatic lesions in each model is also presented. In the second half of this chapter, results of pharmacological studies using the obese animal models for new antiobesity drugs are shown. The pharmacological effects were investigated using both genetic and nongenetic animal models.

2. Obese animal model

2.1. Genetic mouse model

2.1.1. ob/ob mouse

Lep^{ob} mutation on chromosome 6 was discovered at the Jackson laboratory in a multiple recessive stock in 1949 [20], and the Lep^{ob} mutation was subsequently transferred to B6 inbred strain background. Lep^{ob} mutation on the B6 background (ob/ob) mice shows obesity, hyperinsulinemia, and relatively mild hyperglycemia.

Body weights in ob/ob mice significantly increased as compared with those in lean mice at 7 weeks of age (mean values; ob/ob mice, 44.0 g vs. lean mice, 23.1 g). The body weights periodically increased, reaching a maximum level of approximately 55 g at 11 weeks of age. With overt obesity, blood insulin levels in ob/ob mice also significantly increased as compared with those in lean mice. The blood insulin levels in ob/ob mice showed a remarkable increase at 7 weeks of age (mean values; ob/ob mice, 23.7 ng/ml vs. lean mice, 4.2 ng/ml). Blood glucose levels in ob/ob mice increased as compared with those in lean mice from 7 to 11 weeks of age, but the levels decreased with aging and normalized after 12 weeks of age. Since the pancreatic islets in ob/ob mice have a proliferative activity with an increase of blood insulin levels, the hyperglycemia is improved with aging. Moreover, ob/ob mice show the overt fat accumulation with hyperphagia. In ob/ob mice, the *de novo* lipogenesis and the hepatic fatty acid synthesis are significantly elevated [21].

The ob/ob mice fed a standard diet show fatty liver, but do not represent NASH-like lesion. NASH-like lesion is induced in ob/ob mice by methionine-choline deficient (MCD) and high-fat (HF) diets [22, 23].

2.1.2. db/db mouse

In 1966, a recessive *Lepr^{db}* mutation (db/db) was found on chromosome 4 in C57BL KS/J inbred strain [24]. The db/db mouse was produced by backcrossing among the C57BL KS/J inbred strains.

db/db mice show a development of obesity after weaning, but the metabolic abnormalities, including hypeglycemia, are more severe as compared with those in ob/ob mice. Body weights in db/db mice significantly increased as compared with those in lean mice at 7 weeks of age (mean values; db/db mice, 42.4 g vs. lean mice, 28.4 g). The body weights periodically increased, reaching a maximum level of approximately 50 g at 11 weeks of age. The degree of weight gain in db/db mice was mild as compared with that in ob/ob mice. With obesity, the blood insulin levels in db/db mice increased as compared with those in lean mice at 7 weeks of age (mean values; db/db mice, 10.8 ng/ml vs. lean mice, 3.2 ng/ml). However, the insulin levels decreased gradually with aging, and the level in db/db mice at 11 weeks of age was comparable with that in lean mice. Blood glucose level at 7 weeks of age in db/db mice was about 700 mg/dl, and the hyperglycemia is sustained over the life span. The fluctuation in blood insulin and glucose levels is associated with the pancreatic β cell mass in db/db mice.

In examination of renal lesions in db/db mice, the creatinine clearance decreases after 20 weeks of age, and the substantial glomerular changes, such as albuminuria, mesangial area enlargement, and basement membrane thickening, are observed [25]. There are some reports of neuropathy and retinopathy in db/db mice [26, 27]. Impaired motor nerve conduction velocities (MNCV) are observed during the early phase of the diabetic syndrome. In morphological studies, db/db mice show loss or shrinkage of myelinated fibers in sural nerve and ventral root, and axonal atrophy after 25 weeks of age [28]. In the retina, pathological changes, such as loss of pericytes, acellular capillaries, and blood-retinal barrier breakdown, are observed.

The db/db mice fed a standard diet show fatty liver, but do not represent NASH-like lesion. Like ob/ob mice, NASH-like lesion is induced in ob/ob mice by methionine-choline deficient (MCD) and high-fat (HF) diets [29, 30].

2.1.3. KKA^y mouse

KK mouse, which is a spontaneously diabetic model, was established by Kondo et al. [31]. Furthermore, Nakamura et al. established KKA^y mouse, which is an obese diabetic model, by introducing the yellow obese gene (A^y) into the KK mice [32, 33].

In KKA^y mice, metabolic abnormalities, such as obesity, hyperinsulinemia, and hyperglycemia, are observed from 6 weeks of age, but the abnormalities are improved with aging [34].

Glomerular lesions, such as glomerulosclerosis, glomerular basement membrane (GBM) thickening, and nodular-like changes, are observed after 16 weeks of age [35]. Moreover, in retina of KKA^y mice, the apoptosis cell number for retinal neural cells in the ganglion cell layer increased with aging [36].

It is reported that NASH-like lesions are observed in KKA^y mice fed a MCD diet [37].

2.1.4. Tsumura Suzuki obese diabetics (TSOD) mouse

In 1992, two inbred strains: Tsumura Suzuki obese diabetics and Tsumura Suzuki nonobese (TSNO) mice were established by selective breeding of obese mice in ddy strain [38, 39].

In the male TSOD mice, metabolic abnormalities, such as hyperinsulinemia, hyperglycemia, and dyslipidemia, are developed with the increase of body weight. In the examination of pancreatic islets, the hypertrophy is observed with the increase in number of β cells and the degranulation of β cells [38].

In histopathological analyses in kidney, glomerular lesions, such as GBM thickening and mesangial area enlargement, are observed after 18 weeks of age [40]. The sensory neuropathy is observed after 12 months of age, and the motor neuropathy is also shown after 14 months of age. In histological analyses in sciatic nerves, a decrease in the density of nerve fibers is observed after 18 months of age. Moreover, the degenerative changes of myelinated fibers and the separation of myelin sheaths are observed with intralamellar edema and remyelination. Retinal lesions in TSOD mice are not reported.

2.2. Genetic rat model

2.2.1. Zucker fatty (ZF) rat

Zucker rats were originally bred to be a genetic model for research on obesity and hypertension. Two types of Zucker rat: a lean Zucker rat, denoted as the dominant trait (Fa/Fa) or (Fa/fa); and the characteristically obese Zucker rat (ZF) rat, which is actually a recessive trait (fa/fa) of the leptin receptor [41, 42]. ZF rats show overt obesity with hyperphagia (mean ± standard deviation in body weights at 12 weeks of age: ZF rats, 476.4 ± 39.4 g vs. lean rats, 306.9

± 21.9 g; mean ± standard deviation in body weights at 18 weeks of age; ZF rats, 634.8 ± 50.3 g vs. lean rats, 409.9 ± 33.5 g), and hyperinsulinemia (mean ± standard deviation in body weights at 6 weeks of age: ZF rats, 8.9 ± 1.9 ng/ml vs. lean rats, 1.1 ± 0.3 ng/ml; mean ± standard deviation in body weights at 18 weeks of age: ZF rats, 29.8 ± 12.4 ng/ml vs. lean rats, 2.7 ± 1.2 ng/ml). Blood glucose levels in ZF rats were comparable to those in lean mice from 8 to 12 weeks of age, but the glucose levels in ZF rats slightly increased as compared with those in lean rats after 12 weeks of age.

There are some reports of microangiopathy in ZF rats. Renal lesions, such as glomerular area expansion and tubular cast accumulation are observed at 24 weeks of age in ZF rats [43]. Decreased hind limb pressure pain threshold is an early indicator of insulinopenia and neuropathy, and the decreased pressure pain threshold is observed at 10 weeks of age in ZF rats [44]. Histological changes in retina of ZF rats are not reported, but some markers of inflammation, including nuclear factor (NF)-κβ, increased in the retina [45].

There are few reports of NASH-like lesions in ZF rats. Obese and hypertensive SHRSP-ZF rats treated with a high fat diet and carbon tetrachloride show the pathophysiological and histopathological characteristics of NASH [46].

2.2.2. Zucker diabetic fatty (ZDF) rat

Zucker diabetic fatty rats derived from the ZF strain exhibit obesity with diabetes. It is reported that characteristics of the male ZDF rat maintained on Purina 5008 diet include obesity, hyperinsulinemia, and hyperglycemia beginning at 6–7 weeks of age [47]. Also, in our study, obesity and hyperinsulinemia were observed at 6 weeks of age (mean ± standard deviation in body weights: ZDF rats, 221.8 ± 9.3 g vs. lean rats, 157.6 ± 5.0 g; mean ± standard deviation in insulin levels; ZDF rats, 23.1 ± 4.3 ng/ml vs. lean rats, 1.1 ± 0.3 ng/ml). By 14 weeks of age, blood glucose levels steadily increase, reaching an average of approximately 800 mg/dl. Since the ZDF rats develop diabetes, the degree of obesity in ZDF rats is mild as compared with that in ZF rats (body weights at 9 weeks of age: ZDF rats, 314.3 ± 10.7 g vs. ZF rats, 414.6 ± 19.2 g vs. lean rats, 277.6 ± 11.9 g; body weights at 13 weeks of age: ZDF rats, 388.3 ± 17.7 g vs. ZF rats, 572.5 ± 33.2 g vs. lean rats, 352.0 ± 15.8 g).

In examination of renal lesion, pathological changes, such as glomerulosclerosis and tubu-lointerstitial scarring/inflammation are observed. ZDF rats at 8 weeks of age show neither glomerulosclerosis nor evidence of tubulointerstitial lesions. Renal hypertrophy is slightly observed at 12 weeks of age, and the renal hypertrophy is more prominent by 16 weeks of age [48]. Glomerulosclerosis commences after 20 weeks of age, and is associated with glomerular hypertrophy and mild mesangial expansion with podocyte injury [49]. Furthermore, tubu-lointerstitial scarring and inflammation are observed in ZDF rats at 22 weeks of age [50]. In ZDF rats, the retinal capillaries demonstrated hypercellularity, and the retinal capillary basement membrane thickness revealed thicker membrane as compared with lean rats [51, 52]. The blood-retinal barrier is broken at 26 weeks of age in ZDF rats, and the inflammatory state and cell death by apoptosis in retina are observed [53]. In examination of sciatic nerve functions in ZDF rats, motor nerve conduction velocity (MNCV) decreases after 12 weeks of age, and vascular relaxation of sciatic nerve is impaired after 8 weeks of age [54, 55]. In the histological analyses from 24 to 28 weeks of age after the onset of diabetes, ZDF rats do not represent sympathetic neuroaxonal dystrophy [56].

ZDF rats show fatty liver with insulin resistance, but the NASH-like lesions are not reported.

2.2.3. Otsuka Long-Evans Tokusima fatty (OLETF) rat

Otsuka Long-Evans Tokushima fatty rats show an impaired glucose tolerance from 8 weeks of age, and the plasma glucose level becomes higher from 18 weeks of age [57]. In kidney of OLETF rats, pathological changes such as diffuse glomerulosclerosis and nodular lesion are observed [58]. The proliferation in mesangial cells is observed at 25 weeks of age, and the mesangial area enlargement is observed with extracellular matrix accumulation and GBM thickening after 40 weeks of age. Nodular-like lesions are observed after 65 weeks of age, and the lesions expand to the proliferated mesangial area. Tubular interstitial lesions, such as mononuclear cell filtration and fibrosis, are also observed. In the retinal capillaries after 56 weeks of age, the basement membranes are thicker, and the ratio of pericyte area decreases [59]. Regarding cataract, slight lens fiber swelling is observed in the anterior and/or posterior subcapsular regions at 40 weeks of age in OLETF rats [60]. In examination of peripheral nerve functions in OLETF rats, MNCV tends to decrease after about 40 weeks of age as compared with lean rats [61].

In NASH-like lesions of OLETF rats, there are some reports of MCD diet-induced steatohepatitis [62, 63]. The steatohepatitis is accelerated in OLETF rats after 8 weeks fed MCD diet. Furthermore, the MCD + HF diet leads to rapid development of precirrhosis in OLETF rats.

2.2.4. Wistar fatty rat

In Wistar fatty rats, glucose intolerance accompanied by exaggerated insulin secretion and an increase of basal plasma glucose level are observed at 8 weeks of age, and an increase of basal plasma insulin level also increased at 14 weeks of age [64].

Kidney enlargement and glomerular hypertrophy are observed at 20 and 42 weeks of age in Wistar fatty rats [65]. In histopathological analyses, glomerular lesions, including mesangial area enlargement and tubular lesions, are observed. Intercellular adhesion molecular (ICAM)-1 expression on the glomeruli is significantly observed at 15 weeks of age, and progresses further at 29 weeks of age [66]. The other complications, such as retinopathy, neuropathy, and NASH, are not reported in Wistar fatty rats.

2.2.5. Spontaneously Diabetic Torii (SDT) fatty rat

Spontaneously Diabetic Torii fatty rats of both sexes show a significant hyperphagia and obesity after weaning, and especially, the increase of body weight in female rats is remarkable. In the male SDT fatty rats, the blood insulin levels increase after weaning, but the insulin levels decrease after 16 weeks of age. The female SDT fatty rats show hyperinsulinemia from 4 to 8 weeks of age, and the insulin levels decrease with aging. Serum glucose levels in SDT fatty rats of both sexes are elevated from 6 weeks, and the hyperglycemia is sustained for a long time afterwards.

With early incidence of diabetes mellitus, diabetic complications, such as nephropathy, retinopathy, and neuropathy, are observed at younger ages than the SDT rats [67, 68]. In histopathological analyses of the male rats, tubular lesions are observed after 8 weeks of age, and glomerular lesions are also observed after 16 weeks of age [67]. The glomerulosclerosis are observed from 16 weeks of age, and the nodular-like lesions are observed at 40 weeks of age. The renal tubular lesions, such as Armanni-Ebstein lesions and tubular dilation, are observed from 8 weeks of age. In histopathological analyses of the female rats, tubular lesions are observed from 16 weeks of age, and glomerular lesions are also observed from 32 weeks of age [68]. In lens of the male rats, histopathological changes, such as hyperplasia of epithelium and vacuolation of fiber, are observed after 8 weeks of age. Similar changes are observed after 16 weeks of age in the female SDT fatty rats. The male and female SDT fatty rats show the retinal lesions, such as folding and thickening, after 40 weeks of age [67, 68]. The decrease in caudal MNCV is observed at 24 weeks of age in the male SDT fatty rats [67]. In histopathological analyses, the male rats show the decrease in fiber number and the atrophy in myelinated nerve at 40 weeks of age.

It is reported that female SDT fatty rats fed a standard diet develop HASH-like hepatic lesions [4]. Hepatic lipid content significantly increases in female SDT fatty rats from 8 to 32 weeks of age. Histopathologically, severe hepatosteatosis accompanied by inflammation was observed from 8 weeks of age, and fibrosis started to occur at 32 weeks of age (**Figure 1**). Female SDT fatty rats have the potential to become an important animal model of NASH with diabetes and obesity.

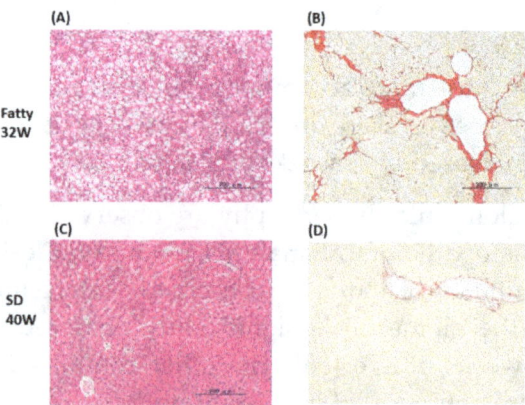

Figure 1. Histological analysis of liver in female Spontaneously Diabetic Torii fatty and Sprague-Dawley (SD) rats[4]. Liver sections are from SDT fatty at 32 weeks of age (A, B) and SD at 40 weeks of age (C, D). Hematoxylin and eosin (HE) stain (A, C) and Sirius Red stain (B, D). Bar = 200 μm.

2.2.6. cp/cp rat

The LA/N-corpulent (LA/N-cp) rat is a normotensive strain derived from Koltesky's original mutant strain of the spontaneously hypertensive rat (SHR). When homozygous for the cp gene (cp/cp), the rats are hyperphagous, obesity, hyperinsulinemia, hyperglycemia, and dyslipidemia [69]. The levels of body weight, systolic blood pressure, serum TG and blood glucose in cp/cp rats being 1.43, 1.65, 25.4, and 1.25 times, respectively, compared with those in control rats, Wistar Kyoto rats at 19 or 20 weeks of age [70].

Renal lesions, including glomerular and tubular changes, are observed in cp/cp rats, from 24 to 36 weeks of age [71]. In light microscopy, cp/cp rats develop glomerular lesions, characterized by glomerular hypertrophy, mesangial expansion, and focal and segmental glomerular sclerosis. Also, interstitial lesions, such as tubular hypertrophy and atrophy, inflammation cell infiltration, and thickening of tubular basal membrane, are prominent. In electron microscopy, thickening of glomerular basal membrane (GBM) and glomerular epithelial injuries, such as pseudocyst formation, vacuolization, detachment from the GBM, podocyte depletion, and foot process effacement are observed. Retinal lesions in cp/cp rats are also reported [72]. In cp/cp rats at 24 weeks of age, partial capillary obstruction and acellular, tortuous, irregular capillaries are observed by light microscope. In electron microscopy, thickening and irregularity of the basement membrane along with remnants of pericytes or so-called ghost pericytes are observed. Neuropathy in cp/cp rats is not reported.

It is reported that cp/cp rats fed a diet of AIN-93G show NASH-like lesions after 23 weeks [73].

2.2.7. WBN/Kob fatty rat

WBN/Kob fatty rat is a new congenic strain for the *fa* allele of the leptin receptor gene, and the homozygous rat provides a model of type 2 diabetes with obesity [74]. Male and female WBN/Kob fatty rats show inflammatory cell infiltration of the pancreas and impaired glucose tolerance at 7 weeks of age. Furthermore, the rats developed diabetes with pancreatitis at 3 months of age. From 7 to 12 weeks of age, the body weight and body mass index (BMI) of male WBN/Kob fatty rats are significantly greater than those of lean rats. Female WBN/Kob fatty rats have a significantly greater body weight and BMI than lean rats from 5 to 32 weeks of age. Male WBN/Kob fatty rats show hyperinsulinemia until 8 weeks of age, but after 8 weeks their insulin levels decrease with the increase of blood glucose levels. There has been no report regarding microangiopathy and NASH.

2.3. Nongenetic rodent model

2.3.1. Diet-induced obese models

Diet-induced obesity (DIO) animal model is a created model to study obesity and its comorbidities, such as insulin resistance, type 2 diabetes, dyslipidemia, hypertension, and atherosclerosis. In this model, an animal is fed a HF diet or HF/high sucrose or fructose diet for long term. As a result, it becomes obese with several glucose and lipid metabolic abnormalities, such as impaired glucose tolerance, increased fasting glucose level, hyperlipidemia, and hyperinsulinemia. The DIO models have become one of the most important tools for understanding the relationship of high-calorie Western diets and the development of obesity [75]. In recent years, Western diet-loaded genetic animal models have investigated to elucidate the pathophysiology of obese related diseases including NAFLD/NASH and pancreatic lesion with diabetes and develop the new therapies of the diseases [76].

HF diet-induced obesity models are commonly used to gain a greater understanding of pathophysiology in obesity and develop antiobesity drugs. When choosing the HF diet, the fat level in diet should be taken into consideration. The low-fat diet has about 10% of the calories coming from fats, while the HF diet has about 30–50% of the calories coming from fats, and the very HF diet contains greater than 50 kcal% fats. When those diets are used to induce obesity, there is a dose response for body weight [77]. The source of dietary fat is also important. The rodents fed diets with fish oil do not gain so much weight and are more insulin sensitive as compared with those fed saturated fats [78]. Moreover, there are variable responses in physiological parameters, such as glucose tolerance, insulin resistance, and blood lipid levels, on strain and gender [79]. HF diet promotes the incidence of diabetes, and induces NASH-like lesions in genetic obese models. It is reported that HF diet-fed db/db mouse shows NASH-like lesions [29].

In rodent models, high-fructose or/and sucrose diets elevates triglyceride and glucose production in liver, and this increased availability of nutrients leads to insulin resistance and hypertriglyceridemia [80]. Unless fed for a prolonged period of time, these high-fructose or/and sucrose diets do not appear to lead to excessive weight gain [81]. Since high-fructose or/and sucrose diets induce the elevation of lipid production in liver, these diets may be more effective to produce NASH-like hepatic lesions.

3. Antiobesity drugs

3.1. Protein tyrosine phosphatase 1B inhibitor

PTP1B is a 50-KD cytosolic tyrosine dephosphorylase consisting of 435 amino acids that are ubiquitously expressed in organs throughout the body. Originally, PTP1B was known to dephosphorylate phosphorylated insulin receptor (IR) β subunit and IR substrate in order to negatively regulate insulin signal transmission [82]. PTP1B is also reportedly related to the negative regulation of leptin signal transmission and to dephosphorylate phosphorylated signal transducer and activator of transcription 3 (STAT3) [83]. Therefore, PTP1B inhibitors are expected to be developed as antiobesity drugs as well as antidiabetes drugs. PTP1B KO mice are protected from diet-induced obesity, and neuronal PTP1B KO mice also show increased leptin signaling in the hypothalamus, reductions in feeding, body weight and adiposity, and increases in energy expenditure [84].

Ito et al. reported the antiobesity effects of JTT-551, which was developed as a novel PTP1B inhibitor [85, 19]. The single administration of JTT-551 and leptin enhanced STAT3 phosphorylation in the hypothalamus of DIO mice, and the food intake resulted in a significant reduction as compared with that in the control group. The food intake in JTT-551 administration without leptin treatment did not result in the reduction. DIO mice at 8 weeks of age were given 10 or 100 mg/kg of JTT-551 contained in food for 6 weeks and the chronic effects were investigated.

In the JTT-551 100 m/kg group, the cumulative calorie intake tended to decrease from 2 weeks after treatment and significantly decreased from 6 weeks after treatment. Body weight in JTT-551 treatment tended to decrease dose-dependently and the decreases in the JTT-551 100 mg/kg group were significant from 5 to 6 weeks after treatment. PTP1B inhibitor is a unique target that shows not only an improvement of glucose metabolism but also an antiobesity effect possibly by enhancement of leptin signaling.

3.2. Microsome triglyceride transfer protein inhibitor

MTP is localized in the endoplasmic reticulum in hepatocytes and enterocytes, and MTP leads the transfer of triglyceride (TG) and cholesteryl ester between membranes [86]. The protein participates in the assembly of TG-rich lipoproteins, such as chylomicron particles in the small intestine and very low-density lipoprotein (VLDL) particles in the liver, thereby also participating in the mobilization and secretion of TG-rich lipoproteins from enterocytes and hepatocytes [87]. Since enteric MTP has been shown to play a critical role in the absorption of fat or cholesterol, the inhibition of MTP in small intestine is expected to induce the potential of weight loss as an antiobesity drug.

Since the *in vivo* effects of MTP inhibitors were reported, it has been pointed out that inhibition of hepatic MTP could lead to the potent blockade of VLDL release, resulting in reduced plasma lipids but inducing fatty liver and hepatic dysfunction [88]. In fact, while the potential benefits of MTP inhibition, such as lowering chylomicron-TG and VLDL-TG levels, are demonstrated in animal experiments and in clinical studies, several major toxicity issues affect the clinical development of MTP inhibitors [89]. In clinical studies of BAY 13-9952 and BMS-201038, for example, hepatotoxicity indicated by the elevation of transaminase level halted their developments. Therefore, the compounds designed to show a high selectively inhibition for intestine-MTP have been developed and lipid-absorption inhibitors are expected to show pharmacological effects, including weight loss, without any hepatotoxicity.

Mera et al. designed the compound, JTT-130, that would be rapidly metabolized during the absorption process to avoid inhibition of hepatic MTP after oral administration [90, 91]. JTT-130 was designed to be rapidly hydrolyzed to its inactive metabolite (M1) by cleavage of ester group in the structures. The IC_{50} values of JTT-130 on MTP inhibitory activities were 0.83 nM for TG transfer and 0.74 nM for cholesteryl ester (CE) transfer, respectively. No inhibitory effect of M1 on MTP was observed at concentrations of M1 increasing up to 30,000 nM. Antiobesity effects were investigated in a DIO model, Sprague-Dawley rat fed a 35% fat diet [15]. JTT-130 treatment decreased body weights with suppression of food intake (**Figure 2A** and **B**). Interestingly, the pharmacological effects were not observed in rats fed with the 3.1% fat diet (**Figure 2C** and **D**), and JTT-130 showed antiobesity effects in a dietary fat-dependent manner. The elevation of plasma levels of gut hormones, such as glucagon-like peptide-1 (GLP-1) and peptide YY (PYY), was observed in DIO rats, and the elevation of gut peptides may be related with body weight loss with JTT-130 treatment. The antiobesity effect of JTT-130 was also investigated using a genetic model, ZDF rat [92]. Male ZDF rats at 7 weeks of age were fed a regular diet with JTT-130 as a food admixture for 6 weeks. JTT-130 treatment decreased the food intake in the ZDF rats throughout the treatment period, resulting in reduction in the body weight in the first 4 weeks of the treatment period. However, the body weights of the JTT-130-treated ZDF rats were comparable to those of the control ZDF rats after 5 weeks of treatment. The body weight change is considered to be induced by the improvement of metabolic abnormalities in whole body with JTT-551 treatment.

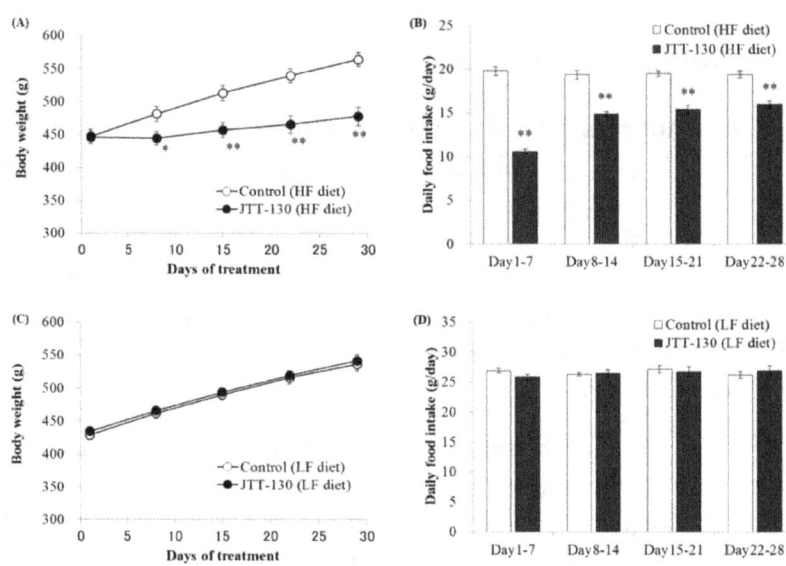

Figure 2. Effects of microsomal triglyceride transfer protein inhibitor, JTT-130 on body weights and food intake in Sprague-Dawley rats on a 35% fat diet (A, B) and a 3.1% fat diet (C, D). Rats in the JTT-130 treatment groups were fed with the drug as a 0.029% food admixture (approximately 10 mg/kg/day), beginning at 10 weeks of age [15]. Data represent mean ± standard deviation (n = 6). *p < 0.05, **p < 0.01: significantly different from control group.

Furthermore, JTT-130 treatment has been reported as ameliorating impaired glucose and lipid metabolism in ZDF rats [92], and attenuates dyslipidemia in hyprlipidemic hamsters and rabbits [93]. It is expected that intestine-specific MTP inhibitors will be useful in treatment of diabetes and atherosclerosis as well as obesity.

3.3. Acyl-CoA: diacylglycerol acyltransferase 1 inhibitor

DGAT1 is an enzyme that catalyzes the final step of TG synthesis, i.e., synthesis of TG from diacylglycerol and fatty acyl-CoA. DGAT1 is expressed in various organs, and is especially highly expressed in the small intestine, fat tissue, and testes [94]. The enzyme is involved in TG absorption from the small intestine and fat accumulation in adipose tissues [95]. Indeed, DGAT1-knockout (−/−) mice show resistance to the antiobesity effects of a HF diet; wherein body weight gain is suppressed, fat weight and TG contents decrease, and energy consumption in the liver and skeletal muscles accelerates, as well as observing improvements in insulin and leptin resistance, in comparison with wild-type mice [96]. Since the inhibition of DGAT1 is expected to result in two kinds of pharmacological effects: (1) inhibition of fat absorption in the small intestine and (2) inhibition of fat synthesis in adipose tissues, DGAT1 inhibitors are likely to become a good therapeutic option for obesity.

Tomimoto et al. reported antiobesity effects with JTT-553, which was discovered as a novel DGAT1 inhibitor [97]. A single administration of JTT-553 inhibited the increase of plasma TG levels after olive oil loading in Sprague-Dawley (SD) rats, suggesting that JTT-553 inhibited fat absorption in the small intestine. Furthermore, JTT-553 suppressed TG synthesis in adipose tissues [98]. The antiobesity effects of JTT-553 were investigated in DIO rats, SD rats fed a 35% fat diet, and a genetic model, the KKAy mouse. In DIO rats, body weight and visceral fat in the JTT-553 administration group decreased dose-dependently; however, the suppressive effects of JTT-553 on body weight were not observed with the 3.1% fat diet. Interestingly, the antifeeding effects of JTT-553 were observed in DIO rats, which was not observed in DGAT1-knockout (−/−) mice. A single administration of JTT-553 decreased food consumption depending on dietary fat content. The difference in appetite between DGAT1 inhibitor-treated and knockout mice remains unknown. In KKAy mice, JTT-553 decreased the food intake and body weight (**Figure 3**). Repeated administration of JTT-553 showed decreases of the liver and fat weights, and the liver TG content. The DGAT1 inhibitor was considered to suppress food consumption via the elevation of levels of gut hormones, such as GLP-1, in plasma [99]. Furthermore, JTT-553 was administrated to DIO mice and antiobesity effects and antidiabetic effects were investigated at the same time [98]. JTT-553 decreased body weight and food consumption, and treatment resulted in improvements in hyperinsulinemia and hyperlipidemia. In the glucose tolerance test, JTT-553 treatment resulted in ameliorations of insulin resistance. In addition, JTT-553 treatment resulted in significant reductions in fat mass, and increased glucose utilization of epididymal adipose tissues in the presence of insulin.

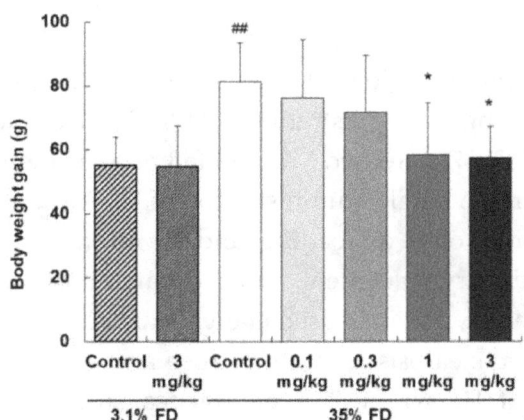

Figure 3. Effects of Acyl CoA: diacylglycerol acyltransferase1 inhibitor, JTT-553 on body weights gain in KKAy mice on a 35% fat diet [98]. JTT-553 was dosed as food admixture to KKAy mice for 5 weeks. Data represent mean ± standard deviation ($n = 7$–8). *$p < 0.05$, **$p < 0.01$: significantly different from 35% control group, #$p < 0.05$, ##$p < 0.01$: significantly different from 3.1% control group.

3.4. Acyl-CoA: monoacylglycerol acyltransferase 2 inhibitor

MGAT2 is an enzyme that catalyzes the esterification of monoacylglycerol (MG), i.e., synthesis of diglycerides from MG and fatty acyl-CoA [100, 101]. The genes encoding three MGATs,

MGAT1, MGAT2, and MGAT3 have been identified [102–104]. MGAT1 is mainly expressed in the heart, lung, skeletal muscle, and pancreas, but not in the small intestine. Both MGAT2 and MGAT3 are mainly expressed in human small intestine, whereas only MGAT2 is expressed in mouse small intestine [102].

MGAT2 is involved in the resynthesis of TG in the intestine, and plays an important role in the assembly and secretion of chylomicrons. In fact, MGAT2 KO mice demonstrate reduced fat uptake in the small intestine and delay in the absorption of fat into circulation [105]. In addition, the elevation of postprandial GLP-1 and not PYY levels are observed in MGAT2 KO mice fed a HF diet [106]. The chronic function of MGAT2 on metabolic disorders is investigated using MGAT2 KO mice. MGAT2 deficient mice are protected from HF diet-induced obesity and glucose intolerance [106]. Moreover, MGAT2 deficiency results in increased metabolic rates, decreased food consumption, and protection from obesity in genetically obese Agouti mice, suggesting that MGAT2 regulates energy balance [106, 107]. The intestinal function of MGAT2 and the effect of this function on obesity are also investigated using intestine-specific MGAT2 KO mice [108]. Intestinal-specific deletion of MGAT2 alters TG metabolism in the small intestine and delays fat absorption. These mice are protected from obesity and impair glucose metabolism when feed a HF diet. Thus, there is considerable interest that inhibition of MGAT2 is a feasible target for obesity and other metabolic disorders caused by excess dietary calories. Although, the physiological role of MGAT2 has been mainly investigated using genetically modified mice, the detailed pharmacological characteristics of MGAT2 inhibitors have not been reported.

Okuma et al. reported the pharmacological profile of JTP-103237, which was discovered as a novel MGAT2 inhibitor. A single administration of JTT-103237 reduced plasma TG after lipid loading. In addition, JTT-103237 increased MG and fatty acid content, which are MGAT2 substrates, in the small intestine. A single administration of JTT-103237 tended to elevate plasma levels of GLP-1 and PYY after olive oil loading, and the antifeeding effect of JTT-103237 was observed independent of dietary fat content. After repeated dosing, JTT-103237 reduced food consumption and body weight, and increased energy expenditure in DIO mice. Furthermore, JTT-103237 reduced hepatic steatosis in high sucrose and very low fat (HSVLF)-fed mice, through the suppression of TG synthesis related genes, such as sterol regulatory element-binding protein (SREBP)-1c, fatty acid synthesis, and stearoyl-CoA desaturase (SCD)-1. The inhibition of hepatic MGAT2 activity is considered to directly reduce hepatic TG synthesis. 2-MG content in the small intestine is considered to increase by administration of MGAT2 inhibitor. The effects of 2-MG on food intake and diarrhea were evaluated and compared with the long-chain fatty acid (LCFA) in rats by intrajejunal infusion [109]. 2-MG did not induce diarrhea under the condition in which it comparably reduced food intake as compared with LCFA, suggesting that 2-MG stimulates satiety without inducing diarrhea, different from LCFA. From these findings, MGAT2 inhibition may prove to be a useful strategy target for treating obesity and related metabolic disorders.

4. Conclusion

Obesity is the consequence of an imbalance between energy intake and energy expenditure, and basic therapies for obesity are appropriate dietary restriction to decrease energy intake and effective exercise to increase energy consumption. However, maintaining these lifestyle modifications, such as diet therapy and exercise, are difficult and therapeutic effects are limited. Medical therapy then becomes a pivotal step.

It is important to elucidate the complex mechanisms of obesity in developing new antiobesity therapies, including the discovery of novel drugs. In particular, investigations using obese animal models are essential to clarify the pathophysiology and develop new antiobesity drugs. Several drug types that target various mechanisms, such as increased satiety with anorexia, inhibition of nutritional absorption, and acceleration of energy consumption, have been developed using various obese animal models including genetic models and nongenetic models. To help develop new antiobesity therapies, including the understanding of pathophysiology of obesity, the importance of the obese animal models will be a constant in the future.

Author details

Takeshi Ohta[1,2*], Yasutaka Murai[1] and Takahisa Yamada[2]

*Address all correspondence to: takeshi.ota@jt.com

1 Japan Tobacco Inc., Central Pharmaceutical Research Institute, Murasaki-cho, Takatsuki, Osaka, Japan

2 Laboratory of Animal Genetics, Graduate School of Science and Technology, Niigata University, Nishi-ku, Niigata, Japan

References

[1] Boulghassoul-Pietrzykowska N, Franceschelli J, Still C. New medications for obesity management: changing the landscape of obesity treatment. Curr Opin Endocrinol Diabetes Obes 2013;20(5):407–11.

[2] Henry RR, Chilton R, Garvey WT. New options for the treatment of obesity and type 2 diabetes mellitus (narrative review). J Diabetes Complications 2013;27(5):508–18.

[3] de Alwis NM, Day CP. Non-alcoholic fatty liver disease: the mist gradually clears. J Hepatol 2008;48 (Suppl 1):S104–12.

[4]   Ishii Y, Motohashi Y, Muramatsu M, Katsuda Y, Miyajima K, Sasase T, et al. Female spontaneously diabetic Torii fatty rats develop nonalcoholic steatohepatitis-like hepatic lesions. World J Gastroenterol 2015;21(30):9067–78.

[5]   Ertle J, Dechêne A, Sowa JP, Penndorf V, Herzer K, Kaiser G, et al. Non-alcoholic fatty liver disease progresses to hepatocellular carcinoma in the absence of apparent cirrhosis. Int J Cancer 2011;128(10):2436–43.

[6]   Fock KM, Khoo J. Diet and exercise in management of obesity and overweight. J Gastroenterol Hepatol 2013;28 (Suppl 4):59–63.

[7]   Halpern A, Mancini MC. Treatment of obesity: an update on anti-obesity medications. Obes Rev 2003;4(1):25–42.

[8]   Ioannides-Demos LL, Proietto J, McNeil JJ. Pharmacotherapy for obesity. Drugs 2005;65(10):1391–418.

[9]   Mori Y. Mazindol. Nihon Rinsho 2011;69 (Suppl 1):683–6.

[10] McClendon KS1, Riche DM, Uwaifo GI. Orlistat: current status in clinical therapeutics. Expert Opin Drug Saf 2009;8(6):727–44.

[11] Simonyi G1, Pados G, Medvegy M, Bedros JR. The pharmacological treatment of obesity: past, present and future. Orv Hetil 2012;153(10):363–73.

[12] Shyh G, Cheng-Lai A. New antiobesity agents: lorcaserin (Belviq) and phentermine/ topiramate ER (Qsymia). Cardiol Rev 2014;22(1):43–50.

[13] Nigro SC, Luon D, Baker WL. Lorcaserin: a novel serotonin 2C agonist for the treatment of obesity. Curr Med Res Opin 2013;29(7):839–48.

[14] Li J, Bronk BS, Dirlam JP, Blize AE, Bertinato P, Jaynes BH, et al. In vitro and in vivo profile of 5-[(4'-trifluoromethyl-biphenyl-2-carbonyl)-amino]-1H-indole-2-carboxylic acid benzylmethyl carbamoylamide (dirlotapide), a novel potent MTP inhibitor for obesity. Bioorg Med Chem Lett 2007;17(7):1996–9.

[15] Hata T, Mera Y, Tadaki H, Kuroki Y, Kawai T, Ohta T, et al. JTT-130, a novel intestine-specific inhibitor of microsomal triglyceride transfer protein, suppresses high fat diet-induced obesity and glucose intolerance in Sprague-Dawley rats. Diabetes Obes Metab 2011;13(5):446–54.

[16] Yamamoto T, Yamaguchi H, Miki H, Shimada M, Nakada Y, Ogino M, et al. Coenzyme A: diacylglycerol acyltransferase 1 inhibitor ameliorates obesity, liver steatosis and lipid metabolism abnormality in KKAy mice fed high-fat or high-carbohydrate diets. Eur J Pharmacol 2010;640(1–3):243–9.

[17] Birch AM, Buckett LK, Turnbull AV. DGAT1 inhibitors as anti-obesity and anti-diabetic agents. Curr Opin Drug Discov Devel 2010;13(4):489–96.

[18] Cho H. Protein tyrosine phosphatase 1B (PTP1B) and obesity. Vitam Horm 2013;91:405–24.

[19] Ito M, Fukuda S, Sakata S, Morinaga H, Ohta T. Pharmacological effects of JTT-551, a novel protein tyrosine phosphatase 1B inhibitor, in diet-induced obesity mice. J Diabetes Res 2014;2014:680348.

[20] Ingalls AM, Dickie MM, Snell GD. Obese, a new mutation in the house mouse. J Hered 1950;41(12):317–8.

[21] Memon RA, Grunfeld C, Moser AH, Feingold KR. Fatty acid synthesis in obese insulin resistant diabetic mice. Horm Metab Res 1994;26(2):85–7.

[22] de Oliveira CP, de Lima VM, Simplicio FI, Soriano FG, de Mello ES, de Souza HP, et al. Prevention and reversion of nonalcoholic steatohepatitis in OB/OB mice by S-nitroso-N-acetylcysteine treatment. J Am Coll Nutr 2008;27(2):299–305.

[23] de Lima VM, de Oliveira CP, Sawada LY, Barbeiro HV, de Mello ES, Soriano FG, et al. Yo jyo hen shi ko, a novel Chinese herbal, prevents nonalcoholic steatohepatitis in ob/ob mice fed a high fat or methionine-choline-deficient diet. Liver Int 2007;27(2): 227–34.

[24] Hummel KP, Dickie MM, Coleman DL. Diabetes, a new mutation in the mouse. Science 1966;153(3740):1127–8.

[25] Sharma K, McCue P, Dunn SR. Diabetic kidney disease in the db/db mouse. Am J Physiol Renal Physiol 2003;284(6):F1138–44.

[26] Midena E, Segato T, Radin S, di Giorgio G, Meneghini F, Piermarocchi S. Studies on the retina of the diabetic db/db mouse. I. Endothelial cell-pericyte ratio. Ophthalmic Res 1989;21(2):106–11.

[27] Robertson DM, Sima AA. Diabetic neuropathy in the mutant mouse [C57BL/ks(db/db)]: a morphometric study. Diabetes 1980;29(1):60–7.

[28] Kim J1, Kim CS, Lee IS, Lee YM, Sohn E, Jo K, et al. Extract of Litsea japonica ameliorates blood-retinal barrier breakdown in db/db mice. Endocrine 2014;46(3):462–9.

[29] Yoo NY, Jeon S, Nam Y, Park YJ, Won SB, Kwon YH. Dietary supplementation of genistein alleviates liver inflammation and fibrosis mediated by a methionine-choline-deficient diet in db/db Mice. J Agric Food Chem 2015;63(17):4305–11.

[30] Takahashi Y, Soejima Y, Kumagai A, Watanabe M, Uozaki H, Fukusato T. Japanese herbal medicines shosaikoto, inchinkoto and juzentaihoto inhibit high-fat diet-induced nonalcoholic steatohepatitis in db/db mice. Pathol Int 2014;64(10):490–8.

[31] Nakamura M, Yamada K. Studies on a diabetic (KK) strain of the mouse. Diabetologia 1967;3(2):212–21.

[32] Nishimura, M. Breeding of mice strains for diabetes mellitus. Exp Anim 1969;18:147–57.

[33] Bultman SJ, Michaud EJ, Woychik RP. Molecular characterization of the mouse agouti locus. Cell 1992;71(7):1195–204.

[34] Iwatsuka H, Taketomi S, Matsuo T, Suzuoki Z. Congenitally impaired hormone sensitivity of the adipose tissue of spontaneously diabetic mice, KK. Validity of thrifty genotype in KK mice. Diabetologia 1974;10 (Suppl):611–6.

[35] Chen LM, Li XW, Huang LW, Li Y, Duan L, Zhang XJ. The early pathological changes of KKAy mice with type 2 diabetes. Zhongguo Yi Xue Ke Xue Yuan Xue Bao 2002;24(1): 71–5.

[36] Ning X, Baoyu Q, Yuzhen L, Shuli S, Reed E, Li QQ. Neuro-optic cell apoptosis and microangiopathy in KKAY mouse retina. Int J Mol Med 2004;13(1):87–92.

[37] Okumura K, Ikejima K, Kon K, Abe W, Yamashina S, Enomoto N, et al. Exacerbation of dietary steatohepatitis and fibrosis in obese, diabetic KK-A(y) mice. Hepatol Res 2006;36(3):217–28.

[38] Suzuki W, Iizuka S, Tabuchi M, Funo S, Yanagisawa T, Kimura M, et al. A new mouse model of spontaneous diabetes derived from ddY strain. Exp Anim 1999;48(3): 181–9.

[39] Hirayama I, Yi Z, Izumi S, Arai I, Suzuki W, Nagamachi Y, et al. Genetic analysis of obese diabetes in the TSOD mouse. Diabetes 1999;48(5):1183–91.

[40] Iizuka S, Suzuki W, Tabuchi M, Nagata M, Imamura S, Kobayashi Y, et al. Diabetic complications in a new animal model (TSOD mouse) of spontaneous NIDDM with obesity. Exp Anim 2005;54(1):71–83.

[41] Kurtz TW, Morris RC, Pershadsingh HA. The Zucker fatty rat as a genetic model of obesity and hypertension. Hypertension 1989;13(6 Pt 2):896–901.

[42] Takaya K, Ogawa Y, Isse N, Okazaki T, Satoh N, Masuzaki H, et al. Molecular cloning of rat leptin receptor isoform complementary DNAs-identification of a missense mutation in Zucker fatty (fa/fa) rats. Biochem Biophys Res Commun 1996;225(1):75–83.

[43] Nakano R, Kurosaki E, Shimaya A, Kajikawa S, Shibasaki M. YM440, a novel hypogly-cemic agent, protects against nephropathy in Zucker fatty rats via plasma triglyceride reduction. Eur J Pharmacol 2006;549(1–3):185–91.

[44] Romanovsky D, Walker JC, Dobretsov M. Pressure pain precedes development of type 2 disease in Zucker rat model of diabetes. Neurosci Lett 2008;445(3):220–3.

[45] Mima A, Qi W, Hiraoka-Yamomoto J, Park K, Matsumoto M, Kitada M, et al. Retinal not systemic oxidative and inflammatory stress correlated with VEGF expression in rodent models of insulin resistance and diabetes. Invest Ophthalmol Vis Sci 2012;53(13): 8424–32.

[46] Kochi T, Shimizu M, Terakura D, Baba A, Ohno T, Kubota M, et al. Non-alcoholic steatohepatitis and preneoplastic lesions develop in the liver of obese and hypertensive rats: suppressing effects of EGCG on the development of liver lesions. Cancer Lett 2014;342(1):60–9.

[47] Katsuda Y, Ohta T, Miyajima K, Kemmochi Y, Sasase T, Tong B, et al. Diabetic complications in obese type 2 diabetic rat models. Exp Anim 2014;63(2):121–32.

[48] Vora JP, Zimsen SM, Houghton DC, Anderson S. Evolution of metabolic and renal
changes in the ZDF/Drt-fa rat model of type II diabetes. J Am Soc Nephrol 1996;7(1):
113–7.

[49] Hoshi S, Shu Y, Yoshida F, Inagaki T, Sonoda J, Watanabe T, et al. Podocyte injury
promotes progressive nephropathy in zucker diabetic fatty rats. Lab Invest 2002;82(1):
25–35.

[50] Chander PN, Gealekman O, Brodsky SV, Elitok S, Tojo A, Crabtree M, et al. Nephropathy in Zucker diabetic fat rat is associated with oxidative and nitrosative stress:
prevention by chronic therapy with a peroxynitrite scavenger ebselen. J Am Soc
Nephrol 2004;15(9):2391–403.

[51] Danis RP, Yang Y. Microvascular retinopathy in the Zucker diabetic fatty rat. Invest
Ophthalmol Vis Sci 1993;34(7):2367–71.

[52] Yang YS, Danis RP, Peterson RG, Dolan PL, Wu YQ. Acarbose partially inhibits
microvascular retinopathy in the Zucker Diabetic Fatty rat (ZDF/Gmi-fa). J Ocul
Pharmacol Ther. 2000;16(5):471–9.

[53] Gonçalves A, Leal E, Paiva A, Teixeira Lemos E, Teixeira F, Ribeiro CF, et al. Protective
effects of the dipeptidyl peptidase IV inhibitor sitagliptin in the blood-retinal barrier
in a type 2 diabetes animal model. Diabetes Obes Metab 2012;14(5):454–63.

[54] Oltman CL, Coppey LJ, Gellett JS, Davidson EP, Lund DD, Yorek MA. Progression of
vascular and neural dysfunction in sciatic nerves of Zucker diabetic fatty and Zucker
rats. Am J Physiol Endocrinol Metab 2005;289(1):E113–22.

[55] Shimoshige Y, Ikuma K, Yamamoto T, Takakura S, Kawamura I, Seki J, et al. The effects
of zenarestat, an aldose reductase inhibitor, on peripheral neuropathy in Zucker
diabetic fatty rats. Metabolism 2000;49(11):1395–9.

[56] Schmidt RE, Dorsey DA, Beaudet LN, Peterson RG. Analysis of the Zucker Diabetic
Fatty (ZDF) type 2 diabetic rat model suggests a neurotrophic role for insulin/IGF-I in
diabetic autonomic neuropathy. Am J Pathol 2003;163(1):21–8.

[57] Kawano K, Hirashima T, Mori S, Saitoh Y, Kurosumi M, Natori T. Spontaneous long-
term hyperglycemic rat with diabetic complications. Otsuka Long-Evans Tokushima
Fatty (OLETF) strain. Diabetes 1992;41(11):1422–8.

[58] Kawano K, Mori S, Hirashima T, Man ZW, Natori T. Examination of the pathogenesis
of diabetic nephropathy in OLETF rats. J Vet Med Sci 1999;61(11):1219–28.

[59] Miyamura N, Bhutto IA, Amemiya T. Retinal capillary changes in Otsuka Long-Evans
Tokushima fatty rats (spontaneously diabetic strain). Electron-microscopic study.
Ophthalmic Res 1999;31(5):358–66.

[60] Kubo E, Maekawa K, Tanimoto T, Fujisawa S, Akagi Y. Biochemical and morphological changes during development of sugar cataract in Otsuka Long-Evans Tokushima fatty (OLETF) rat. Exp Eye Res 2001;73(3):375–81.

[61] Nakamura J, Koh N, Sakakibara F, Hamada Y, Wakao T, Sasaki H, et al. Diabetic neuropathy in sucrose-fed Otsuka Long-Evans Tokushima fatty rats: effect of an aldose reductase inhibitor, TAT. Life Sci 1997;60(21):1847–57.

[62] Ota T, Takamura T, Kurita S, Matsuzawa N, Kita Y, Uno M, et al. Insulin resistance accelerates a dietary rat model of nonalcoholic steatohepatitis. Gastroenterology 2007;132(1):282–93.

[63] Uno M, Kurita S, Misu H, Ando H, Ota T, Matsuzawa-Nagata N, et al. Tranilast, an antifibrogenic agent, ameliorates a dietary rat model of nonalcoholic steatohepatitis. Hepatology 2008;48(1):109–18.

[64] Ikeda H, Shino A, Matsuo T, Iwatsuka H, Suzuoki Z. A new genetically obese-hyperglycemic rat (Wistar fatty). Diabetes 1981;30(12):1045–50.

[65] Velasquez MT, Kimmel PL, Michaelis OE 4th. Animal models of spontaneous diabetic kidney disease. FASEB J 1990;4(11):2850–9.

[66] Matsui H, Suzuki M, Tsukuda R, Iida K, Miyasaka M, Ikeda H. Expression of ICAM-1 on glomeruli is associated with progression of diabetic nephropathy in a genetically obese diabetic rat, Wistar fatty. Diabetes Res Clin Pract 1996;32(1–2):1–9.

[67] Matsui K, Ohta T, Oda T, Sasase T, Ueda N, Miyajima K, et al. Diabetes-associated complications in Spontaneously Diabetic Torii fatty rats. Exp Anim 2008;57(2):111–21.

[68] Ishii Y, Ohta T, Sasase T, Morinaga H, Ueda N, Hata T, et al. Pathophysiological analysis of female Spontaneously Diabetic Torii fatty rats. Exp Anim 2010;59(1):73–84.

[69] Russell JC, Amy RM. Myocardial and vascular lesions in the LA/N-corpulent rat. Can J Physiol Pharmacol 1986;64(10):1272–80.

[70] Kawai K, Sakairi T, Harada S, Shinozuka J, Ide M, Sato H, et al. Diet modification and its influence on metabolic and related pathological alterations in the SHR/NDmcr-cp rat, an animal model of the metabolic syndrome. Exp Toxicol Pathol 2012;64(4):333–8.

[71] Nangaku M, Izuhara Y, Usuda N, Inagi R, Shibata T, Sugiyama S, et al. In a type 2 diabetic nephropathy rat model, the improvement of obesity by a low calorie diet reduces oxidative/carbonyl stress and prevents diabetic nephropathy. Nephrol Dial Transplant 2005;20(12):2661–9.

[72] Kim SH, Chu YK, Kwon OW, McCune SA, Davidorf FH. Morphologic studies of the retina in a new diabetic model; SHR/N:Mcc-cp rat. Yonsei Med J 1998;39(5):453–62.

[73] Omagari K, Kato S, Tsuneyama K, Hatta H, Sato M, Hamasaki M, et al. Olive leaf extract prevents spontaneous occurrence of non-alcoholic steatohepatitis in SHR/NDmcr-cp rats. Pathology. 2010;42(1):66–72.

[74] Akimoto T, Nakama K, Katsuta Y, Zhang XJ, Ohsuga M, Ishizaki M, et al. Characterization of a novel congenic strain of diabetic fatty (WBN/Kob-Lepr(fa)) rat. Biochem Biophys Res Commun 2008;366(2):556–62.

[75] Wang CY, Liao JK. A mouse model of diet-induced obesity and insulin resistance. Methods Mol Biol 2012;821:421–33.

[76] Kubo K, Shimada T, Onishi R, Tsubata M, Kamiya T, Nagamine R, et al. Puerariae flos alleviates metabolic diseases in Western diet-loaded, spontaneously obese type 2 diabetic model mice. J Nat Med 2012;66(4):622–30.

[77] Ghibaudi L, Cook J, Farley C, van Heek M, Hwa JJ. Fat intake affects adiposity, comorbidity factors and energy metabolism of sprague-dawley rats. Obes Res 2002;10(9):956–63.

[78] Buettner R, Parhofer KG, Woenckhaus M, Wrede CE, Kunz-Schughart LA, Schölmerich J, Bollheimer LC. Defining high-fat-diet rat models: metabolic and molecular effects of different fat types. J Mol Endocrinol 2006;36(3):485–501.

[79] Levin BE, Dunn-Meynell AA, Balkan B, Keesey RE. Selective breeding for diet-induced obesity and resistance in Sprague-Dawley rats. Am J Physiol 1997;273(2 Pt 2):R725–30.

[80] Daly ME, Vale C, Walker M, Alberti KG, Mathers JC. Dietary carbohydrates and insulin sensitivity: a review of the evidence and clinical implications. Am J Clin Nutr 1997;66(5): 1072–85.

[81] Chicco A, D'Alessandro ME, Karabatas L, Pastorale C, Basabe JC, Lombardo YB. Muscle lipid metabolism and insulin secretion are altered in insulin-resistant rats fed a high sucrose diet. J Nutr 2003;133(1):127–33.

[82] Wu X, Hardy VE, Joseph JI, Jabbour S, Mahadev K, Zhu L, et al. Protein-tyrosine phosphatase activity in human adipocytes is strongly correlated with insulin-stimulated glucose uptake and is a target of insulin-induced oxidative inhibition. Metabolism 2003;52(6):705–12.

[83] Zabolotny JM, Bence-Hanulec KK, Stricker-Krongrad A, Haj F, Wang Y, Minokoshi Y, et al. PTP1B regulates leptin signal transduction in vivo. Dev Cell 2002;2(4):489–95.

[84] Elchebly M, Payette P, Michaliszyn E, Cromlish W, Collins S, Loy AL, et al. Increased insulin sensitivity and obesity resistance in mice lacking the protein tyrosine phosphatase-1B gene. Science 1999;283(5407):1544–8.

[85] Fukuda S, Ohta T, Sakata S, Morinaga H, Ito M, Nakagawa Y, et al. Pharmacological profiles of a novel protein tyrosine phosphatase 1B inhibitor, JTT-551. Diabetes Obes Metab 2010;12(4):299–306.

[86] Lin MC, Gordon D, Wetterau JR. Microsomal triglyceride transfer protein (MTP) regulation in HepG2 cells: insulin negatively regulates MTP gene expression. J Lipid Res 1995;36(5):1073–81.

[87] Wetterau JR, Gregg RE, Harrity TW, Arbeeny C, Cap M, Connolly F, et al. An MTP inhibitor that normalizes atherogenic lipoprotein levels in WHHL rabbits. Science 1998;282(5389):751–4.

[88] Xie Y, Newberry EP, Young SG, Robine S, Hamilton RL, Wong JS, et al. Compensatory increase in hepatic lipogenesis in mice with conditional intestine-specific Mttp deficiency. J Biol Chem 2006;281(7):4075–86.

[89] Shiomi M, Ito T. MTP inhibitor decreases plasma cholesterol levels in LDL receptor-deficient WHHL rabbits by lowering the VLDL secretion. Eur J Pharmacol 2001;431(1): 127–31.

[90] Mera Y, Odani N, Kawai T, Hata T, Suzuki M, Hagiwara A, et al. Pharmacological characterization of diethyl-2-({3-dimethylcarbamoyl-4-[(4'-trifluoromethylbiphenyl-2-carbonyl)amino]phenyl}acetyloxymethyl)-2-phenylmalonate (JTT-130), an intestine-specific inhibitor of microsomal triglyceride transfer protein. J Pharmacol Exp Ther 2011;336(2):321–7.

[91] Hata T, Mera Y, Ishii Y, Tadaki H, Tomimoto D, Kuroki Y, et al. JTT-130, a novel intestine-specific inhibitor of microsomal triglyceride transfer protein, suppresses food intake and gastric emptying with the elevation of plasma peptide YY and glucagon-like peptide-1 in a dietary fat-dependent manner. J Pharmacol Exp Ther 2011;336(3):850–6.

[92] Hata T, Mera Y, Kawai T, Ishii Y, Kuroki Y, Kakimoto K, et al. JTT-130, a novel intestine-specific inhibitor of microsomal triglyceride transfer protein, ameliorates impaired glucose and lipid metabolism in Zucker diabetic fatty rats. Diabetes Obes Metab 2011;13(7):629–38.

[93] Mera Y, Kawai T, Ogawa N, Odani N, Sasase T, Miyajima K, et al. JTT-130, a novel intestine-specific inhibitor of microsomal triglyceride transfer protein, ameliorates lipid metabolism and attenuates atherosclerosis in hyperlipidemic animal models. J Pharmacol Sci 2015;129(3):169–76.

[94] Cases S, Smith SJ, Zheng YW, Myers HM, Lear SR, Sande E, et al. Identification of a gene encoding an acyl CoA:diacylglycerol acyltransferase, a key enzyme in triacylglycerol synthesis. Proc Natl Acad Sci U S A 1998;95(22):13018–23.

[95] Buhman KK, Smith SJ, Stone SJ, Repa JJ, Wong JS, Knapp FF Jr, et al. DGAT1 is not essential for intestinal triacylglycerol absorption or chylomicron synthesis. J Biol Chem 2002;277(28):25474–9.

[96] Smith SJ, Cases S, Jensen DR, Chen HC, Sande E, Tow B, et al. Obesity resistance and multiple mechanisms of triglyceride synthesis in mice lacking Dgat. Nat Genet 2000;25(1):87–90.

[97] Tomimoto D, Okuma C, Ishii Y, Akiyama Y, Ohta T, Kakutani M, et al. Pharmacological characterization of [trans-5'-(4-amino-7,7-dimethyl-2-trifluoromethyl-7H-pyrimido[4, 5-b][1,4]oxazin-6-yl)-2',3'-dihydrospiro(cyclohexane-1,1'-inden)-4-yl]acetic acid mono-

benzenesulfonate (JTT-553), a novel acyl CoA:diacylglycerol transferase (DGAT) 1 inhibitor. Biol Pharm Bull 2015;38(2):263–9.

[98] Tomimoto D, Okuma C, Ishii Y, Kobayashi A, Ohta T, Kakutani M, et al. JTT-553, a novel Acyl CoA:diacylglycerol acyltransferase (DGAT) 1 inhibitor, improves glucose metabolism in diet-induced obesity and genetic T2DM mice. J Pharmacol Sci 2015;129(1):51–8.

[99] Ables GP1, Yang KJ, Vogel S, Hernandez-Ono A, Yu S, Yuen JJ, et al. Intestinal DGAT1 deficiency reduces postprandial triglyceride and retinyl ester excursions by inhibiting chylomicron secretion and delaying gastric emptying. J Lipid Res 2012;53(11):2364–79.

[100] Senior JR, Isselbacher KJ. Direct esterification of monoglycerides with palmityl coenzyme a by intestinal epithelial subcellular fractions. J Biol Chem 1962;237:1454–9.

[101] Yen CL, Farese RV Jr. MGAT2, a monoacylglycerol acyltransferase expressed in the small intestine. J Biol Chem 2003;278(20):18532–7.

[102] Yen CL, Stone SJ, Cases S, Zhou P, Farese RV Jr. Identification of a gene encoding MGAT1, a monoacylglycerol acyltransferase. Proc Natl Acad Sci U S A 2002;99(13):8512–7.

[103] Cao J, Cheng L, Shi Y. Catalytic properties of MGAT3, a putative triacylgycerol synthase. J Lipid Res 2007;48(3):583–91.

[104] Tsuchida T, Fukuda S, Aoyama H, Taniuchi N, Ishihara T, Ohashi N, et al. MGAT2 deficiency ameliorates high-fat diet-induced obesity and insulin resistance by inhibiting intestinal fat absorption in mice. Lipids Health Dis 2012;11:75.

[105] Okawa M, Fujii K, Ohbuchi K, Okumoto M, Aragane K, Sato H, et al. Role of MGAT2 and DGAT1 in the release of gut peptides after triglyceride ingestion. Biochem Biophys Res Commun 2009;390(3):377–81.

[106] Yen CL, Cheong ML, Grueter C, Zhou P, Moriwaki J, Wong JS, et al. Deficiency of the intestinal enzyme acyl CoA:monoacylglycerol acyltransferase-2 protects mice from metabolic disorders induced by high-fat feeding. Nat Med 2009;15(4):442–6.

[107] Gao Y, Nelson DW, Banh T, Yen MI, Yen CL. Intestine-specific expression of MOGAT2 partially restores metabolic efficiency in Mogat2-deficient mice. J Lipid Res 2013;54(6):1644–52.

[108] Nelson DW, Gao Y, Yen MI, Yen CL. Intestine-specific deletion of acyl-CoA:monoacylglycerol acyltransferase (MGAT) 2 protects mice from diet-induced obesity and glucose intolerance. J Biol Chem 2014;289(25):17338–49.

[109] Okuma C, Ohta T, Ito M, Tadaki H, Oda T, Kume S, et al. Intrajejunal infusion of 2-monoacylglycerol reduced food intake without inducing diarrhea in rats. J Pharmacol Sci 2016;130(2):136–8.

Permissions

The contributors of this book come from diverse backgrounds, making this book a truly international effort. This book will bring forth new frontiers with its revolutionizing research information and detailed analysis of the nascent developments around the world.

We would like to thank all the contributing authors for lending their expertise to make the book truly unique. They have played a crucial role in the development of this book. Without their invaluable contributions this book wouldn't have been possible. They have made vital efforts to compile up to date information on the varied aspects of this subject to make this book a valuable addition to the collection of many professionals and students.

This book was conceptualized with the vision of imparting up-to-date information and advanced data in this field. To ensure the same, a matchless editorial board was set up. Every individual on the board went through rigorous rounds of assessment to prove their worth. After which they invested a large part of their time researching and compiling the most relevant data for our readers.

The editorial board has been involved in producing this book since its inception. They have spent rigorous hours researching and exploring the diverse topics which have resulted in the successful publishing of this book. They have passed on their knowledge of decades through this book. To expedite this challenging task, the publisher supported the team at every step. A small team of assistant editors was also appointed to further simplify the editing procedure and attain best results for the readers.

Apart from the editorial board, the designing team has also invested a significant amount of their time in understanding the subject and creating the most relevant covers. They scrutinized every image to scout for the most suitable representation of the subject and create an appropriate cover for the book.

The publishing team has been an ardent support to the editorial, designing and production team. Their endless efforts to recruit the best for this project, has resulted in the accomplishment of this book. They are a veteran in the field of academics and their pool of knowledge is as vast as their experience in printing. Their expertise and guidance has proved useful at every step. Their uncompromising quality standards have made this book an exceptional effort. Their encouragement from time to time has been an inspiration for everyone.

The publisher and the editorial board hope that this book will prove to be a valuable piece of knowledge for researchers, students, practitioners and scholars across the globe.

List of Contributors

Canan Nebigil
CNRS-University of Strasbourg, (UMR 7242), Illkirch, France

Ibrahim Akin and Uzair Ansari
University Mannheim, Mannheim, Germany

Christoph A. Nienaber
Royal Brompton Hospital and Harefield Trust, London, UK

Andrea Ramalho
Micronutrients Research Center (NPqM), Institute of Nutrition Josué de Castro (INJC) of the Federal University of Rio de Janeiro (UFRJ), Rio de Janeiro, Brazil
Social Applied Nutrition Department, Institute of Nutrition Josué de Castro (INJC) of the Federal University of Rio de Janeiro (UFRJ), Rio de Janeiro, Brazil
Medical Clinic Program, Faculty of Medicine, UFRJ, Rio de Janeiro, Brazil

Adryana Cordeiro
Micronutrients Research Center (NPqM), Institute of Nutrition Josué de Castro (INJC) of the Federal University of Rio de Janeiro (UFRJ), Rio de Janeiro, Brazil
Medical Clinic Program, Faculty of Medicine, UFRJ, Rio de Janeiro, Brazil

Henrique Nascimento, Alice Santos-Silva and Luís Belo
UCIBIO\REQUIMTE, Department of Biological Sciences, Laboratory of Biochemistry, Faculty of Pharmacy, University of Porto, Porto, Portugal

Susana Coimbra
UCIBIO\REQUIMTE, Department of Biological Sciences, Laboratory of Biochemistry, Faculty of Pharmacy, University of Porto, Porto, Portugal

CESPU, Institute of Research and Advanced Training in Health Sciences and Technologies (IINFACTS), Gandra-PRD, Portugal

Carla Rêgo
Children and Adolescent Centre, CUF Hospital, Center for Health Technology and Services Research (CINTESIS), Faculty of Medicine, University of Porto, Porto, Portugal

Tomás Cerdó
EURISTIKOS Excellence Centre for Paediatric Research, University of Granada, Granada, Spain
Department of Paediatrics, School of Medicine, University of Granada, Granada, Spain
Centre for Biomedical Research, University of Granada, Granada, Spain

Cristina Campoy
EURISTIKOS Excellence Centre for Paediatric Research, University of Granada, Granada, Spain
Department of Paediatrics, School of Medicine, University of Granada, Granada, Spain
Centre for Biomedical Research, University of Granada, Granada, Spain
CIBERESP: National Network of Research in Epidemiology and Public Health, Institute Carlos III, Valencia, Spain

Alicia Ruiz
EURISTIKOS Excellence Centre for Paediatric Research, University of Granada, Granada, Spain
Centre for Biomedical Research, University of Granada, Granada, Spain

Emilio González-Jiménez
Department of Nursing, Faculty of Health Science, University of Granada, Spain

Milton-Omar Guzmán-Ornelas and Fernanda-Isadora Corona-Meraz
Institute for Rheumatology Research and MuscleSkeletal System, CUCS, University of Guadalajara, Guadalajara, Jalisco, Mexico
UDG-CA-701, Research Group on Immunometabolism and Emerging Diseases, Health Sciences School, Guadalajara, Jalisco, Mexico

Rosa-Elena Navarro-Hernández
Institute for Rheumatology Research and MuscleSkeletal System, CUCS, University of Guadalajara, Guadalajara, Jalisco, Mexico
UDG-CA-701, Research Group on Immunometabolism and Emerging Diseases, Health Sciences School, Guadalajara, Jalisco, Mexico
UDG-CA-817, Research Group on Genomics and Biomedicine, Department of Farmacy and Biology, University of Guadalajara, Exact Sciences and Engineering School, Marcelino García Barragán Boulevard, Guadalajara, Jalisco, Mexico
Department of Molecular Biology and Genomics, University of Guadalajara, Health Sciences

Efrain Chavarria-Avila
Institute for Rheumatology Research and MuscleSkeletal System, CUCS, University of Guadalajara, Guadalajara, Jalisco, Mexico
UDG-CA-701, Research Group on Immunometabolism and Emerging Diseases, Health Sciences School, Guadalajara, Jalisco, Mexico
Deparment of Philosophical, Methodological, and Instrumental Disciplines, University of Guadalajara, Health Sciences School, Guadalajara, Jalisco, Mexico School, Guadalajara, Jalisco, Mexico
Department of Molecular Biology and Genomics, University of Guadalajara, Health Sciences

Mónica Vázquez-Del Mercado
Institute for Rheumatology Research and MuscleSkeletal System, CUCS, University of Guadalajara, Guadalajara, Jalisco, Mexico

Department of Molecular Biology and Genomics, University of Guadalajara, Health Sciences
Rheumatology Service PNPC 004086, CONACyT, Internal Medicine Division, Civil Hospital Dr. Juan I. Menchaca, Guadalajara, Jalisco, Mexico
UDG-CA-703, Research Group on Immunology and Rheumatology, University of Guadalajara, Health Sciences School, Guadalajara, Jalisco, Mexico

Sandra-Luz Ruíz-Quezada
UDG-CA-701, Research Group on Immunometabolism and Emerging Diseases, Health Sciences School, Guadalajara, Jalisco, Mexico
UDG-CA-817, Research Group on Genomics and Biomedicine, Department of Farmacy and Biology, University of Guadalajara, Exact Sciences and Engineering School, Marcelino García Barragán Boulevard, Guadalajara, Jalisco, Mexico

Darren Henstridge and Kiymet Bozaoglu
Baker IDI Heart and Diabetes Institute, Melbourne, VIC, Australia

Stefano Stagi, Martina Bianconi, Maria Amina Sammarco and Maurizio de Martino
Health Sciences Department, University of Florence, Anna Meyer Children's University Hospital, Florence, Italy

Rosangela Artuso and Sabrina Giglio
Genetics and Molecular Medicine Unit, Anna Meyer Children's University Hospital, Florence, Italy

Yasutaka Murai
Japan Tobacco Inc., Central Pharmaceutical Research Institute, Murasaki-cho, Takatsuki, Osaka, Japan

Takeshi Ohta
Japan Tobacco Inc., Central Pharmaceutical Research Institute, Murasaki-cho, Takatsuki, Osaka, Japan

Laboratory of Animal Genetics, Graduate School of Science and Technology, Niigata University, Nishi-ku, Niigata, Japan

Takahisa Yamada
Laboratory of Animal Genetics, Graduate School of Science and Technology, Niigata University, Nishi-ku, Niigata, Japan

Index